Key Concepts and Issues in Nursing Ethics

P. Anne Scott · Shane M. Scott
Editors

Key Concepts and Issues in Nursing Ethics

Second Edition

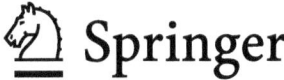

Editors
P. Anne Scott
University of Galway
Galway, Co Galway, Ireland

Shane M. Scott
Public Policy Practitioner
London, UK

ISBN 978-3-031-54107-0   ISBN 978-3-031-54108-7 (eBook)
https://doi.org/10.1007/978-3-031-54108-7

© The Editor(s) (if applicable) and The Author(s), under exclusive license to Springer Nature Switzerland AG 2017, 2024
This work is subject to copyright. All rights are solely and exclusively licensed by the Publisher, whether the whole or part of the material is concerned, specifically the rights of translation, reprinting, reuse of illustrations, recitation, broadcasting, reproduction on microfilms or in any other physical way, and transmission or information storage and retrieval, electronic adaptation, computer software, or by similar or dissimilar methodology now known or hereafter developed.
The use of general descriptive names, registered names, trademarks, service marks, etc. in this publication does not imply, even in the absence of a specific statement, that such names are exempt from the relevant protective laws and regulations and therefore free for general use.
The publisher, the authors and the editors are safe to assume that the advice and information in this book are believed to be true and accurate at the date of publication. Neither the publisher nor the authors or the editors give a warranty, expressed or implied, with respect to the material contained herein or for any errors or omissions that may have been made. The publisher remains neutral with regard to jurisdictional claims in published maps and institutional affiliations.

This Springer imprint is published by the registered company Springer Nature Switzerland AG
The registered company address is: Gewerbestrasse 11, 6330 Cham, Switzerland

If disposing of this product, please recycle the paper.

To John, Rebecca, and the four new members of our family—Emily, Adel (Addy), Aiden John (AJ) and Ryan

Foreword to the First Edition

Since its establishment in the late 1960s, modern bioethics has been dominated by a focus on respect for rational and autonomous persons as the pivotal actors in medicine and healthcare. This focus reflects the influence of the Kantian philosophy of autonomous human beings, able to identify and prescribe universal ethical standards to themselves, entirely rational and free from any heterogeneous reinforcement. It also mirrors Mill's appreciation of the high value of human freedom of individuals, only to be restricted when it confines the freedom of others.

The prioritisation of respect for autonomy in modern bioethics has radically changed the perspective in which patients are regarded within healthcare. For millennia, patients were seen as fundamentally incapacitated by pain, suffering, ignorance and disease, thus justifying a paternalistic approach in medicine. In contemporary healthcare—at least in most Western countries—patients are now seen as being fundamentally on an equal footing with physicians. As a positive consequence of the stellar status of autonomy in contemporary bioethics, medical paternalism has lost its justification as the default approach of physicians. On the flipside however, because of its narrow emphasis on autonomy, bioethics has not been giving the phenomenon of human vulnerability its fair share of recognition for quite some time. This is especially problematic, if we accept the claim that "[…] vulnerability is the general predicament of humans, while autonomy is the exception" (Ten Have 2016, 2).

Without attempting anything near to a substantiation of the above claim, it could easily be argued that *Homo sapiens* is one of the most vulnerable species around. *Homo sapiens*, for example, is the only species that after birth needs years and years of continuous care and attention from its parents to be able to survive. At the end of life, many humans are again heavily dependent on others for long stretches of time because of chronic illnesses, neurodegenerative diseases and fragility. So at first glance, vulnerability seems to be an essential human trait, anthropologically on a par with autonomy.

This observation notwithstanding, in bioethics the notion of vulnerability has stood in the shadow of the concept of autonomy for a long period of time. The idea of vulnerability made its bioethical entrée in the Belmont Report in 1978. Here it was applied in the context of research with human participants. The document warned of the danger that "vulnerable subjects" might be disproportionately targeted for research purposes as a "special instance of injustice" (Belmont Report 1978, 19).

After this landmark publication, the role of the concept of vulnerability in bioethics continued to be confined to the research context, until it was solidly advanced as an all-round European ethical principle some 20 years later in the BIOMED II project "Basic Ethical Principles in European Bioethics and Biolaw" (1995–1998) (see Rendtorff and Peter 2000). Not only did this European project elevate the idea of vulnerability to the status of an independent ethical principle, equal to the principle of respect for autonomy, it also broadened its application beyond the realm of research.

In 2005, the bioethical status of vulnerability was further enhanced to that of a universal ethical principle in the UNESCO *Universal Declaration on Bioethics and Human Rights*. Article 8 of this document solemnly states: "In applying and advancing scientific knowledge, medical practice and associated technologies, human vulnerability should be taken into account. Individuals and groups of special vulnerability should be protected and the personal integrity of such individuals respected" (UNESCO 2005) (see Ten Have (2016) for a more elaborate history of the concept of vulnerability in bioethics).

Unlike the average bioethicist—indeed even in contrast to physicians—nurses have always had abundant exposure to the full plethora of patients' vulnerabilities. That may be the reason why in nursing literature the concept of vulnerability already started to figure in a prominent position in the 1970s. McGilloway, for example, distinguished two traits of the patient's predicament relevant to nursing: "The first is that the patient's dependency places him in a vulnerable situation, and second that his situation is such as to make rational judgement difficult for him" (McGilloway 1976, 229).

More recently, Sellman (2011) used the concept of vulnerability as central for the understanding of the aims of nursing. He distinguished between "ordinary and extra-ordinary vulnerability" (Sellman 2011, 51). While human beings in general are susceptible to a variety of harms, some are significantly more susceptible than others. This particular susceptibility might be such that they need care and assistance from others in ways that are normally not necessary for persons with only ordinary vulnerability. Nursing can accordingly be understood "as a response to the additional human vulnerability that comes with being a patient" (Sellman 2011, 51). As extraordinary vulnerability involves reduced chances for human flourishing, the true aim of nursing can thus be regarded as "[…] the promotion of flourishing for more-than-ordinarily vulnerable persons" (Sellman 2011, 51).

At the start of this stimulating volume on nursing ethics, Anne Scott rightly refers to Sellman's understanding of nursing in terms of vulnerability. This sets the tone in her introductory chapter exploring the ethical aspects of nursing in general. The following six chapters focus on a number of key concepts in nursing ethics. This is followed by four chapters that analyse nursing from the perspective of a selection of established ethical theories: principlism, utilitarianism, virtue ethics and care ethics. The remaining chapters then focus on a variety of crucial topics in nursing ethics salient in nursing in particular contexts.

As indicated above, nurses can tap into a rich and exclusive experiential background. This gives them a privileged position as contributors to bioethics debates.

Their perspective on vulnerability is only one case in point. They have never neglected this phenomenon to the extent that it was overlooked in mainstream bioethics. The lucky readers of this thought-provoking volume will encounter many other examples of the ethical significance of the distinctive nursing perspective.

References

McGilloway FA (1976) Dependency and vulnerability in the nurse/patient situation. J Adv Nurs 1(3):229–236

National Commission for the Protection of Human Subjects of Biomedical and Behavioral Research (1978) The Belmont report: Ethical principles and guidelines for the protection of human subjects of research. https://videocast.nih.gov/pdf/ohrp_belmont_report.pdf. Accessed 31 Oct 2016

Rendtorff JD, Peter K (2000) Basic ethical principles in European bioethics and biolaw. Volume I. Autonomy, dignity, integrity and vulnerability. Centre for Ethics and Law, and InstitutBorja de Bioetica, Copenhagen/Barcelona

Sellman D (2011) What makes a good nurse: why the virtues are important for nurses. Jessica Kingsley Publishers, London

Ten Have H (2016) Vulnerability: challenging bioethics. Routledge.

UNESCO (United Nations Educational Scientific and Cultural Organisation) (2005) Universal Declaration on Bioethics and Human Rights. UNESCO, Paris. http://unesdoc.unesco.org/images/0014/001461/146180e.pdf . Accessed 31 Oct 2016

Institute of Ethics, Dublin City University   Bert Gordijn
Dublin, Ireland

Foreword to the Second Edition

This second edition of *Key Concepts and Issues in Nursing Ethics* builds of the success of the first edition, offering a timely and welcome opportunity to gain a better understanding of what good nursing practice involves. Anne Scott, in the opening chapter of this collection, provides an important and refreshing read that examines the ethical dimension of nursing practice. Through a wonderful variety of authors this stimulating volume takes in several perspectives enabling exploration of the integrated ethical and clinical aspects of the modern-day nursing role.

Florence Nightingale's philosophy and teachings emphasise that nurses must use their brains, heart and hands to create healing environments to care for the patient's body, mind and spirit. While not far from the reality of what is actually required to deliver safe, quality care, it is probably fair to say even Florence Nightingale could not have anticipated the complexity of today's healthcare environment or the scale of need. This book begins with an important focus across a range of topics in nursing ethics. With significant relevance to today's world the text addresses complexities, such as moral injury, that must be understood and addressed to achieve workforce well-being and ultimately quality care. Professor Scott begins with three fundamental chapters addressing the ethical domain of practice, a modern view of advocacy and nursing, and the very current issue of resourcing and rationing in nursing.

The backdrop of the COVID-19 pandemic threaded throughout the book provides an important context. Practising during the pandemic challenged so many aspects of nursing and patient care. Despite many decisions, conflicting with the core values of the profession at times, to deliver care based on the greater good, it also forced a visibility and understanding of nursing value, practice and impact not seen before. Nursing fulfilled its broader role across society at this time, highlighting the responsibility that comes with becoming a more autonomous profession.

Nursing has always been able to adopt to meet patient care needs. The chapters in this book provide an important reminder that the proximity to the patient, across a range of care areas, uniquely positions nurses to see and understand how practice impacts patients and communities. As Chief Nursing Office immersed in policy development during the reforms of the last decade, as well as during a global pandemic, I can attest to the value of evidence-based policy, as an important frame to support and lead quality care, that should not be underestimated. This volume brings together many aspects of practice that can and should influence policy development.

Whether decisions are required over time to support system-wide reform or quickly, such as during the pandemic, the profession's real success comes as a result of being able to inform and influence the care required and demonstrate the impacts of that care for patients. Driving and developing practice and patient care through evidence-based policy provides structure built on knowledge, science and principles for good practice that grasps the crossover of ethical and clinical practice. The flexibility this provides helps navigate the delivery of 'good" practice in a dynamic, unpredictable and complex system. Nursing policies in the Irish context, such as the *Safe Nurse Staffing and Skills Mix Framework* (DoH 2016) and *Graduate to Advance Practice* (DoH 2019) are a testament to this; developed in 'normal times' to address patient need they survived and thrived during the pandemic.

Ensuring that nursing remains part of policy development and implementation remains a challenge we must embrace. Post COVID the context for practice remains challenging. A global shortage of nurses, growing technology-led care, increasingly complex patient needs, and a more constrained financial time will require more supports for good practice and safety which chapters in this volume captured so well.

The correlation between the nursing resource and quality care is well demonstrated through the literature, and this is further strengthened through the evidence in recent years of nursing policy implementation. Policy, particularly evidence-rich policy, has been proven to secure investment, which in turn enables the development of care solutions for complex needs and delivery of that care with adequate resources; thus enabling nurses to also care for and manage themselves.

Ireland is on the cusp of major reform, moving from a hospital-centric system to more community-based care that will integrate people, care and environments. This volume clearly sets out the crossover of ethics and clinical practice, and, relevant to today, it does so across different populations or care groups, providing thought-provoking insights into a more integrated future and the ethical challenges ahead. Reform will require the profession to continue to evolve at pace. Evidence-based policy is a key enabler for the profession to embrace the ethical responsibilities associated with being highly skilled professionals, carrying out safety-critical roles that can significantly impact population health. Indeed, no local or global health agenda can be realised without sustained efforts to maximise the contributions of the nursing workforce and their respective roles within inter-professional health teams. It is in this context that this book provides a powerful, practical and compelling read.

Department of Health   Rachel Kenna
Dublin, Ireland

Preface

The idea for the first edition of this book took some time to come to fruition! When AS started to teach healthcare ethics to nursing and medical students in the mid-1980s, there were very few texts on healthcare ethics available in Ireland, or the UK, and almost none dedicated to nursing. This has changed remarkably in the intervening years, and there are now many such texts to choose from. Nonetheless, feedback on the first edition of *Key Concepts and Issues in Nursing Ethics* has been resoundingly positive and usage suggests that, particularly in the post COVID-19 pandemic world of healthcare, a second edition of this text would be both welcome and of value.

The COVID-19 pandemic has had a profound impact on nursing, and the nursing role continues to develop, change, and become increasingly complex; with consequent impacts on the ethical dimension of nursing practice. In our experience, many students find nursing ethics a challenging and somewhat obtuse subject. Those of us engaged in teaching ethics to nursing students can struggle to convince students of the value of the subject matter, and to engage them effectively in discussion and analysis of the ethical dimension of their practice. It seems to be important, to student understanding of the topic, that the approach to teaching nursing ethics is well grounded in a description of nursing that students can recognise, accept, and engage with. This is apparently even more so since the onset of the COVID-19 pandemic, the impact on nurses of working during the pandemic, and the aftermath that many nurses and other healthcare practitioners continue to live with and practice through. For this reason, through the use of short case studies, each chapter of this book uses examples of nursing practice that are based on, and informed by, actual experiences of receiving and/or giving nursing care. Many of the chapters and case studies in this second edition are directly or indirectly influenced by the context of practising during the pandemic.

In recent years pre-, during, and post-pandemic, we have witnessed the publication of a number of reports and inquiries on both the nursing workforce and on patient care. These reports have had some very strong messages for nurses, policy makers, and health service managers, regarding the quality, value, and impact of nursing care—on both the patients' experiences of care and the outcomes of that care. Some of these reports articulate, in a very powerful way, the deeply intertwined nature of the ethical and the clinical aspects of nursing practice, and the provision of nursing care. Many of the chapters of this book make direct reference to the findings and analyses of these reports.

Good nursing, nursing that is explicitly and consciously rooted in a clear understanding of the ethical dimension of nursing practice, is essential to safe, humane patient care; never more so than in situations of significant pressures on the healthcare resource.

This book provides an opportunity, and an invitation, to examine the ethical dimension of nursing practice; through a variety of theoretical lenses, across a number of patient care situations, and at different stages of the human life span. It also tries to strike a balance between a recognition and articulation of the ethical responsibilities of the individual nurse to provide humane, sensitive, and competent care to their patients, and the responsibility of the organisation within which nurses work to support nursing staff in providing this care.

Galway, Ireland P. Anne Scott
London, UK Shane M. Scott

Acknowledgements

As with the first edition, this book would not have been written without the contributions of many people. It has been a privilege to work with the contributing authors over a two year period. Thank you for your thoughtful contributions and willingness to engage in discussion, debate, and review. Additionally, a number of colleagues generously gave of their time providing comments on and/or reviewing chapters for this second edition—in particular, we would like to thank Anna-Marie Greaney, Janet Holt, Michael Igoumenidis, Kate Irving, Alan J Kearns, Marcia Kirwan, Anne Matthews, Joan McCarthy, Dónal O'Mathúna, and Evridiki Papastravou.

John Scott and Emily Burt have been there whenever, and for whatever, required. A.J provided the joy of watching a son and grandson develop through his first two years of life, and Becky and Addy provided the excitement and fun of their wedding, and more recently the birth of their baby boy Ryan to keep us all on our toes! We are deeply grateful.

We also wish to express our thanks to Nathalie Lhorset-Poulain and Aruna Sharma of Springer; to Nathalie for encouraging us to initiate this project in the first place and and then to work on this second edition; to Aruna for her advice, follow-up and support.

Finally, AS would like to thank all her students over the years, in Ireland, Scotland, England, and Kenya, for their engagement, insights, and stimulating, challenging discussions.

Contents

Part I Nursing and Ethics: Some Key Concepts

1 Nursing and the Ethical Dimension of Practice 3
P. Anne Scott
Introduction 4
Nursing and the Ethical Domain of Practice 6
Nurse-Patient Interaction: The Nurse-Patient Relationship
(Including a Case Study) 8
Conclusion 15
References 16

2 Advocacy and Nursing 19
P. Anne Scott
Introduction 20
   Case Study 1: Safe Staffing Framework 21
Advocacy in Recent Nursing Literature 22
The Patient Experience 23
   Case Study 2: Alice 23
   Case Study 3: Mr. S 23
Some Arguments in Favour of an Advocacy Role for Nurses 26
Some Common Arguments Against an Advocacy Role for Nurses 29
Conclusion 31
References 33

3 Resource Allocation and Rationing in Nursing Care 37
P. Anne Scott
Introduction 38
Resource Allocation and Rationing: Some Definitions 40
Rationing in Nursing: Design or Default? 44
Cases to Consider 46
   Alice 46
   Ms. P 47
Conclusion 49
References 50

4	**Moral Injury and Nursing Practice**........................	53
	Anto Čartolovni, Minna Stolt, Riitta Suhonen, and P. Anne Scott	
	Case Study	54
	Introduction..	55
	Conceptual and Terminological Conundrums.....................	58
	Contributing Factors to the Occurrence of Moral Injury	60
	How to Prevent, Reduce, and Recover from Moral Injury	62
	Conclusion	64
	References..	65
5	**Values-Based Nursing and Fitness to Practice Issues**	69
	Julie-Ann Hayes	
	Introduction (Including Case Study)..............................	69
	Case Study	70
	What Is Value-Based Nursing?...................................	70
	Moral and Personal Values	71
	Conflicting Values..	72
	Professional Values...	72
	Values of the NHS..	73
	Professionalism..	73
	Understanding Fitness to Practise................................	74
	What Does Fitness to Practise Actually Mean?	76
	'Good' Character and Integrity...................................	78
	'Good' Character	78
	Integrity..	79
	Conclusion	82
	References..	83
6	**Patient Autonomy in Nursing and Healthcare Contexts**............	85
	Anna-Marie Greaney and Dónal P. O'Mathúna	
	Introduction: Autonomy and the 'Patient'	86
	Defining Autonomy in Nursing and Healthcare Contexts	87
	Autonomy in Context: Bronagh's Story	89
	Autonomy and Interference: Are they Compatible for Professional Carers?	90
	Autonomy, Capacity, and the Law	94
	Autonomy and Others: Relational Autonomy......................	96
	Autonomy Solutions in Contemporary Healthcare Practice...........	97
	Conclusion: Autonomy, Accountability, and Bronagh	101
	References..	102

Part II Theoretical Approaches to Ethical Analysis and Decision-Making

7	**Principles and Nursing Ethics**.................................	107
	Alan J. Kearns	
	Introduction...	107
	Ethical Positions of Consequentialism, Deontology, and Virtue	108

	Framework of Principles.................................	110
	Case Study	111
	Ethical Questions and Discussion.........................	112
	Conclusion	115
	References...	115
8	**Utilitarianism: A Nursing Perspective**	117
	Michael Igoumenidis	
	Introduction and Case Study.............................	118
	Main Concepts and Theories.............................	119
	Brief History of Utilitarianism	120
	Variants of Utilitarianism	122
	Criticisms Against Utilitarianism	124
	Utilitarianism in Practice	125
	General Applications...............................	125
	Applications in Health Care	126
	Utilitarian Perspectives in Nursing........................	127
	Dilemmas Related to Nursing Ideals	127
	Pandemic Policies from a Utilitarian Point of View	129
	Conclusion	132
	References...	133
9	**Virtue Ethics and Nursing Practice**.........................	135
	Derek Sellman	
	Introduction...	135
	Case Study	137
	What Is Virtue Ethics?	137
	Some Background Regarding the Idea of Virtue and the Idea of Virtue Ethics..	139
	Eudaimonia......................................	140
	Phronesis..	140
	Virtue Ethics and Nursing...............................	141
	The Situationist Argument Against Character	143
	Using the Situationist Critique to Enhance the Development of Character..	144
	Conclusion	144
	References...	146
10	**Care Ethics and Nursing Practice**	147
	Ann Gallagher	
	Introduction...	147
	The Evolution of Care Ethics	148
	The Core of Care Ethics	150
	Claim 1	151
	Claim 2	151
	Claim 3	151
	Claim 4	152
	Perspectives on Care Ethics: Joan Tronto....................	152

Perspectives on Care Ethics: Chris Gastmans. 155
A Practice Situation: Case Study 157
Care Ethics and Nursing Ethics: Strengths and Limitations. 158
Conclusion 159
References. 160

Part III Ethical Issues in Caring for Specific Groups, and in Specific Contexts

11 Ethical Issues at the Beginning of Life 165
Janet Holt
Introduction (Including Case Study). 165
When Does Life Begin? 166
When Does Life Begin to Matter? 168
Assisted Conception 169
Prenatal Diagnosis 171
Saviour Siblings 173
Choosing Children 174
Abortion 175
The Future. 176
Conclusion 177
References. 178

12 Ethical Issues in Mental Health Nursing 181
Grahame Smith
Introduction. 182
The Context of Mental Health Nursing 182
The Moral Domain of Practice 185
Ethical Challenges 187
A Case Study. 189
Conclusion 192
References. 193

13 Ethical Issues in Caring for Older People 195
Riitta Suhonen and Minna Stolt
Case Study 196
Introduction. 196
Autonomy and Dignity as Fundamental Ethical Issues 199
"Seeing Individuals" as an Ethical Issue. 201
Ethical Issues in Using Technology in Caring for Older People 203
Conclusions. 204
References. 205

14 Ethical Issues at the End of Life 209
Janet Holt
Introduction. 210
The Concept of a Good Death (Including Case Study) 210

	Advance Care Planning.	212
	Withdrawing Treatment	213
	Assisted Dying: Suicide and Physician-Assisted Suicide.	216
	Physician-Assisted Suicide.	217
	Assisted Dying: Dignitas	219
	Assisted Dying: Euthanasia	220
	Conclusion	223
	References.	224
15	**Pandemic Ethics and Nursing Practice: When Will We Learn?**	227
	Dónal P. O'Mathúna	
	Introduction.	228
	Lack of Preparation.	230
	Humanitarian Ethics for Nursing in Pandemics	232
	From Individual Ethics to Public Health Ethics	232
	Emotions and Ethics	234
	Social Justice.	235
	Solidarity.	236
	Resistance Humanitarianism.	237
	Conclusion	239
	References.	240
16	**The Ethics of Communication Technologies in the Provision**	
	of Remote, Home-Based Nursing Care.	243
	Alan J. Kearns	
	Introduction.	243
	Communication Technologies for Remote Care.	245
	Telemedicine, Telehealth and Telenursing	246
	Ethical Concerns and Questions	247
	Principle of Equivalence of Care	250
	Technomoral Virtues.	251
	Technomoral Virtue of Honesty	251
	Technomoral Virtue of Humility.	252
	Technomoral Virtue of Justice	252
	Technomoral Virtue of Care	252
	Technomoral Virtue of Practical Wisdom	253
	Case Study	253
	Questions to Consider.	254
	Conclusion	254
	References.	255
17	**Ethical Issues and Principles in Nursing and Healthcare**	
	Research.	257
	P. Anne Scott	
	Introduction.	257
	Some Important Considerations	259
	Respect for the Human Person	259

Informed Consent 260
Beneficence and Non-maleficence 262
Justice (Including Case Study) 263
Working It Through: Ethical Issues and the Stages of the Research
Process 265
Ethics and Data Analysis 268
Ethics and the Relationship with Research Participants.............. 268
Ethics and Dissemination of Research 269
Conclusion 269
References... 270

Authors and Contributors

About the Authors

Bert Gordijn   is Professor and Director, Institute of Ethics, Dublin City University, Dublin, Ireland (Email: bert.gordijn@dcu.ie).

Anto Čartolovni   is an Assistant Professor at the School of Medicine at the Catholic University of Croatia in Zagreb. He teaches nursing and medical students nursing ethics and philosophy, bioethics and medical humanities. His main research areas are bioethics, nursing ethics, philosophy of medicine, ethics of emerging technologies (AI, big data), and philosophy of technology. He has published extensively on various topics in bioethics, philosophy, nursing ethics, and ethics of emerging technologies. He is currently involved in several international and national projects and has been engaged as an ethics expert in several ethical committees and IRB boards (Email: anto.cartolovni@unicath.hr).

Catholic University of Croatia, Zagreb, Croatia.

Ann Gallagher   is Professor and Head of the Department of Health Sciences at Brunel University, London. She has extensive experience as a nurse, ethicist, teacher, researcher, and editor of the international journal *Nursing Ethics*. Ann has researched areas such as dignity in residential care, compassion in the NHS, professionalism in paramedic practice, ethical aspects of professional regulation, and ethics education in social care. She trained as a general nurse at the Royal Victoria Hospital in Belfast during 'the troubles' and as a psychiatric nurse at West Park Hospital Epsom, Surry. Ann's most recent single authored book is *Slow Ethics and the Art of Care* (Gallagher 2020) and co-edited book is *Nursing Practice and Education: Aspiring to Excellence Through Seven Pillars of Learning* (Gallagher A, Deering K and De Luca E (2024)) (Ann.Gallagher@brunel.ac.uk).

Brunel University, London, England, UK.

Anna-Marie Greaney   is a registered nurse who practised clinically primarily in nephrology and renal dialysis. She currently lectures on ethics and professional issues in the Department of Nursing and Healthcare Sciences at Munster Technological University. Anna-Marie is an inaugural member, and previous chair, of the Research Ethics Committee in her host institution. She is engaged in research, publication, supervision, and consultancy in the area of healthcare ethics. Anna-Marie most recently acted as a member of the steering group for the HSE National Policy for Consent in Health and Social Care Research (2023). Research interests centre on autonomy, decision-making, and professional ethics. In 2022, Anna-Marie led an Irish National Forum funded project: Professional Ethics at MTU: Giving Voice to Values in an Irish Context (2022). This project sought to support ethics teaching and learning through engagement with a Giving Voice to Values (GVV) approach to ethical leadership (Gentile 2010). This project continues to evolve (Email: Anna.Marie.Greaney@mtu.ie).

Department of Nursing and Healthcare Sciences, Munster Technological University, Tralee, Ireland.

Julie-Ann Hayes is a Senior Lecturer within the Faculty of Education, Health and Community at Liverpool John Moores University. She is a registered nurse with experience ranging from general medicine and surgery to intensive care and high dependency nursing. Her teaching expertise is within medical law and ethics. Julie teaches across several programmes within the Faculty and is a module leader on the BSc and MSc programmes. Julie completed her PhD in 2016. Her study utilised simulated Fitness to Practice (FtP) panels across three professional groups: nursing, paramedic practice, and social work practice, in order to improve current understanding of the factors that influence decision-making processes involved in FtP. This is a novel research approach to an under-researched area of practice (Email: j.nicholson@ljmu.ac.uk).

Liverpool John Moores University, Liverpool, England, UK.

Janet Holt has recently retired as Associate Professor in Healthcare Ethics in the School of Healthcare at the University of Leeds and now holds the position of Visiting Associate Professor at Leeds and Visiting Professor at Shifa Tameer-E-Millat University (STMU) in Islamabad, Pakistan. At STMU, Janet was part of the team that developed the PhD in Nursing programme, and now she teaches the Nursing Philosophy course and supervises student research projects on this programme. She is a registered nurse with a BA (Hons) in Philosophy from the University of Leeds, an MPhil in Applied Philosophy from the University of Manchester and a PhD in Psychology from the University of Leeds. Janet has had an extensive career in teaching and research in Healthcare Ethics and Nursing Philosophy with a national and international profile and numerous publications in these disciplines. During her career, Janet has served as the Royal College of Nursing representative on the British Medical Association Medical Ethics Committee, Chair of the NHS Research Ethics Committee, Ethics Advisor to two EU horizon 2020 Marie Sklodowska-Curie Innovative Training Networks and Chair of the International Philosophy of Nursing Society (Email: hcsjh@leeds.ac.uk).

University of Leeds, Leeds, England, UK.

Michael Igoumenidis has studied Nursing (BSc) and Philosophy (BA) at the University of Athens. He holds an MA in Healthcare Ethics and Law and a PhD from the University of Manchester, School of Law. He has published several articles related to healthcare with an emphasis on ethical issues, and his research interests mainly lie with the allocation of health resources, nurses' moral competence, and teaching methods in nursing ethics. Michael has taught at graduate and postgraduate level in various institutions. He currently holds the position of Assistant Professor of Nursing Ethics and Deontology in the Department of Nursing at the University of Patras, Greece (Email: Igoum@upatras.gr).

University of Patras, Patras, Greece.

Alan J. Kearns is a Lecturer in Ethics at Dublin City University (DCU), Ireland, and a member of the DCU Institute of Ethics. He has a range of scholarly publications in the area of ethics and nursing. As well as having been involved in a number of ethics committees, Alan has extensive experience in teaching ethics and delivering healthcare ethics talks and courses in hospitals (Email: alan.kearns@dcu.ie).

Dublin City University, Dublin, Ireland.

Rachel Kenna is the Chief Nursing Officer (CNO) for Ireland and was appointed to the post in June 2020. She is a Registered Children's and General Nurse (RCN/RGN) and has extensive clinical and managerial experience, spanning 30 years in Ireland and the UK, across a wide variety of clinical areas. The CNO role is as important strategic leadership and influencing role providing professional policy direction and evidence-based expert advice for Government on nursing, midwifery, and general health policy development. As an Assistant Secretary in the Department of Health, the CNO, in addition to nursing and midwifery policy has a wide health policy portfolio including the National Patient Safety Office, professional regulation and strategic workforce planning and reform. Rachel is educated in a wide range of areas to support her in her role and holds an MSc in Child Protection and Welfare and a BSc in Nursing Management. Rachel's other educational qualifications include a Higher Diploma in Professional Practice, Critical Care Nursing, Leadership and Quality in Healthcare, a Diploma in Human Rights and Equality, and a Professional Diploma in Governance. Rachel is also a Florence Nightingale Leadership graduate (Email: rachel_kenna@health.gov.ie).

Department of Health, Government of Ireland, Dublin, Ireland.

Dónal P. O'Mathúna is Associate Professor in the College of Nursing and Associate Director of Research in the Centre for Bioethics at The Ohio State University (OSU), Columbus, Ohio, USA. Dónal has two main areas of research interest: healthcare ethics and evidence-based practice. He is the Director of the Cochrane Affiliate at the OSU Fuld National Institute for Evidence-Based Practice in Nursing and Healthcare and a member of the Executive Committee of the Cochrane US Network. Dónal's research in ethics focuses on ethical issues in disasters, pandemics, and humanitarian crises. He is particularly interested in research ethics for One Health projects and during emergencies and violent conflicts (Email: Omathuna.6@osu.edu).

Ohio State University, Columbus, OH, USA.

P. Anne Scott is Professor Emerita University of Galway, Ireland. She was previously Professor and Vice President for Equality and Diversity, National University of Ireland, Galway. Anne is a nurse and philosopher. She has worked as a nurse and academic in Ireland, England, Kenya, and Scotland. Her main research and scholarly interests are in the philosophy and ethics of healthcare, judgement and decision-making, and the health workforce. Anne was recently part of a COST Action project on rationing of nursing care: RANCARE. CA15208 (Email: anne.scott@universityofgalway.ie).

University of Galway, Galway, Ireland.

Shane M. Scott is a practitioner with a background in public policy, focusing on prudential and communications regulation. His interests include the ethical implications of public policy development and implementation, with a particular focus on resource allocation and nursing input into policy development (Email: shanescott91boe@gmail.com).

London, UK.

Derek Sellman was, until retirement, an Associate Professor at the Faculty of Nursing, University of Alberta, Canada. His academic interests included nursing ethics, philosophy of nursing, and education for professional practice. Derek served as Editor-in-Chief of the international journal *Nursing Philosophy* for 12 years and is the author of *What Makes a Good Nurse: Why the Virtues are Important for Nurses*.

University of Alberta, Edmonton, Canada.

Grahame Smith is a mental health nursing academic, a Reader (Associate Professor) in Mental Health Innovation, and founder and centre lead for the Centre for Collaborative Innovation in Dementia at Liverpool John Moores University. Grahame continues to practice, research, and publish within the mental health nursing field. His specific interests include living well with dementia, user-centric innovation (health), and mental health ethics. As a methodological pragmatist, Grahame has used a number of research methodologies within a co-production context, participatory action research being his main methodological approach (Email: g.m.smith@ljmu.ac.uk).

Liverpool John Moores University, Liverpool, England, UK.

Minna Stolt, PhD is Professor (acting) in the Department of Nursing Science at the University of Turku, Finland and Satakunta Wellbeing Services County. Minna is a podiatrist by professional background. Her main research interests are in functional health and quality of care, as well as ethics of healthcare and rehabilitation. She is a Fellow of the European Academic of Nursing Science (FEANS) and Fellow of the Royal College of Physicians and Surgeons of Glasgow (FFPM RCPS Glasg.). Currently, she is involved in many international and national projects in nursing science (Email: minna.stolt@utu.fi).

Department of Nursing Science, University of Turku, Turku, Finland.

Riitta Suhonen is Professor in Nursing Science, Gerontological Nursing, in the University of Turku, Finland and the Director of the Doctoral Programme in Nursing Science. Riitta has two main areas of research interest and leads two research programmes: Older Individuals' Health, Nursing and Science, and Ethical Healthcare and Nursing. Riitta is a Director of Nursing in Turku University Hospital, The Wellbeing Services County of Southwest Finland. She is a Member of the Academia Europea and a Fellow of the European Academy of Nursing Science. Riitta is interested in the values base in caring for older people, patients' rights, individualised nursing care, and organisational and leadership ethics (Email: riisuh@utu.fi).

Department of Nursing Science, University of Turku, Turku, Finland.

Contributors

Anto Čartolovni School of Medicine, Catholic University of Croatia, Zagreb, Croatia

Ann Gallagher Department of Health Sciences, Brunel University London, London, UK

Anna-Marie Greaney Department of Nursing and Healthcare Sciences, Munster Technological University, Tralee, Co. Kerry, Ireland

Julie-Ann Hayes School of Nursing and Allied Health, Liverpool John Moores University, Liverpool, UK

Janet Holt School of Healthcare, University of Leeds, Leeds, UK

Michael Igoumenidis University of Patras, Patras, Greece

Alan J. Kearns School of Theology, Philosophy, and Music, Dublin City University, Dublin, Ireland

Dónal P. O'Mathúna College of Nursing, The Ohio State University, Columbus, OH, USA

P. Anne Scott University of Galway, Galway, Co Galway, Ireland

Derek Sellman Edmonton, AB, Canada

Grahame Smith School of Nursing and Allied Health, Liverpool John Moores University, Liverpool, UK

Minna Stolt Department of Nursing Science, University of Turku, Turku, Finland
Wellbeing Services County of Satakunta, Pori, Finland

Riitta Suhonen Department of Nursing Science, University of Turku, Turku, Finland
Turku University Hospital, Wellbeing Services County of Southwest Finland, Turku, Finland

Part I

Nursing and Ethics: Some Key Concepts

Nursing and the Ethical Dimension of Practice

P. Anne Scott

Abstract

Nurses are important to patients. Nurses touch people's lives during some of the peaks and troughs of human existence. Therefore it is important that we think carefully about nurses and nursing. What do our patients require from nurses, and how do we, as a society, as nurses, and as health service leaders, meet patient need? A first step in thinking about nurses and nursing is to observe that nursing is an important health service resource that needs to be recognised, supported, and protected.

It is also important to recognise that nursing, as a practice, has moral values at its core. The nurse-patient relationship, which is central to the provision of nursing care, has ethical importance and is of ethical significance.

Additionally, it is noted that the context within which nurses practice can shape, and be shaped by, the moral values of nursing. These moral values form what can be termed the ethical dimension of nursing. It is therefore important that we explore and examine these moral values. Codes of conduct are examples of the nursing profession's collective attempt to express its underlying values. The institutions within which nurses work help, or hinder, the actual expression of these values in nursing practice and patient care.

The interplay of these various factors needs to be recognised, in order to ensure that we as nurses, as potential patients, and as members of society understand what good nursing practice means, what it looks like in practice, and how it can be supported. This chapter sets out to identify the ethical dimension of nursing practice and signal its relevance for good nursing care and a safe, supportive patient experience. The chapters which follow provide theoretical and

P. A. Scott (✉)
University of Galway, Galway, Co Galway, Ireland
e-mail: anne.scott@universityofgalway.ie

conceptual lenses through which to identify, analyse, and discuss ethical issues in nursing practice, with a view to providing tools for the nurse to practice in an ethically sensitive and appropriate manner.

Keywords

Ethical domain · Nurse-patient relationship · Nursing ethics · Patient-centred care · Codes of conduct · Values · Moral values

Introduction

The COVID-19 pandemic has had a profound impact on the nursing workforce internationally (Buchan and Catton 2023). Levels of burnout and psychological distress among nurses are unprecedented, and many nurses have retired earlier than planned and/or have left their nursing positions as a direct result of the overwhelming pressures placed on them while caring for patients during the pandemic (Buchan et al. 2022; ICN 2023). These pressures have exacerbated the nursing shortages experienced in many health systems for a variety of reasons including lack of investment in, and lack of adequate planning for, nursing workforce requirements in the years leading up to the pandemic (Buchan et al. 2022; Gurková et al. 2022).

The pandemic also highlighted to the public the important role nursing plays in health systems and patient care internationally (Gurková et al. 2022; Buchan and Catton 2023). However, the impact of the nursing shortages, both pre-pandemic and pandemic-induced, may be changing the way nurses think about nursing and about themselves as practicing nurses. Mandal (2020), a systematic review examining rationing of nursing care, indicates that such rationing is pervasive, built structurally into our health systems, and is in grave danger of increasing risks to patient safety and undermining the philosophical foundations of nursing, for example. Scott et al. (2020), in an editorial on missed care and the appropriate use of the nursing resource, make a very similar point:

> *Of equal concern is the reality that inadequate nurse staffing levels, at the sharp end of care delivery, forces and perpetuates models of hollowed out, reduced, incomplete conceptions of nursing practice and patient care. This may ultimately change the nature of nursing, both as a practice and as a values-based, humane, self-reflective, practice discipline.* (Scott et al. 2020, e12288)

However, the pre-pandemic, pandemic, and post-pandemic experience of being ill, vulnerable, and needing care and support has not changed for the patients for whom nurses care (Scott et al. 2014; Avallin et al. 2020). What can and what should nurses do in light of the realities of patient care needs and the practice environment? These questions have ethical as well as professional import. Nurses are important to patients: to their experience of illness, disease, treatment, care, and recovery (Institute of Medicine (IoM) 2011; Scott et al. 2014; Dall'Ora et al. 2022). For example, in a systematic review exploring the impact of nurse staffing levels on patient outcomes Dall'Ora et al. (2022, e104311) concluded that "Higher registered nurse staffing levels reduced the risk of patient death in acute care settings." Nurses can touch people's lives during some of the peaks and troughs of human existence. Nurse education curricula, the nursing literature, and codes of professional conduct for nurses provide some insight into both professional and societal expectations of nurses. Much of these insights and expectations centre around the professional skills and competence and the personal characteristics and engagement of the individual nurse (Scott et al. 2014).

Professional codes of conduct such as those published by the Nursing and Midwifery Council (NMC) (2015), the Nursing and Midwifery Board of Ireland (NMBI) (2021), and the International Council of Nurses (ICN) (2021) are examples of the profession's collective attempt to express the underlying values of the nursing profession. Many of the values expressed in professional codes for nurses are moral values. As a further example in the 2023 annual report for International Nurses Day, "Our Nurses, Our Future", the ICN states the following:

> *The promotion of equity, social justice and respect for human rights are fundamental principles of nursing ethics. Nurses play a vital role in ensuring that these principles are upheld in health systems' design and delivery to provide equitable and non-discriminatory care to all patients. ... One way to protect vulnerable populations is by promoting health equity. This can be achieved by addressing the root causes of health disparities such as poverty, discrimination and lack of access to health care. Nurses can advocate for policy changes that address these issues and ensure that health care services are accessible to all.*
> (International Council of Nurses 2023, p. 37)

However, as indicated above, nursing practice also happens within a context. This context is the health service of the relevant institution, locality, region, or country. It is necessary to acknowledge, as well as to fully appreciate, the impact that this context has on the individual practitioner's ability to practice to the best of their ability, including providing ethically sensitive care. Certain expectations of nurses are expressed, for example, in the nursing literature, education programmes, and codes of conduct. With this back drop, in addition to the increasingly urgent call from the ICN and the World Health Organisation (WHO) to recognise the current world-wise nursing shortage as a "global health emergency" (Buchan et al. 2022,; Buchan and Catton 2023, p. 4) and recognising the impact of the context of nursing practice on the nurse's ability to provide good (competent, sensitive, respectful) nursing care, it is important that we explore and examine the morally relevant aspects (in other words the moral dimension) of nursing practice.[1]

---

[1] The terms moral and ethical, while having roots in the Latin and Greek languages respectively, will be used interchangeably throughout this text.

Nursing and the Ethical Domain of Practice

The ethical domain of human life relates to how we behave towards each other and the reasons we do so. As the American scholar Martha Levine, writing for practising nurses in the 1970s, succinctly and powerfully states:

> *Ethical behaviour is not the display of one's moral rectitude in times of crisis. It is the day-to-day expression of one's commitment to other persons and the ways in which human beings relate to one another in their daily interactions.* (Levine 1977, p. 845)

The way we relate to one another, behave towards one another, the attitudes we display to other people—whether strangers, neighbours, patients or clients—are moral actions, behaviours, and attitudes. These behaviours, actions, and attitudes are based on personal, as well as professionally socialised, attitudes, judgements, and decisions. This implies, for example, that despite a difficult working environment, there is personal responsibility on the individual nurse for the care they provide (NMBI 2021; Kearns 2020). The nurse may be very busy and stressed by work load; however, how they receive the newly admitted patient, or respond to a patient's call for help, is in part a personal ethical decision and behaviour. Being fully and continuously aware of this ethical dimension of nursing care is a topic that deserves some attention. Likewise, also deserving of attention is the topic of what it is reasonable to expect from nursing staff, in situations where the work environment of the nurse is unsupportive of good nursing and detrimental to safe, humane patient care.

A growing evidence base indicates the detrimental impacts of a poor work environment on nurses and on patient care (Scott et al. 2014; Dall'Ora and Saville 2021; Dall'Ora et al. 2022; Gurková et al. 2022). Such situations arose during the recent COVID-19 pandemic where nurses were placed in direct risk to their health due to the shortage/unavailability of personal protective equipment (PPE) or vaccinations for staff. It was also the case where dramatic increase in demand for care overwhelmed the limited nursing resource in hospitals (Lavoi-Tremblay et al. 2022) and care homes (Hillestad et al. 2023). However, there was evidence of this type of detrimental environment on nurse and patient outcomes prior to the pandemic (Jones et al. 2015; Tønnessen et al. 2020). There is recognition, for example, of corporate responsibility, in addition to individual responsibility, in situations such as those reported in Mid Staffordshire (Francis 2010, 2013) or maternity care (Ockenden 2022), for a lack of humane, competent nursing/midwifery care.

The COVID-19 pandemic has heightened or exacerbated these issues – including very significant impacts on the nursing workforce (Buchan et al. 2022). The recognition of corporate/organisational responsibility is also articulated in an explicit manner. For example, in an analysis of the impact of the COVID-19 pandemic on practising nurses worldwide, Buchan and Catton (2023, p. 27) state:

> *The key point that emerges from these surveys and reviews is that the scale of actual and potential trauma and burnout in the nursing workforce is huge. This is extremely concerning, because nurse burnout is both an issue of personal health and well-being, and a risk to*

> *service quality and health system recovery and rebuild. In addition, policy makers must recognise that nurses are individuals with non-work commitments and that, during the pandemic, their concerns extended beyond their own personal experiences, to include responsibilities for their families. ... Traditionally, burnout is viewed as an individual issue. However, reframing burnout as an organisational and collective phenomenon affords the broader perspective necessary to address nurse burnout.*

In a similar vein, the European Commission expert panel on the mental health of the health workforce during the pandemic emphasised the need to "immediately support the mental health and alleviate the consequences of stress, fear, and moral injury." The expert panel go on to highlight that "The organisation, as opposed to the individual worker, is to be held publicly accountable for worker well-being" (European Commission, Directorate-General for Health and Food Safety 2021, pp. 9–10).

Health worker well-being, in this case nurse well-being, is directly correlated with patient outcomes; i.e., nurse burnout is directly correlated with adverse patient outcomes such as increased risk to patient safety and adverse events, such as medication errors, infections, and falls (Dall'Ora and Saville 2021). Employers have a duty of care to their workers. This duty of care has both moral and legal elements (in some countries this is enshrined in legislation, in other countries, such as England, it is supported via case law). It can be argued that nurses are an important part of the healthcare workforce and, as health service employees, are a vital contributor to safe, humane patient care and positive patient outcomes. Nurses' ability to provide safe, humane care for patients/clients is significantly influenced by their work environment (including leadership, culture, and resourcing). Therefore health service employers have a moral duty to support nurses in the provision of safe, humane patient care, by ensuring a supportive work environment.

In nursing we interact with human beings made *more than ordinarily vulnerable* (Sellman 2011, p. 67) by illness, disease, or other life circumstances. These human beings need our professional help and care. Good nursing practice therefore requires us to engage at a human as well as a professional level. Patients assume professional competence, until we prove them wrong (Scott 2014). They seek kindness and compassion as the basis of developing confidence and trust that they are "in good hands." They seek to be cared about as individuals, as well as being cared for, by the nurses they encounter. We, the nurses responsible for the care of these patients, may show kindness and compassion through many ordinary interactions and interventions that acknowledge the individuality and human context of the patient – or we may choose not to do so. These choices are at the heart of the ethical domain of our nursing practice.

The ability to recognise the need of the patient: to relate to, respond to, and to recognise those who are "more than ordinarily vulnerable" (Sellman 2011, p. 67) suggests the ability, in the nurse, to develop a basic connection as human being with another human being. In developing this connection, we are setting the foundations for a nurse-patient relationship. This is the vehicle through which we provide engaged, connected, and patient-led care. Nurse-patient interaction and engagement, as manifest through the nurse-patient relationship, are at the heart of the moral domain of nursing practice.

Nurse-Patient Interaction: The Nurse-Patient Relationship (Including a Case Study)

The American nurse scholar Janice Morse (1991) argues that the relationship between the patient and the nurse is not only the basis and frame within which nursing care happens: the patient-nurse relationship is a direct outcome of a series of interactions, observations, and engagements between the patient and nurse. The nurse-patient and patient-nurse relationship is a negotiated and evolving reality for the duration of the patient-nurse contact. Morse (1991) in her seminal study of the nurse-patient relationship identified four different types of relationship: the clinical relationship, the therapeutic relationship, the connected relationship, and the over-involved relationship. The type of relationship that develops, Morse argues, depends:

> *on the durations of the contact between the nurse and the patient, the needs of the patient, the commitment of the nurse and the patient's willingness to trust the nurse…* (Morse 1991, p. 455).

We might add to this list a fifth dependency, which is the basic support and resource, such as nursing time, which the healthcare institution provides to the nurse to enable such engagement with patients (Buchan and Catton 2023; ICN 2023).

The clinical relationship, as described by Morse, is that which is appropriate when the contact is short, functional, and the needs of the patient very discreet – such as the removal of sutures as an outpatient or the dressing of a minor wound. The therapeutic relationship, which Morse suggests is the most often encountered, goes somewhat deeper than the clinical relationship – contact between the nurse and patient is still relatively brief, patient need is relatively minor, and care is given quickly and effectively. In this type of relationship, the patient expects to be treated as a patient and has family and friends to meet other psychosocial support needs. Morse suggests that within the context of this type of relationship, some degree of testing of the relationship will occur from the patient's perspective, to see if the patient can "trust" the nurse to look after them properly, until they can care for themselves again. This can involve ringing the call bell for a minor matter to see if the nurse will answer or observing a nurse to see if they will actually return when they have indicated to the patient that they will get back to them on a specific issue. This is likely to be the most common form of nurse-patient relationship encountered in modern acute care settings. However, for very dependent and acutely ill individuals, their needs require the nurse to be able to flex between the therapeutic and connected forms of the nurse-patient relationship.

The connected relationship either evolves over time, as patient and nurse get to know each other over an extended care period, or is stimulated by the ability of a nurse to respond to the intensity of the patient's need. Morse suggests that:

in this relationship, the patient believes that the nurse 'has gone the extra mile', respects the nurse's judgement and feels grateful, the nurse believes that her care has made a difference to the patient. (Morse 1991, p. 458)

In the over-involved relationship, the nurse treats the patient as a person and friend first and a patient second. The nurse can become territorial over the patient believing she/he is the only one who can care properly for this patient. The nurse may become over-extended, lose a sense of balance, and suffer impaired judgement. This kind of scenario can lead to impaired patient care and burnout.

The case study below will help bring focus to our discussion of the nurse-patient relationship and provide some insight into its importance in understanding the ethical domain of practice, in addition to its potential significance to a patient's experience. This case study involves a nursing academic and former colleague (CN) who had been diagnosed with breast cancer.[2] CN kept a diary as she confronted and experienced biopsy, diagnosis, surgery, and prepared for radiotherapy. Her diary provides important insights into both the nurse-patient relationship, and nursing care, from the perspective of an informed patient:

Being 'prepped' consisted of having my breast, axilla, and back painted. The sensation was pleasant; the last pleasant sensation there would be for a breast that had, in its time, been appreciated by baby and lover alike. There was no avoiding the issue, this was what I was going to lose. The nurse and I didn't talk. She didn't fill the moment with idle chit chat or pseudo empathy, which I would have found offensive and would have demanded social responses from me that I would have struggled to make. The nurse treated the task and thus me and my soon to be no more breast, with respect. While sharing none of the horrors of pubic shaving, this preoperative preparation was an activity that called for high calibre nursing skills. I was very grateful for the way it was managed; it preserved my dignity, did not exacerbate an intrinsically distressing situation and gave me a sense of, literally, 'being in good hands'. (CN)

The nurse described here is observant, respectful of her patient, competent, and "managed" the interaction with CN and the required nursing intervention, in a calm, professional, and respectful manner. It seems reasonable to suggest that the above scenario portrays the "therapeutic" relationship described by Morse:

On return from theatre it was trained staff who washed me, made me comfortable, gave me iced water to drink while checking heart rate, blood pressure, oxygen saturation, drain, and wound. The sense of being completely cared for, when I was in that post anaesthesia dependency state was wonderfully comforting and reassuring. For a short while I was completely in their hands and their competence was very obvious. Each task done well reinforced the sense of that competence. So it was as important that the water from the face cloth didn't run down my front as that the drain wasn't pulled or the wound exposed, forcing me to look at it rather than letting me choose my moment. These demonstrations of hands-on competence created a climate of confidence in the nurses' expertise. (CN)

---

[2] This narrative is used in a paper published in *Nursing Philosophy* (Niven and Scott 2003), to explore the role of the patient's voice in determining the appropriate distribution of the nursing resource. I wish to express my thanks to *Nursing Philosophy* for enabling its reproduction in this chapter.

Again, in this diary extract, CN describes examples of therapeutic relationships. The nurses remain nameless, part of the effective, competent, caring team. CN then goes on to describe the patient experience and the missed opportunities when that therapeutic engagement is lacking:

> *In contrast the first postoperative shower was the domain of the nursing assistant. Of course this cannot be combined with cardio-vascular monitoring in the way that bed-based care can be. And it is a low level activity, with the focus of concern on not letting the patient stumble, get scalded or the wound get wet. Even though at this level the task was completed competently and kindly, my sense, as a patient and as a nurse, is that this first postoperative shower is a key nursing activity, not one to be 'given away' to a nursing assistant. As a nurse I recognise the opportunity for proper monitoring of the wound and drain, and much more crucially of the patient's psychological state. Is she afraid to look and, if so, how best should this be managed? Does she want to talk about it; get information, reassurance that her thoughts and feelings are normal? How does it feel, is hypo or hypersensitivity present, to what extent; how should it be accommodated while showering and dressing? These assessments can be more completely made in the shower than in the bed; and they can be inferred from the patient's behaviour without the need for intrusive, insensitive, premature questioning. For the patient, the first post-op shower represents her most vulnerable moment, naked, only one breast, a huge wound, a drain, a newly improved view of one's flabby bits. Not only is the patient confronting this sight for the first time, she is exposing herself to someone else's view in, for many, a rehearsal of showing her husband or partner. That degree of vulnerability demands a professional's response. It is the nurse, not her assistant, who has the biological, psychological and sociological knowledge that enables her to deal with the situation appropriately.* (CN)

CN's comments here have ethical as well as clinical relevance. Exposure of the patient to this first post-operative shower has ethical as well as clinical salience and shows a potential lack of ethical sensitivity in the delegation of this task to the care assistant. We then find, in CN's account of her interactions with the Clinical Nurse Specialist in Oncology, an excellent description of Morse's "connected" relationship:

> *E's skill and respect for me as a patient were evident in a number of ways, on this occasion and on all succeeding occasions. I told her I was scared, I would have told anyone but she made it easy to say to her and her reaction, which was minimal, didn't make me feel foolish. Her behaviour made it entirely clear that she had understood my terror and was reacting accordingly. E knew I was an academic before she met me, so her conversation during the biopsy, clearly designed to distract me, utilised that knowledge. She told me about her Master's degree and the essay she stayed up all night word processing and which had got lost. The topic was familiar enough to hold my attention and to remind me of situations in which I was a competent 'grown up' person; thus boosting my self-esteem and confidence. I nearly passed out at one point. Her skill in dealing with that was very evident – position, comfort, maintaining the circumstances which allowed the biopsy to continue; afterwards a glass of really cold water; keeping someone with me when she had to go. And everything done in a way which allowed me to maintain my dignity. E's behaviour during the biopsy established the basis for my total trust in her. This was vital when she became the person to communicate the confirmed diagnosis and the options for surgery.* (CN)

An essential element here may be to make the invisible visible. CN struggles to articulate the ways in which E had provided such vital care:

The sense of unlimited time and a depth of knowledge about a huge range of vital things – surgery, recovery, side-effects and how best to manage them, the individual differences, the emotional consequences, the hands-on skills and her availability for anything – to be with you the first time you looked, when you got your prosthesis, for my husband, for my daughter, for me when I want, not according to a schedule. … I have seen E many times now and her skills are always impressive but it's at times of shock and distress – diagnosis, admission, post-operatively – that they are most evident. It's like the matching pieces of a jigsaw – what she provides fits your needs so well that it makes something approaching a whole. (CN)

This is a really powerful narrative about good nursing and a real accolade to a number of nurses but particularly to E; a nurse who clearly provided excellent nursing care and a vital, enriching supportive relationship at a very bewildering and difficult time in a patient's life. The narrative also demonstrates the intertwined nature of the ethical and clinical domains of nursing practice, as manifest in the provision of nursing care.

As this narrative demonstrates, nurse-patient interactions and the provision of nursing care are formed by, and essentially exist as, attitudes, behaviours, and actions, the latter often being highly skilled. This is integral to the very essence of nursing. How one behaves with a patient, how one responds to the patient's need for care, is as much about the nurse's ethical response, ethical behaviour towards another human being who is vulnerable (Sellman 2011), or suffering, as it is about the nurse's clinical response. Indeed many authors, including Nortvedt (2001), argue that it is not possible to divide the clinical from the ethical in many nursing care activities and interventions.[3] From a position of recognising the ethical as well as the clinical response of the nurse, it is a short step to argue that nursing practice, and consequently nursing care, has an important ethical element or dimension. In other words the ethical is inherent in nursing practice and thus to the provision of nursing care (Tønnessen et al. 2020). So how does this play out in the context of patient care? What does the ethical dimension of nursing care and nursing practice actually look like?

From the perspective of the patient, and their families, they seem to want reasonably consistent things from their nursing and medical carers: kindness, compassion, competence, consideration, information, communication, and care (Scott et al. 2014). This does not seem an extreme or unreasonable demand from well-educated professionals in a health system of the twenty-first century, in a developed and relatively well-resourced society. It is also entirely consistent with the conception of nursing that is articulated clearly in our codes of practice. The core values expressed in the NMC (2015) code are the following:

(a) Prioritise people.
(b) Practice effectively.
(c) Preserve safety.
(d) Promote professionalism and trust.

---

[3] Grahame Smith in Chap. 12 of this book also holds this position.

The NMBI (2021) *Code of Professional Conduct and Ethics* describes the following five principles as the core principles that should underlie nursing care in the Irish healthcare context:

1. Respect for the dignity of the person.
2. Professional responsibility and accountability.
3. Quality of practice.
4. Trust and confidentiality.
5. Collaboration with others.

A reader of the text of these two codes of practice would discover significant similarities in the values being expressed, the description of good nursing, and the types of behaviours and attitudes required of the professional nurse in their interactions with both patients/clients and colleagues.

The codes, as indicated above, are examples of the profession's collective attempt to express what good nursing practice looks like. These descriptions of good nursing practice are firmly rooted in moral values and a language that expresses the underlying ethical dimension of nursing practice. The codes provide a clear recognition of the reality that nurses can have a profound impact on their patients/clients. Nursing registration and regulatory bodies demand that this impact is beneficial (good) for the patient. In the context of illness and disease, patients frequently experience heightened vulnerability. They are in need of nursing care and attention. This increased vulnerability of the patient combined with the inherent ability of the nurse to assist, support, and nurture the patient/client or to snub, injure, or neglect the patient/client throws the ethical dimension of nursing into sharp relief. How should recognition of, and insight into, this ethical reality of practice be supported in our everyday nursing care?

We have an extensive nursing literature that claims the importance, or centrality, of care and caring in nursing practice (Karlsson and Pembrant 2020). This is often mirrored in nursing rhetoric and educational texts. Empirical studies exploring nursing support a conceptualisation of nursing care that includes psychosocial support and a recognition of the patient/client as a whole person, with psychological, social, and physical care needs (Ausserhofer et al. 2014; Scott et al. 2014). Care is, however, only one of the ethically relevant concepts used in descriptions of nursing practice. de Raeve (2002) considers the importance of trust and integrity in the provision of appropriate patient care. Nortvedt (2001) and Scott (2019) speak of the need to be sensitive to the personhood of the patient in order to really come to understand what the patient requires from the nurse.

This description of patient need, as well as the appropriate nursing response, not only assumes an understanding of the patient as a human being who presents both unique and anticipated responses to their illness and circumstances; it also assumes a description and understanding of nursing that sees the nurse as responsive and equipped to meet these needs. A description and articulation of nursing as a practice capable of meeting such needs is the beginning of a theory of nursing practice. As the above would indicate, this is a theory of nursing practice that sees the good for patients and nurses' ability to help provide some of these goods, as central to nursing practice.

The good in healthcare frequently has psychological, social, spiritual, as well as physical dimensions. Recognising the human being who is a patient/client in need in this manner suggests (1) that practitioners must be sensitive to more than the physical domain of patient experience; and (2) this broader sensitivity calls on the involvement of the practitioner, as person, in a distinct way. The clinician and ethicist Søren Holm expresses this latter point thus:

> *When you meet the patient you meet another human being who is vulnerable, who trusts you, and whose life you can influence in a significant way. This creates a specific responsibility towards this other human being, which can be difficult to understand for outsiders, but which nevertheless plays a significant role in the deliberation of health care professionals. In their minds it is both related to the power they have, and to the respect they have to show.* (Holm 1997, p. 127)

The respect and the power over another, which nurses and other practitioners have, and the trust and confidence which patients can be enabled to feel are mediated, normally, through the specific relationship the practitioner has with the patient. Working out what the nurse-patient/client relationship should be takes thought, reflection, and a recognition that different patient-practitioner interactions may require differing responses depending on the clinical context and patient care needs, as we can see from CN's narrative above. Nursing care should therefore be patient-led and patient-focused (Scott 2014).

However, as indicated in the introduction to this chapter, nursing and the nurse-patient relationship take place in a context. This context is that of the particular healthcare institution, in the local, regional, and national arena of health service provision. At a micro level, the nurse practices in a ward or community context. The structure of care delivery, the resourcing, and the leadership in this context can have a significant influence on the nurse's ability and motivation to provide patient-sensitive, patient-led, and patient-focused nursing care. If structures, leadership (institutional and nursing leadership), and resourcing are not supportive of good nursing, the efforts of individual nurses will be undermined, nursing morale will gradually deteriorate, and nurses will become ill or leave. High staff turnover leads to lack of engagement and commitment and deteriorating patient care (Buchan and Catton 2023):

> *There is also growing evidence that the elements of nursing care most frequently left undone or missed are the so-called "basic" and "softer" elements of care, such as patient hygiene, comfort care, patient education, and discharge planning. These are elements of care that make the patient feel better, feel cared for. These elements of care lead to patients perceiving that they are "in good hands" - that is, they are being cared for by competent, caring staff. It can be argued that care that helps the patient feel better, feel cared for, is care that is rooted in ethically sound practice - recognising what is good for the patient from a care perspective* (Tønnessen et al. 2020, p. 1396).

It is the case that the context of nursing practice has changed quite dramatically over the past decade or so in many countries, with the length of patient stay in the acute hospital sector being significantly reduced, leading to increasing numbers of very dependent patents, increased churn, and little or no "downtime" for nursing staff (Cho et al. 2014). This is a situation dramatically impacted and augmented by the COVID-19 pandemic. This means that the amount of time and opportunities that the nurse has to interact with and get to know the patient is also substantially reduced. This has implications for the way we think about nursing and the nurse-patient relationship.

While we, as nurses and as ordinary members of the public, have been upset, even scandalised, by reports of poor care (Francis 2010; Vale of Leven 2014; HIQA 2015; Ockenden 2022), we should also carefully consider potential barriers to providing good nursing care and remove such barriers where there is the possibility to do so. We thus must make the resourcing,[4] context, organisation, and culture of nursing practice visible in order that ethically appropriate practice is not deemed to be the exclusive responsibility of the individual nurse.

These are sentiments shared by a number of scholars and policymakers in recent reports (Buchan et al. 2022; Buchan and Catton 2023; ICN 2023). Judge Francis, for example, in his reports, emphasises how inadequate staffing, lack of leadership, and low staff morale ultimately led to a breakdown of acceptable norms and nursing care (Francis 2010, 2013). Lord MacLean, author of the report from the Vale of Leven Hospital inquiry, draws on both his experience as a patient who contracted Clostridium difficile in, and on his overall review of, the Vale of Leven Hospital:

> *It has to be emphasised that good nursing care lies at the very heart of the appropriate management of patients who contract CDI. ... Many patients were exposed unnecessarily to CDI*[5] *and had to suffer the humiliation and distress often associated with the infection. ... A lack of strong management as well as personal and system failures contributed to the development of a culture in the VOLH that had lost sight of what is of the very essence of a hospital – a caring and compassionate environment dedicated to the provision of the highest possible level of care.*—Vale of Leven Hospital Inquiry (2014), Executive Summary (pp. 5–6).

From this report it is evident that patient safety, personal dignity, and the quality of care patients received was compromised in this hospital over the specified period of time. This inadequate care resulted in the deaths of 28 elderly people in situations of significant distress and discomfort. The experience of seeing vulnerable elderly relatives in such a state also brought considerable distress to relatives of these patients. Lord MacLean's sentiments, expressed in the report of the Vale of Leven Hospital inquiry, echo the findings and recommendations of many other reports on failures in the health service and among health service staff. See, for example, Francis (2013), HIQA (2015), and Ockenden (2022).

---

[4] See Chap. 3 for an introduction to resource allocation and rationing in nursing and healthcare.
[5] Clostridium difficile infection.

These reports emphasise the vital importance of competent, engaged, and compassionate nursing to both the experience of care and, ultimately, to the survival of very vulnerable patients who find themselves incapacitated by illness and very dependent for care and support on the strangers who are healthcare and nursing staff. In these reports the ethical and clinical domains of nursing are inextricably intertwined, as is the need for supportive organisational structures and systems to enable, challenge, and engage nurses in the provision of ethically sensitive, high quality patient care.

Conclusion

This introductory chapter sets out to begin an exploration of the ethical dimension of nursing practice, many elements of which will be taken up by other authors and developed in the other chapters in this book. A key point developed in this chapter is that the ethical and clinical domains of nursing overlap significantly and are deeply intertwined. Ethically sensitive, clinically competent care humanises the patient experience and is a vital element in safe effective care. However, the ability to provide competent, humanising care is either enabled, enhanced, or inhibited by the organisational structure and culture within which nurses practice.

The fact that nurses, as well as the institutions within which nurses work, can do patients/clients good or ill as persons and human beings link us directly into the ethical domain of nursing practice. It raises questions about what we, as nurses, as members of the public, and as potential patients, mean by "good nursing care". What are the similarities and differences in how we should nurse the infant who needs our care, the young child, the adolescent, the cognitively intact adult, the cognitively impaired but functioning adult, the memory impaired adult, those living with dementia, the frail elderly, the terminally ill, the dying person? The answers to these questions are at the heart of ethical, humane, competent nursing practice.

The remainder of the chapters in this book will help us explore potential answers to the questions "What is good nursing from an ethics perspective?" and "How is ethically praiseworthy nursing enacted?" within the context of particular organisations, patient circumstances, and experiences.

We begin (Chaps. 2, 3, 4, 5, and 6) by considering a number of key concepts in nursing ethics – such as advocacy, resource allocation, moral injury, values, fitness to practice, and autonomy in nursing and healthcare. We then move in Chaps. 7 through 10 to discuss a number of theoretical lenses via which an examination of the ethical domain of nursing practice may be developed. Chapters 11 and 14 explore ethical issues at the beginning and end of life. Mental health nursing contexts give rise to some unique ethical issues, as described in Chap. 12. This is followed in Chaps. 13, 15 and 16, by an exploration of ethical issues that may arise in the care of older people, nursing in emergency situations such as pandemics and in the use of communication technologies for the provision of remote, home-based nursing care. The book closes with a brief consideration of some of the ethical issues requiring consideration when engaged in nursing and healthcare research.

Key Learning Points
- The ethical aspect of human behaviour refers to how we interact with and treat other people.
- Nursing practice and, consequently, nursing care has an important ethical dimension.
- The ethical and clinical domains of nursing practice are deeply intertwined.
- Codes of conduct are the nursing professions collective attempt to articulate the ethical domain of nursing practice.
- The nurse-patient relationship which is central to providing nursing care is also central to the ethical domain of nursing practice.
- The organisations within which nurses work can enable, enhance, or inhibit good nursing.
- Health service employers have a moral duty to support nurses in the provision of safe, competent, humane patient care.

References

Ausserhofer D, Zander B, Busse R, Schubert M, De Geest S, Rafferty AM, Ball J, Scott PA, Kinnunen J, Heinen M, Strømseng Sjetne I, Moreno-Casbas T, Kózka M, Lindqvist R, Diomidous M, Bruyneel L, Sermeus W, Aiken L, Schwendimann R (2014) Prevalence, patterns and predictors of nursing care left undone in European hospitals: results from the multicountry cross-sectional RN4CAST study. BMJ Qual Saf 2(23):126–135. Available online 11 Nov 2013. http://qualitysafety.bmj.com/cgi/content/full/bmjqs2013-002318 . Accessed 30 July 2016

Avallin T, Muntlin AÅ, Björck M, Jangland E (2020) Using communication to manage missed care: a case study applying the fundamentals of care framework. J Nurs Manag 28(8):2091–2102

Buchan J, Catton H (2023) Recover to build: investing in the nursing workforce for health system effectiveness. International Council of Nurses (ICN), Geneva

Buchan J, Catton H, Shaffer FA (2022) Sustain and retain in 2022 and beyond: the global nursing workforce and the COVID-19 pandemic. ICNM. International Centre for Nurse Migration, Philadelphia

Cho SH, Park M, Jeon SH, Chang HE, Hong HJ (2014) Average hospital length of stay nurses' work demands and their health and job outcomes. J Nurs Scholarsh 46(3):199–206

Dall'Ora C, Saville C, Rubbo B, Turner L, Jones J, Griffiths P (2022) Nurse staffing levels and patient outcomes: a systematic review of longitudinal studies. Int J Nurs Stud 134:104311

Dall'Ora C, Saville C (2021) Burnout in nursing: what have we learnt and what is still unknown? Nurs Times 117(2):43–44

deRaeve L (2002) Trust and trustworthiness in the nurse-patient relationship. Nurs Philos 3(2):152–162

European Commission Director-General for Health and Food Safety (2021) Supporting mental health of the health workforce and other essential workers. Publications Office of the European Union. https://doi.org/10.2875/80970. Accessed 29 July 2023

Francis R (2010) Independent inquiry into care provided by Mid Staffordshire NHS Foundation Trust January 2005–March 2009, vol 1. Chaired by Robert Francis QC, Stationary Office, London

Francis R (2013) Report of the mid Staffordshire NHS Foundation Trust Public Inquiry. Chaired by Robert Francis QC, Stationary Office, London

Gurková E, Mikšová Z, Šáteková L (2022) Missed nursing care in hospital environments during the COVID-19 pandemic. Int Nurs Rev 69(2):175–184

Hillestad AH, Rokstad AM, Tretteteig S, Julnes SG, Lichtwarck B, Eriksen S (2023) Nurses' ethical challenges when providing care in nursing homes during the COVID-19 pandemic. Nurs Ethics 30(1):32–45

HIQA Regulation Directorate (2015) Compliance monitoring inspection report designated centres under the Health Act 2007 as amended. https://static.rasset.ie/documents/news/4910-14-january-2015.pdf. Accessed 11 September 2023

Holm S (1997) Ethical problems in clinical practice: the ethical reasoning of health care professionals. Manchester University Press, Manchester

Institute of Medicine (IoM) (2011) The future of nursing: leading change, advancing health. Committee on the Robert Wood Johnson Foundation Initiative on the future of nursing at the Institute of Medicine. The National Academies Press, Washington, DC

International Council of Nurses (ICN) (2021) The ICN code of ethics for nurses. https://www.icn.ch/resources/publications-and-reports/code-ethics-nurses. Accessed 11 September 2023

International Council of Nurses (ICN) (2023) International nurses day 2023: our nurses, our future. International Council of Nurses, Geneva

Jones TL, Hamilton P, Murry N (2015) Unfinished nursing care, missed care, and implicitly rationed care: State of the science review. Int J Nurs Stud 52(6):1121–1137

Karlsson M, Pennbrant S (2020) Ideas of caring in nursing practice. Nurs Phil 21(4):e12325

Kearns AJ (2020) "Ought implies can" & missed care. Nurs Philos 21(1):e12272

Lavoie-Tremblay M, Gélinas C, Aubé T, Tchouaket E, Tremblay D, Gagnon MP, Côté J (2022) Influence of caring for COVID-19 patients on nurse's turnover, work satisfaction and quality of care. J Nurs Manag 30(1):33–43

Levine M (1977) Nursing ethics and the ethical nurse. Am J Nurs 77(5):845–849

Mandal L, Seethalakshmi A, Rajendrababu A (2020) Rationing of nursing care, a deviation from holistic nursing: a systematic review. Nurs Philos 21(1):e12257. https://doi.org/10.1111/nup.12257

Morse J (1991) Negotiating commitment and involvement in the nurse-patient relationship. J Adv Nurs 16:455–468

Niven CA, Scott PA (2003) The need for accurate perception and informed judgement in determining the appropriate use of the nursing resource: hearing the patient's voice. Nurs Philos 4(3):201–210

Nortvedt P (2001) Clinical sensitivity: the inseparability of ethical perceptiveness and clinical knowledge. Sch Inq Nurs Pract 15(1):25–43

Nursing and Midwifery Board of Ireland (2021) Code of professional conduct and ethics for registered nurses and midwives. Nursing and Midwifery Board of Ireland, Blackrock, Dublin. http://www.nmbi.ie/NMBI/media/NMBI/Code-of-Professional-Conduct-and-Ethics.pdf. Accessed 11 September 2023

Nursing and Midwifery Council (2015) The Code: professional standards of practice and behaviour for nurses and midwives. Updated 2018. Nursing and Midwifery Council, Portland Place, London. https://www.nmc.org.uk/globalassets/sitedocuments/nmc-publications/nmc-code.pdf. Accessed 11 September 2023

Ockenden D (2022) Ockenden report—final: findings, conclusions and essential actions from the independent review of maternity services at The Shrewsbury and Telford Hospital NHS trust. Open Government licence V3.0 Crown Copyright: https://www.ockendenmaternityreview.org.uk/wp-content/uploads/2022/03/FINAL_INDEPENDENT_MATERNITY_REVIEW_OF_MATERNITY_SERVICES_REPORT.pdf. Accessed 11 September 2023

Scott PA (2014) Character and nursing. Guest editorial. Int J Nurs Stud 51(2):177–180

Scott PA (2019) Niven and Scott (2003): sixteen years of hindsight. Nurs Philos 20(3):e12250

Scott PA, Matthews A, Kirwan MP (2014) What is nursing in the 21st century and what does the 21st century health service require from nurses? Nurs Philos 15:23–34

Scott PA, Suhonen R, Kirwan M (2020) Missed care, care left undone: organisation ethics and the appropriate use of the nursing resource. Nurs Philos 21(1):e12288

Sellman D (2011) What makes a good nurse: why the virtues are important for nurses. Jessica Kingsley Publishers, London

Tønnessen S, Scott PA, Nortvedt P (2020) Safe and competent nursing care: an argument for a minimum standard? Nurs Ethics 27(6):1396–1407

Vale of Leven Hospital Inquiry Report (2014) Chaired by Rt Hon Lord MacLean. Published on behalf of the Vale of Leven Hospital Inquiry by APS Group. www.valeoflevenhospitalinquiry.org. Accessed 3 Aug 2016

Advocacy and Nursing

P. Anne Scott

Abstract

The nurse's role as an advocate for the patient appears to be a taken-for-granted aspect of nursing in the twenty-first century; in both the nursing literature and in the British, Irish, and international nursing practice contexts. The focus on the advocacy role of the nurse is predominantly located in the context of hospital-based care and at the level of the individual patient, as opposed to the wider sociopolitical context. However, there are some signs that the greater focus on primary care, globalisation, and the implementation of legislation such as the Assisted Decision-Making (Capacity) Act (ADMA) (https://www.irishstatutebook.ie/eli/2015/act/64/enacted/en/html. Accessed 11 August 2023) will broaden this focus in future.

While many nurse scholars, nursing registration bodies, professional organisations, and practising nurses are comfortable with the rhetoric of "nurse as patient advocate", this is not an uncontroversial stance. A number of authors have challenged both the basis for the claim that nurses should be patient advocates and the possibility of such a role for nurses.

Given that claims to the advocacy role for nurses are continuing to appear both in our literature and in our codes of practice, it seems relevant to ask what the notion of nurse advocacy means and what are the relative strengths and weaknesses of claims for and against an advocacy role for nurses.

P. A. Scott (✉)
University of Galway, Galway, Co Galway, Ireland
e-mail: anne.scott@universityofgalway.ie

© The Author(s), under exclusive license to Springer Nature Switzerland AG 2024
P. A. Scott, S. M. Scott (eds.), *Key Concepts and Issues in Nursing Ethics*,
https://doi.org/10.1007/978-3-031-54108-7_2

Keywords

Advocacy · Nurse advocacy · Nursing role · Codes of practice · Patient advocate · Public policy · Health policy

Introduction

There is a well-established acceptance of the importance of the advocacy role of the nurse, among practising nurses, nurse regulatory bodies, professional organisations, and in the nursing literature over the past 30 years (Allmark and Klarznski 1992; Spenceley et al. 2006; American Nurses Association (ANA) 2015; Nsiah et al. 2019; Nursing and Midwifery Board of Ireland (NMBI) 2021; Heck et al. 2022; Cole et al. 2022).

However, this claim of the advocacy role for nurses is not uncontroversial. Several authors have challenged both the basis for the claim that nurses should be patient advocates and indeed the possibility of such a role for nurses, given, for example, nurses' perceived position of relative powerlessness within the hierarchy of health professions. See, for example, Allmark and Klarzynski (1992) and Cole et al. (2022).

It is also noteworthy that while the World Health Organisation (WHO) (2017) has actively underlined the key role of nurses and midwives in the development of health policy, as a means of ensuring high-quality care for patients, to date nursing literature and nursing education focus almost entirely on advocacy as embedded in and limited to the domain of the individual patient-nurse relationship. While there are signs that this focus may broaden in the future, as a result of greater emphasis in nurse education curricula on, for example, primary care, population health, and the potential impact of nursing in implementing the 17 United Nations (UN) Social Development Goals (SDGs) (UN 2015), nurses and the nursing profession internationally are struggling to rise to these political/leadership challenges (Fields et al. 2021). It is of crucial importance that we recognise that keeping the focus on a conceptualisation of advocacy that is embedded in and limited to the domain of the patient-nurse relationship ignores the important role nurse have, and should have, in the development of health policy (Spenceley et al. 2006; WHO 2017; Chiu et al. 2021; Scott and Scott 2021). Maintaining a focus on advocacy as embedded in the individual nurse-patient relationship and the needs of individual patients at specific points in their care places all the responsibility on the individual nurse for enactment of the advocacy role, as integral to the provision of good patient care. While this type of patient advocacy is legitimate and important, it is only part of the picture. Such focus may absolve nursing leaders, health service managers, nursing organisations, and governments from ensuring that resources are in place to enable appropriate patient care and the provision of competent, ethically sensitive nursing.

We have argued elsewhere (Scott and Scott 2021) that if nurses are to influence the quality of healthcare effectively, they must engage with policymakers to get nursing care and issues of access to adequate nursing resources onto the policymaking agenda. Effective use of the growing evidence base regarding what is required to support an adequate nursing workforce, as well as the provision of high-quality nursing care, is an important part of the required dialogue with health policymakers.

Case Study 1: Safe Staffing Framework

Nursing care left undone emerges as a salient issue in acute hospitals in Ireland due to several factors: (i) serious resource constraints post the 2008 financial crash and subsequent austerity measures imposed on the health service (Burke et al. 2014), *(ii) growing understanding of a link between nurse staffing and patient outcomes* (Aiken et al. 2014), *and (iii) increasing concerns regarding patient neglect* (HIQA 2012).

As a result of widespread dissemination of relevant research findings (Aiken et al. 2014; Scott et al. 2013), *interest and support from the Office of the Chief Nursing Officer in the Department of Health, and pressure from nursing unions, among other issues, the Department of Health (DoH) set up a taskforce on nurse staffing and skills mix in September 2014:*

> The stimulus to establish the Taskforce included the recommendations from: (1) an increasing number of high profile health inquiry reports such as the Report of the Mid Staffordshire NHS Foundation Trust Public Inquiry (Francis 2013) and the HIQA Tallaght Hospital report ((2012), and (2) the increasing body of research evidence linking components of the nursing resource to patient outcomes. Simultaneously, the Irish health service was and continues to undergo some of the most radical reforms in its history, and collectively these changes and evidence acted as the catalyst to the establishment of the Taskforce (DoH 2018, p. 4).

A framework for safe staffing and skills-mix in general and specialist medical and surgical settings in Irish acute hospitals was developed. The framework for safe staffing and skills mix was then implemented in six pilot wards across three acute general hospitals, selected for variations in size and complexity, commencing in June 2016. The final report and recommendations of the Taskforce was published in April 2018 (DoH 2018).

The Framework for Safe Staffing and Skills Mix in General and Specialist Medical and Surgical Care Settings is currently being implemented across acute hospitals in Ireland (DoH 2023), *supported by a 3-year programme of research. This work was impacted significantly by the COVID-19 pandemic. A further phase of the framework has been developed and tested, with a view to implementation in Accident and Emergency departments throughout the Irish acute hospital sector* (DoH 2022).

If one takes the role of patient advocacy seriously, and as core to the nursing role, two things are required of nurses and nursing organisations worldwide. We must:

1. Broaden the conceptualisation of patient advocacy beyond the individual patient to the system of healthcare provision.

2. Recognise that systemic change is as important a matter as change at the bedside, with and for the individual patient (Chiu et al. 2021; Scott and Scott 2021).

The advocacy role of the nurse at the health system and health policy level is rooted in the mandate nurses have with society since the time of Florence Nightingale. Part of this mandate is to protect the health of the public, work to ensure adequate understanding of the social determinants of health, and lobby for equity of access to healthcare provision (ICN 2023). It is also completely in alignment with recent versions of codes of practise for nurses internationally, which underline a population and public health-focused conceptualisation of the nursing role—e.g., ICN (2021), NMC (2015), NMBI (2021).

Advocacy in Recent Nursing Literature

In order to begin to explore the advocacy role of the nurse and to assess the relative strengths and weaknesses of arguments for and against, it is useful to look at how the term "advocacy" is used in the nursing literature. Recent conceptualisations of advocacy that dominate nursing literature claim advocacy as inherent in the role of the nurse and are understood variously as protecting patients and patient rights (including the right to autonomy), being the patient's voice, ensuring the provision of high-quality care, and educating patients (Davoodvand et al. 2016; Nsiah et al. 2019; NMBI 2021; Heck et al. 2022). Cole et al. (2022, p.154) suggests that:

Despite the importance of advocacy, there's however, no consensus about what advocacy is and how precisely it should be practised.

According to Paley (1996), we can only come to a reasonable level of clarity regarding what "advocacy" means if we locate the term within a particular theory. For example, this might be a theory of nursing—or nursing interventions—or caring or patient need. If we accept that one of the foundations of nursing is the requirement to provide safe, humane, holistic, good-quality care to our patients (Scott et al. 2014), then it seems important to ask what our patients may require in terms of advocacy, from the nurses who care for them.

Recent work continues to focus almost exclusively on the acute care setting in discussions and descriptions of the advocacy role of the nurse, to the detriment of effective consideration of nurse advocacy as an inherent part of the social mandate of nursing; in terms of what nurses/nursing organisations owe the public or a particular population.

It does seem important that the potential for and importance of nurse advocacy at a population and health policy level is recognised, facilitated, and supported (WHO 2017; Chiu et al. 2021; Scott and Scott 2021), as many countries, including Ireland

and the countries of the UK, work to reform their hospital-dominated health services and move to invest in and develop public health and primary care provision:

> *If nurses believe that nursing is important for good patient care and positive patient outcomes, and if nurses accept professional autonomy, then advocating and lobbying for such care, at a public policy level [as portrayed in Case Study 1 above] (Text in [..] is my addition.), is an important element of the nursing role - as important an aspect of the role as educating the next generation of nurses, and essential to growing and applying the evidence base to support good nursing practice. Without influencing the policymaking process, and impacting on agenda-setting in particular, nurses can find themselves making seemingly illogical/distressing decisions with regard to patient care and resource allocation (Peter et al. 2022; Iheduru-Anderson 2021) in order to comply with rules and expectations made without nurses' objectives and priorities in mind. In summary, practising nurses as expert clinicians, as members of an autonomous profession and as patient advocates have a duty to engage with public policy (Scott and Scott 2021, p. 727).*

The Patient Experience

Case Study 2: Alice

Alice, a 12-year-old girl, is admitted to her local paediatric hospital with a history of "pins and needles" and loss of power in her right hand and right leg. Staff observation reveals apparent loss of power and sensation in the girl's right hand and arm. She also has reduced sensation and power in her right leg which she tends to "drag" when she is encouraged to walk.

Following a number of examinations by various specialists, a battery of blood tests, X-rays and ultrasound, which required the removal of the brace from Alice's teeth, the initial diagnosis of multiple sclerosis, followed by a variety of other neurological conditions, are ruled out, and "functional disorder of unknown origin" is the working diagnosis.

Alice's immediate family—14-year-old brother and parents—are very concerned and attentive and visit regularly. Alice is frightened. She has no idea what is wrong with her or what is happening. The nurses pop into her room a few times a day—to make her bed, take her temperature, and so on. The doctors come and go. The physio has also been to assess Alice. The only person who really talks to her from the hospital is the very kind lady who brings the food. She recognised pretty quickly what Alice does and does not like to eat and saves Alice little treats and the peach yogurt that Alice loves. Alice feels homesick and no one seems to know when she will get home.

Case Study 3: Mr. S

A middle-aged man is admitted to the medical unit via the emergency department (ED) with severe dyspnoea, coughing, and distress. The patient is 6 days post-transurethral prostatectomy (TURP). His surgery and immediate post-operative period were uneventful, and Mr. S was discharged home on the third post-operative day. Over the following days, he becomes increasingly breathless and is referred by his GP to the ED as an emergency. The GP suspects that Mr. S has developed a pulmonary embolism (PE).

Following initial assessment in ED, Mr. S is given IV antibiotics, placed on oxygen via nasal catheters, and eventually transferred to the medical ward to await a scan; to confirm the initial diagnosis of PE, Mr. S is accompanied by his wife. Shortly after arrival on the ward, Mr. S is admitted by a pleasant nurse and told that the doctor would be along to see him. As it is now 9.30 pm, he will not be sent for the scan until tomorrow (Saturday).

Approximately 30 min later, the Registrar arrives, and following a cursory conversation and "look" at Mr. S, the Registrar says that probably Mr. S has a "clot on your lung" and he will "put" Mr. S on warfarin. Mr. S's elderly uncle, who lives in Scotland and who had been on warfarin for many years, has just been taken off warfarin and put on a newer drug that his doctors said was more effective and had fewer side effects. Therefore in response to the Registrar's comment that he will put Mr. S on warfarin, Mr. S and his wife ask what exactly the warfarin is for and if there is not alternative, newer drugs with fewer side effects? The Registrar indicates again that Mr. S likely has a clot and that this needs to be treated. Mr. S and his wife explain that they just want more information about warfarin and what the alternatives are. The Registrar says that this is fine, he will speak with the Consultant, and come back to Mr. S.

Sometime later the night, nurse comes around and speaks to Mr. S as she is doing the nightly medicine round. She says "I hear you have refused medication". Mr. S tries to explain that he has not refused medication and he has simply asked for information on warfarin and what the alternatives are. The following morning the Consultant comes to visit Mr. S. She has also been told that Mr. S has refused his medication...

Regarding the dominant conceptualisation of the advocacy role of the nurse as articulated in the nursing literature—that rooted in the individual nurse-patient relationship—"patient" is taken to refer to an individual hospitalised or in institutional/primary care due to health education deficits, maternity service requirements, mental or physical illness, or disabilities. These clients/patients are, for example, people like Alice and Mr. S described in case studies two and three above. One might usefully ask "Why would such an individual need an advocate?"

It seems that there are at least three possible reasons that a hospitalised patient might need someone to fulfil an advocacy role:

1. Illness is likely to cause an individual distress, increased vulnerability, and dependency. Knowledge deficits and/or institutional structures and processes may also mean that the capacity of the individual to make informed decisions regarding appropriate treatment is curtailed or undermined. These kinds of issues are clearly at play when one considers the types of situations Alice and Mr. S find themselves in.

2. A second reason that a patient may be perceived as requiring a patient advocate to work on their behalf is the power imbalance within the practitioner-patient relationship and the fear that this imbalance will result in an undermining of patient autonomy. The more powerful clinician, guided by the principle of beneficence (doing good/working in the patient's best interests), may fail to recognise that the nature and content of "good" may be understood differently from the practitioner and patient perspectives. There is increasing evidence that patients and practitioners may differ both in perceptions and priorities regarding patient care (Papastavrou et al. 2011). What a clinician perceives to be in the patient's best interests, from a health perspective, may not be accepted by the patient as being in his/her overall best interests: something which a smoker or a mountain climber might readily accept for example.
3. The enactment of the Assisted Decision-Making (Capacity) Act (ADMA) (2015) in Ireland, and similar legislation in other jurisdictions, points to another reason for advocacy, which links with the second reason highlighted above. This third reason is to meet legislative requirements to support decision-making in those persons whose decision-making capacity may be, or may become, compromised for a variety of reasons – such as acquired brain injury, enduring mental health difficulties, age-related cognitive decline, and so forth. Legislation supporting assisted decision-making has implications for all healthcare practitioners, including nurses, and is a significant cultural shift away from a paternalistic and "best interests" approach to an approach which supports rights of choice, control, and consent. It confirms all persons with the right to be central to decisions about what will happen to them. Access to the supports available under the ADMA will become a new feature of healthcare, and healthcare practitioners will interact with decision support structures and roles enabled under the Act.

Because of the power imbalance in the practitioner-patient relationship, the patient's voice may not be either sought or listened to. This is particularly, but not only, the case for those people whose decision-making capacity is compromised. Thus the patient may have little ability to influence their care or treatment, unless they have recourse to a patient advocate. Again this power imbalance does seem to be a factor in both the scenarios describing Alice and Mr. S's experience of hospitalisation. Alice is young, isolated, lonely, and homesick. There is no sense from the case study that any nurse has developed a relationship with her or is helping Alice understand what is planned for her care, discharge, and so on. Mr. S and his wife simply want information and a clear explanation regarding why warfarin is the drug of choice in his case. Yet their entirely reasonable concerns are not being addressed—or are being misunderstood. Mr. S is being labelled as "refusing treatment". The need and right which both Alice and Mr. S have for information regarding their treatment and care is being ignored—as is their need and right to participate in decision-making about their care. Having access to information and being enabled to participate in choosing options and decisions regarding his/her care are key elements of respecting patient autonomy.[1]

It seems that concerns regarding (a) the lack of recognition and support for patient autonomy expressed in the cases above, in combination with (b) the findings from recent investigations and reports from both the Department of Health in England and Wales (Francis 2013; Ockenden 2022) and the Irish Health Information and Quality Authority (HIQA 2012, 2013), give sufficient reasons to accept that the need for a patient advocate may be a reality, for at least some patients within the healthcare setting.

The question then arises as to who would make an effective patient advocate? A further question is "Why do many nurses and nursing bodies (e.g. ANA 2015; NMBI 2021) suggest patient advocacy is an aspect of the nursing role?"

Some Arguments in Favour of an Advocacy Role for Nurses

There are arguments presented in the literature both for and against nurse advocacy. Among those cited in favour of the nurse as appropriate advocate for the patient are the following:

1. *Patient rights need protecting. Part of the nursing role is to support, sustain, and protect patients* (Davoodvand et al. 2016; Nsiah et al. 2019; Heck et al. 2022). However, considering this claim, even if one were to accept that patient rights need protecting, it is a large leap to move from the position that part of the nursing role is to support and protect patients (presumably in certain situations, for particular reasons and against particular sets of circumstances), to the claim that nurses are therefore the natural protectors of patients in all situations (Hewitt 2002; Mahlin 2010). In terms of this latter position, it needs to be noted that, unfortunately, there is a growing evidence base that graphically describes many occasions where the relevant nurses do not rise to the requirement (Conlon 2013; Francis 2013; HIQA 2012; RTE 2014; Ockenden 2022).
2. *Doctors do not always behave in a responsible, accountable manner towards patients. Patients need a knowledgeable supporter to intervene on their behalf with medical staff.* The nurse, because of the nursing role and relationship with the patient, is the most suitable person to bridge the gap between the doctor's behaviour and the patient's needs (Nsiah et al. 2019).

   In considering this particular argument in relation to the advocacy role of the nurse, the following can be said: (a) it is the case that not all doctors behave in a responsible, accountable manner, as many medical scandals in both Ireland and the UK attest—for example Harding Clark (2006), Francis (2013), Ockenden (2022). (b) It is also the case that nurses frequently input/perceive that they input very relevant information regarding a patient's understanding, wishes, home

---

[1] For in-depth discussion of issues related to patient/client autonomy, please see Chap. 6 of this text.

situation, and so forth into case discussions and doctors rounds (Tomaschewski-Barlem et al. 2015).

However, there are difficulties in moving from an acceptance of points (a) and (b) above to the conclusion that nurses are appropriate patient advocates. The first obvious difficulty is that irresponsible, inappropriate patient care is clearly not the exclusive preserve of medicine—cases such as those reported by the Care Quality Commission (2011), the Francis Report (Francis 2013), Conlon (2013), HIQA (2012, 2013), RTE (2014), and Ockenden (2022) attest to this fact. This suggests that nurses may be no more appropriate to function as patient advocates than doctors, because some nurses, like some doctors, may abuse the power of their role. They may undermine patient rights and provide inappropriate or detrimental care to patients. Therefore if patient rights and the standard of patient care are in danger of being undermined by the professionals providing that care, patients do need advocates. However, it appears that these advocates cannot be reliably found among healthcare professionals involved in the provision of care to the particular patient concerned.

The second difficulty with moving from an acceptance of (a) and (b) above to a conclusion that the nurse is an appropriate patient advocate is as follows: it is the case that some nurses do input into doctors' rounds and case conferences, and such input may be relevant to advocacy. However, currently there is little evidence that all nurses make such an input or that nurses do so consistently. In fact there is evidence that some nurses, in some contexts, do not do so at all—even when they feel very strongly that a patient is receiving inappropriate treatment (Barlem et al. 2012; Tíscar-González et al. 2019).

Such evidence appears to suggest that the foundation for an advocacy function within the nursing role may rest on very shaky ground indeed. Conlon's (2013) work on PRN analgesia administration would support this suggestion. Conlon explores nursing perceptions and practice in the provision of analgesia to children in their care. She found very variable practice and little evidence of child-centred care.

3. *A third argument that is frequently offered in support of the advocacy role of the nurse is that nurses are the healthcare professionals with the most sustained contact with patients.* They see patients usually over an 8- to 12-h shift, and nurses are with the patients over the 24-h cycle, for the entire period of patients' hospitalisation. Nurses are therefore in a much better position than any other healthcare professional to get to know a patient and to come to understand their patients' perspective (Hewitt 2002; Mahlin 2010).

This argument does seem to hold some weight in terms of supporting an advocacy role for nurses. Moving from the acute general hospital environment to the context of mental health and community care provision adds further strength to the claims of a legitimate advocacy role for nurses. In the mental health environment patient, practitioner contact and consequent growth in knowledge of a patient may extend over months and years. Such sustained and lengthy patient contact must create the potential for a nurse to develop a real understanding and knowledge of a patient.

However, it is also the case that in the acute physical healthcare sector contact with patients is for much shorter periods of time than those encountered in either community mental health or public health nursing. Nonetheless by the end of one shift, a nurse will have had the opportunity to gain insights into a patient's perspective that a member of medical staff may not have had. A doctor may spend approximately 30 min "admitting" the patient and perhaps another 10 min involved in patient examination, treatment, or consultation. The importance of the nurse's role in patient monitoring and observation and in knowing the patient and the patient's responses is well established from the time of Florence Nightingale and is a recurring theme in the nursing literature—for example, Scott et al. (2014).

It is also the case that the nurse is the one member of the healthcare team that is likely to see the full patient care picture, with the patient at the centre of that care. Hospital nurses organise the context within which the patient receives and experiences healthcare. Nurses are the practitioners who not only provide nursing care to a patient but who also witness, facilitate, and support the provision of care and treatment to the patient, from all other practitioners on the healthcare team.

However, the changing role of the nurse in acute hospital care is likely to impact on this ability to know the patient and thus be an effective patient advocate. Many of our connections with patients resulted from spending time with them providing basic care—feeding and washing patients, for example. Much of this care is now provided by care assistants. In some contexts, such as the Irish acute hospital sector, nursing shift patterns may also mitigate against being an effective patient advocate. A nurse may do three 12-h shifts in a row and then have a week off duty. With reduced lengths of stay, this may mean the nurse who knows the patient best is not around for key meetings, discharge planning, and so forth. This underlines differences between nursing in the acute and community care contexts with regard to the advocacy role of the nurse.

Nonetheless the co-ordinating role of the nurse remains an important part of patient care (Scott et al. 2014). This might mean that a nurse, therefore, is in a better position to understand and represent a patient's views than other members of the healthcare team. This would seem to suggest a particular and unique nursing contribution to patient care, an element of which practising nurses term "advocacy".

What the literature, as well as some empirical evidence, suggests is that from the perspective of practising nurses, patient advocacy is a continuum, a continuum from pleading a case on behalf of a patient to helping a dying person find comfort and meaning in their experience. To use the words of Woodrow (1997, p. 229):

> ... *advocacy need not be a reactive process in the case of major crises, but can be proactive in the case of less sensational quality issues such as:*

- *Encouraging patient involvement in planning care.*
- *Giving information to enable informed decision making by patients.*
- *Removing restrictive visiting times in any institutional settings.*
- *Avoiding disturbing patients routinely in the early morning.*

The first two elements in the list above could, for example, ease the situations for Alice and Mr. S and make their hospital experience less frightening and frustrating.

To return to Paley (1996), advocacy means different things depending on the particular theory driving the particular intervention under consideration. From the perspective of a theory of nursing that focuses on holistic patient care and sees nurses as organisers of the patient care context, the notion of a patient advocacy role for the nurse seems entirely coherent.

Therefore, in summary, of three common arguments cited in the nursing literature in favour of an advocacy role for nurses, *argument three* above appears to provide the most coherent position in support of such a role. An advocacy role for nurses, based on sustained contact with, and thus understanding of the patient and patient care context, is also completely aligned with assisted decision-making legislation where in Ireland, for example, nurses are recognised as having a key role in enactment of ADMA (2015), which involves supporting the recognition and realisation of the persons "will and preferences" (ADMA 2015, Part Two: Guiding Principles: 7(b).

Some Common Arguments Against an Advocacy Role for Nurses

One common argument against the advocacy role for nurses is that nurses do not have sufficient power within the healthcare system to advocate for patients. In the context of the hierarchical organisation of the health service nurses, being part of the less powerful levels of the hierarchy, have insufficient power to challenge medical authority. To ask nurses to do so potentially places the nurse in an untenable position where standing up for a patient or for appropriate patient care results in nurses being disciplined, victimised, and ultimately potentially out of work (Tíscar-González et al. 2019; Cole et al. 2022).

There are however at least two pertinent issues to consider here:

1. If, as suggested, advocacy should be seen as a continuum, then it is not appropriate to assume that advocating for a patient will always or inevitably bring the nurse into conflict with powerful members of the medical staff. Advocating on behalf of a patient may simply mean (a) bringing an issue to the attention of the medical team (this would be helpful to Mr. S in his search for more information on the prescribed medication and available alternatives and to Alice as she tries to understand what is happening and when she can go home), (b) raising the patient's concern/issue at the appropriate moment and/or (c) raising the patient's concern in a context that highlights the importance, or relevance, of an issue to the patient involved (as described by Conlon (2013), Tomaschewski-Barlem et al. (2015)). While conflict and the potential for conflict clearly exists between all members of the healthcare team, sometimes in issues of patient care, there is strength in focusing on a common "enemy" (Shields et al. 2022). Therefore it seems important not to trivialise the potentially multifaceted needs for advocacy

that may face our patients, by describing advocacy in terms of a turf war between nursing and medicine. The fact that attempts at patient advocacy may, on occasion, degenerate into such a turf war is not an indication that there are no real advocacy needs from a patient's perspective. Nor is it evidence that nurses cannot be effective patient advocates.

2. Given that patient advocacy may at least occasionally place extreme demands on the nurse, the second issue that deserves attention here is "What does this imply?". Does the reality of these extreme demands mean that nurses should not be asked to advocate for patients? Or, conversely, does the existence of such extreme risks for nurses imply that the registration body for nurses, health service managers, and/or society as a whole should take their corporate responsibility more seriously? Should there be measures that ensure certain protections for nurses who provide appropriate advocacy for patients—measures that ensure protection from unfair treatment? This latter position seems to be the position evidenced in the Irish and UK health systems (HSE 2018; NHS 2021).

A second argument against an advocacy role for nurses is that patients do not normally choose their nurses, and nurses do not generally choose their patients— they are more likely to be allocated patients.

It is true that a patient generally chooses their general practitioner and it is more a matter of luck or chance what particular nurse a patient ends up with. This is the case whether one is part of a primary nursing system in an acute hospital setting or receiving the care of a community mental health nurse or a public health nurse. The nurse is therefore in some sense "imposed" on the patient, rather than chosen. However, this distinction, even if relevant, can only be taken so far. For example, in looking for a lawyer, my choice may be restricted by my ability to pay, my ability to travel to search for a lawyer, geography, the availability of more than one lawyer in a practice, the case load of those lawyers available, and so forth. This also holds true for my choice of general practitioner. Therefore while nurses are "imposed" on patients and GPs and lawyers are "chosen", one's ability to choose is likely to be limited by any number of factors. Also in most systems of organising the delivery of nursing care, there is still the possibility for a patient to choose to develop a trusting relationship with one nurse rather than another. The patient may divulge certain relevant information to one nurse rather than another and seek help and support from one nurse rather than another. This is the case whether the patient finds themselves on a ward with a staff of 20 nurses, or being cared for at home by a mental health home care team.

A third argument against an advocacy role for nurses is that nurses, as part of the system, are by definition part of the problem. Unfortunately there is clear evidence that nurses can indeed be part of the problems that make patient advocacy necessary. As indicated above work such as that of Francis (2013), Conlon (2013), HIQA (2013), RTE (2014), and Tiscar-González et al. (2019) show this clearly. If this is the case, then it would appear that such nurses cannot provide effective advocacy for the patients involved. Recourse to another form of advocacy is required. In some systems lay advocates are employed by the health service to meet this eventuality. An example is the Patient Advocacy Service in Ireland: https://www.patientadvocacyservice.ie. This service, and the equivalent in other jurisdictions, is likely to expand and be influenced, for example, by implementation of ADMA (2015). However, the fact that nurses may be part of the problem that confronts patients and undermines their care does not mean that this is always the case and thus does not automatically rule out an advocacy role for nurses.

Therefore it does appear that while arguments against an advocacy role for nurses have some strengths and raise issues that require to be addressed if nurses are to function as effective patient advocates, ultimately such arguments do not provide sufficient reason to undermine the coherence of an advocacy role for nurses. However, these arguments do suggest that patient advocacy is not the exclusive preserve of nurses.

Conclusion

Nurses are an important health service resource and vital to good patient experience, including positive patient outcomes (Dall'Ora et al. 2022). We need to recognise as a profession, as members of the public, and as current or potential patients that there is a growing evidence base for the kinds of inputs and resources that are required for good patient and good nursing outcomes (Aiken et al. 2014; DoH 2018). For example, there is now an evidence base, which has been generated and accepted internationally, on the important impact of factors such as nurse education, nurse-patient ratios, and minimum ratios of registered nurses to healthcare assistants, on patient outcomes (Rafferty et al. 2007; Aiken et al. 2014). Such research has influenced the development of a safe staffing framework in Ireland—see "Case Study 1" above. Evidence is also being generated on the impact of nursing and the cost of nursing-sensitive patient outcomes (Murphy et al. 2021). Such evidence should inform both policy development and health service resourcing decisions. Nurses and nurse-researchers, as those "in-the-know", must make sure that information on this type of evidence is appropriately disseminated, to ensure that nursing organisations, nurse leaders, and health policymakers have such information at their fingertips. This evidence is an important component in ensuring sufficient resources at both the macro national level and at the micro level of the individual ward/unit/health centre. It is thus an important component is ensuring good nursing care and positive patient outcomes.

Taxpayers' money has contributed to funding the underpinning research/evidence base. Where we as a profession/nurse researchers know what is needed we have a responsibility to the taxpayer, to patients, to future patients, and to practising nurses to advocate for the development of the required policy to facilitate the required outcomes. This is the type of advocacy required of nurses and nursing organisations at the policy level (Spenceley et al. 2006; Chiu et al. 2021; Scott and Scott 2021).

However, as case studies two and three above indicate, systems problems and policy deficits are not the only type of problem that patients encounter within the health service, nor are they the only instances where advocacy is required. Issues of patient rights to autonomy, choice, and consent, including for people experiencing decision-making capacity compromise, are central to the enactment of the assisted decision-making legislation internationally. Many of the problems encountered by patients are issues nurses, and other healthcare staff, could help with effectively, by working to understand the patient context, patient experience, and developing greater insight into the needs, preferences, and wishes of the patient, rather than assuming that the practitioner knows what those needs and wishes are. These matters are, in many ways, at the heart of the practitioner-patient relationship[2] and now feature centre stage in assisted decision-making legislation such as ADMA (2015) in Ireland.

Current health services are complex, multifaceted organisations. Due to the level of complexity and the numerous demands placed on practitioners within the service, more than one form of advocacy is likely to be required by patients both within our health services and at the national policy level. It seems that nurses, due to their unique organisational, co-ordinating, interconnecting position within the delivery of that health service, can effectively advocate for patients and should do so—at both the level of the health system and that of the bedside. In certain circumstances the nurse may be the only practitioner with sufficient knowledge of the patient's desires and wishes, to advocate effectively for a patient. It follows therefore that nurses should advocate for patients, both at the individual and the population levels, when it is appropriate that they do so. This argument of course does not support an advocacy role that is unique to nurses. Many healthcare workers may have such a role, as indicated, for example, in ADMA (2015). The important thing is that patients can connect with a caregiver and that that caregiver has the skills, confidence, and authority to advocate if required. It is less about who advocates for the patient and more about making sure it gets done.

> **Key Learning Points**
> - The role of the nurse as patient advocate is very well accepted in both nursing practice contexts internationally and in the nursing literature. There is also support for the advocacy role of nurses in assisted decision-making legislation.
> - There are reasons, such as increased vulnerability when one is ill and the natural power imbalance in the practitioner-patient relationship, why patients may need an advocate.
> - However, in practice, an advocacy role for nurses is not uncontroversial, and there are arguments both in favour and against such a role for nurses.
> - An analysis of nursing practice and the function of the nurse does support an advocacy role for nurses—but such a role, in the healthcare context, is not exclusive to nurses.
> - The most important thing is that patients should receive the support they need to participate in and understand their care. This support may be provided by a nurse or other relevant practitioner, depending on the particular circumstances and the particular patient need.
> - The advocacy role of nurses, however, is not restricted to the individual patient in a specific care context. Nurses also have an important role to advocate at the level of the health system and health policy development.

References

Aiken LH, Sloane DM, Bruyneel L, Van den Heede K, Griffiths P, Busse R, Diomidous M, Kinnunen J, Kózka M, Lesaffre E, McHugh MD, Moreno-Casbas MT, Rafferty AM, Schwendimann R, Anne SP, Carol T, van Achterberg T, Walter S (2014) Nurse staffing and education and hospital mortality in nine European countries: a retrospective observational study. Lancet 383(9931):1824–1830. https://doi.org/10.1016/S0140-6736(13)62631-8

Allmark P, Klarzynski R (1992) The case against nurse advocacy. Br J Nurs 2(1):33–36

American Nurses Association (ANA) (2015) Code of ethics for nurses with interpretive statements. Silver Spring, MD. http://www.nursingworld.org/practice-policy/nursing-excellence/ethics/code-of-ethics-for-nurses. Accessed 5 July 2023

Assisted Decision-Making (Capacity) Act (2015). https://www.irishstatutebook.ie/eli/2015/act/64/enacted/en/html. Accessed 11 August 2023

Barlem ELD, Lunard VL, Lunard GL, de Lima DG, Tomaschewshi JG (2012) The experience of moral distress in nursing: the nurses' perception. Rev Esc Enferm USP J School Nurs USP 46(3):678–685. http://pubmed.ncbi.nlm.nih.gov/22773490/. Accessed 8 July 2023

Burke S, Thomas S, Barry S, Keegan C (2014) Measuring, mapping and making sense of Irish health sector performance in the recession. A working paper for the Resilience Project. The Centre for Health Policy and Management, School of Medicine Trinity College Dublin: https://www.tcd.ie/medicine/health_policy_management/assets/pdf/Resilience-working-paper-March-2014.pdf. Accessed 8July 2023

Care Quality Commission (2011) Dignity and nutrition inspection programme: national overview. www.cqc.org.uk . http://www.cqc.org.uk/sites/default/files/media/documents/20111007_dignity_and_nutrition_inspection_report_final_update.pdf. Accessed 9 July 2023

Chiu P, Cummings GG, Thorne S, Schick-Makaroff K (2021) Policy advocacy and nursing organizations: a scoping review. Policy Polit Nurs Pract 22(4):276–296. https://doi.org/10.1177/15271544211050611

Cole C, Mummery J, Peck B (2022) Empowerment as an alternative to traditional patient advocacy roles. Nurs Ethics 29(7–8):1553–1561. https://doi.org/10.1177/09697330211020434

Conlon J (2013) Children in pain: "subjects" of the system (PhD thesis). Dublin City University, Dublin

Dall'Ora C, Saville C, Rubbo B, Turner L, Jones J, Griffiths P (2022) Nurse staffing levels and patient outcomes: a systematic review of longitudinal studies. Int J Nurs Stud 134:104311. https://doi.org/10.1016/j.ijnurstu.2022.104311

Davoodvand S, Abbaszadeh A, Ahmadi F (2016) Patient advocacy from the clinical nurses' viewpoint: a qualitative study. J Med Ethics Hist Med 9:5. https://www.ncbi.nlm.nih.gov/pmc/articles/PMC4958925/. Accessed 12 September 2023

DoH (2018) Framework for safe staffing and skills mix in general and specialist medical and surgical setting in acute hospitals in Ireland. Department of Health, Dublin. https://www.gov.ie/pdf/?file=https:/assets.gov.ie/1011/ela93e955329405694bb7b16aea50b98.pdf#page=null. Accessed 7 July 2023

DoH (2022) Framework for safe nurse staffing and skill mix in adult emergency care settings in Ireland. Department of Health, Dublin. https://www.gov.ie/en/publication/e4419-framework-for-safe-nurse-staffing-and-skill-mix-phase-2/. Accessed 7 July 2023

DoH (2023) Update on implementation of the Framework on safe nurse staffing and skills mix in general and specialist medical and surgical units in acute hospitals in Ireland (phase 1). Department of Health, Dublin. https://www.gov.ie/en/publication/671f3-framework-for-safe-nurse-staffing-and-skill-mix-phase-1/. Accessed 7 September 2023

Fields L, Perkiss S, Dean BA, Moroney T (2021) Nursing and the sustainable development goals: a scoping review. J Nurs Scholarsh 53(5):568–577. https://doi.org/10.1111/jnu.12675

Francis R (2013) Report of the Mid Staffordshire NHS Foundation Trust Inquiry. Chaired by Robert Francis QC. Stationary Office, London. https://assets.publishing.service.gov.uk/government/uploads/system/uploads/attachment_data/file/279124/0947.pdf. Accessed 8 July 2023

Harding Clark M (2006) The Lourdes Hospital inquiry: an inquiry into peripartum hysterectomy at Our Lady of Lourdes Hospital, Drogheda. Report of Judge Maureen Harding Clark S.C., The Stationary Office, Dublin. http://www.lenus.ie/handle/1014/42922. Accessed 9 September 2023

Heck LO, Carrara BS, Mendes IAC, Arena Ventura CA (2022) Nursing and advocacy in health: an integrative review. Nurs Ethics 29(4):1014–1034. https://doi.org/10.1177/09697330211062981

Hewitt JA (2002) A critical review of the arguments debating the role of the nurse advocate. J Adv Nurs 37(5):439–445

HIQA (2013) Patient safety investigation into services at University Hospital Galway (UHG) and as reflected in the care provided to Savita Halappanavar. Health Information and Quality Authority, Dublin. https://www.hiqa.ie/reports-and-publications/key-reports-and-investigations/patient-safety-investigation-report. Accessed 8 July 2023

HIQA (Health Information and Quality Authority) (2012) Report of the investigation into the quality, safety and governance of care provided by the Adelaide and Meath Hospital, Dublin incorporating the National Children's Hospital (AMNCH) for patients who require admission. Health Information and Quality Authority. https://www.hiqa.iw/sites/default/files/2017-01/Tallaght-Hospital-Investigation-Report.pdf. Accessed 8 July 2023

HSE (Health Service Executive) (2018). Protected disclosures procedures: https://www.hse.ie/eng/about/who/protected-disclosures/hse-protected-disclosures-procedures.pdf. Accessed 8 July 2023

ICN (2023) International nurses day 2023 report: our nurse, our future. International Council of Nurses, Geneva

ICN (International Council of Nurses) (2021) The ICN code of ethics for nurses. International Council of Nurses, Geneva. https://www.icn.ch/sites/default/files/inline-files/ICN_Code-of-Ethics_EN_web.pdf. Accessed 8 July 2023

Iheduru-Anderson K (2021) Reflections on the lived experience of working with limited personal protective equipment during the COVID-19 crisis. Nurs Inq 28(1):e12382. https://doi.org/10.1111/nin.12382

Mahlin M (2010) Individual patient advocacy collective responsibility and activism within professional nursing associations. Nurs Ethics 17(2):247–254. https://doi.org/10.1177/0969733009351949

Murphy A, Griffiths P, Duffield C, Brady NM, Scott PA, Ball J, Drennan J (2021) Estimating the economic cost of nurse sensitive adverse events amongst patients in medical and surgical settings. J Adv Nurs 77(8):3379–3388. https://doi.org/10.1111/jan.14860

National Health Service (2021) NHS constitution. https://www.gov.uk/government/publications/the-nhs-constitution-for-england/the-nhs-constitution-for-england . Accessed 8 July 2023

Nsiah C, Siakwa M, Ninnoni JPK (2019) Registered Nurses' description of patient advocacy in the clinical setting. Nurs Open 6(3):1124–1132. https://doi.org/10.1002/nop2.307

Nursing and Midwifery Board of Ireland (NMBI) (2021) Code of professional practice and ethics for registered nurses and midwives. Nursing and Midwifery Board of Ireland, Dublin. http://www.nmbi.ie/NMBI/media/NMBI/Code-of-Professional-Conduct-and-Ethics.pdf. Accessed 5 July 2023

Nursing and Midwifery Council (2015) The code: professional standards of practice and behaviour for nurses and midwives. Nursing and Midwifery Council, Portland Place, London. https://www.nmc.org.uk/globalassets/sitedocuments/nmc-publications/nuc-code.pdf. Accessed 5 July 2023

Ockenden D (2022) Ockenden report final:findings, conclusions and essential actions from the independent review of maternity services at The Shrewsbury and Telford Hospital NHS Trust. Open Government Licence V3.0 Crown Copyright: https://www.ockendenmaternityreview.org.uk/wp-content/uploads/2022/03/FINAL_INDEPENDENT_MATERNITY_REVIEW_OF_MATERNITY_SERVICES_REPORT.pdf. Accessed 5 July 2023

Paley J (1996) How not to clarify concepts in nursing. J Adv Nurs 24(3):572–578

Papastavrou E, Efstathiou G, Charalambous A (2011) Nurses and patients' perceptions of caring behaviours: quantitative systematic review of comparative studies. J Adv Nurs 67(6):1191–1205

Peter E, Mohammed S, Killackey T, MacIver J, Variath C (2022) Nurses' experiences of ethical responsibilities of care during the COVID-19 pandemic. Nurs Ethics 29(4):844–857. https://doi.org/10.1177/09697330211068135

Rafferty AM, Clarke SP, Coles J, Ball J, James P, McKee M, Aiken LH (2007) Outcomes of variation in hospital nurse staffing in English hospitals: cross-sectional analysis of survey data and discharge records. Int J Nurs Stud 44(2):175–182. https://doi.org/10.1016/j.ijnurstu.2006.08.003

RTE (2014) RTE prime time investigates Aras Attracta (December 2014): inside bungalow three: https://www.dailymotion.com/video/x2cadd5. Accessed 8 September 2023

Scott SM, Scott PA (2021) Nursing advocacy and public policy. Nurs Ethics 28(5):723–733. https://doi.org/10.1177/0969733020961823

Scott PA, Kirwan M, Matthews A, Morris R, Lehwaldt D, Staines A (2013) Report of the Irish RN4CAST study 2009–1011: a nursing workforce under strain. Dublin City University, Dublin. https://doras.dcu.ie/19344. Accessed 8 July 2023

Scott PA, Matthews A, Kirwan MP (2014) What is nursing in the 21st century and what does the 21st century health service require from nurses? Nurs Philos 15:23–34

Shields HM, Pelletier SR, Zambrotta ME (2022) Agreement of nurses' and physicians' attitudes on collaboration during the Covid-19 Pandemic using the Jefferson scale of attitudes toward physician-nurse collaboration. Adv Med Educ Pract 13:905–912

Spenceley SM, Reutter L, Allen MN (2006) The Road Less Traveled: Nursing Advocacy at the Policy Level. Policy Polit Nurs Pract 7(3):180–194. https://doi.org/10.1177/1527154406293683

Tíscar-González V, Gea-Sánchez M, Blanco-Blanco J, Moreno-Casbas MT, Peter E (2019) The advocacy role of nurses in cardiopulmonary resuscitation. Nurs Ethics 27(2):333–347

Tomaschewski-Barlem JG, Lunardi VL, Barlem ELD, Ramos AM, Figueria AB, Fornari NC (2015) Nursing beliefs and actions in exercising patient advocacy in a hospital context. Rev Esc Enferm USP J School Nurs USP. https://doi.org/10.1590/S0080-623420150000500015

United Nations (2015) The sustainable development agenda. https://www.un.org/sustainabledevelopment/development-agenda/. Accessed 12 August 2023

WHO (2017) Nursing and midwifery in the history of the World Health Organisation 1948–2017. World Health Organisation, Geneva

Woodrow P (1997) Nurse advocacy: is it in the patient's best interest? Br J Nurs 6(4):225–229

Resource Allocation and Rationing in Nursing Care

3

P. Anne Scott

Abstract

Public discussion of resourcing in healthcare tends to compound ideas of resource allocation and rationing. Public debate also tends to focus on situations of scarcity such as lack of kidneys or hearts for transplantation, or heated arguments regarding whether the latest very expensive new drug should be made available, regardless of cost, to treat certain condition such as cystic fibrosis or a particular type of cancer. The idea that nursing or medical time is an important healthcare resource that needs to be allocated with care rarely gets an effective airing in public debate.

I argue in this chapter that it is important in the healthcare context to differentiate resource allocation from rationing, on the basis that if we assume we are rationing healthcare as our starting point we may miss opportunities to examine more and less effective ways of allocating the healthcare resource. This is particularly important in nursing care where failure to examine carefully how the nursing resource is allocated, and supported, is leading to covert rationing of nursing time and suboptimal patient care in hospitals across Europe.

Keywords

Resource allocation · Rationing · Care left undone · Covert rationing · Nursing care

---

P. A. Scott (✉)
University of Galway, Galway, Co Galway, Ireland
e-mail: anne.scott@universityofgalway.ie

© The Author(s), under exclusive license to Springer Nature Switzerland AG 2024
P. A. Scott, S. M. Scott (eds.), *Key Concepts and Issues in Nursing Ethics*,
https://doi.org/10.1007/978-3-031-54108-7_3

Introduction

The COVID-19 pandemic has ensured that the public, patients, and healthcare staff have become increasingly aware of issues of resource allocation, and the need to ration scarce healthcare resources in times of public health crises. As the pandemic unfolded across the world, there were regular discussions, interviews in the media with stressed clinicians, and inputs from experts all trying to decide how best to use the limited resources available to look after, most effectively, the overwhelming number of patients presenting to clinicians. 'How best to distribute the limited number of ventilators (Savulescu et al. 2020)?' 'Who to treat when all cannot receive treatment (Yip et al. 2022)?' 'How to deal with the physical, psychological and moral distress of those working on the front line in our hospitals and nursing homes, trying to cope and care for patients and residents, in an impossible situation (Turale et al. 2020; Peter et al. 2022; Hillestad et al. 2023)?' Concerns regarding the good of the public versus that of the individual, including the over-riding of patient/resident rights (Hillestad et al. 2023), and the implications of these discussions for healthcare practice feature heavily in the healthcare literature over the recent past.

Public health experts and governments focused initially on how to obtain and distribute limited personal protective equipment (PPE), how to test most effectively for the virus, and then later, once vaccines became available, attention shifted to who should be vaccinated first and according to what criteria (EU 2021).

Even in so-called normal times, resource allocation in health and nursing care raises a number of important political, social, and ethical issues. As populations increase, population demographics change, and/or demand for health and nursing care outstrips supply, this moves us either to make a decision to increase investment in healthcare, redistribute resources from lower priority services to those of higher priority, and/or limit access to the services that exist—the latter is called rationing of healthcare.

Decisions regarding resource allocation and rationing in healthcare, though potentially highly emotive, are important political and social decisions and thus should receive careful attention, analysis, and consideration. This chapter aims to explore issues of resource allocation and rationing, within the context of nursing practice and the provision of nursing care.

Healthcare resource-related discussions, which reach the public domain, often focus on headline-grabbing issues such as whether a particular life-saving treatment should be provided by the relevant national health system (e.g. the National Health Service (NHS) in the UK or the Health Service Executive (HSE) in Ireland) regardless of cost (e.g. Shanahan (2017), on access to the drug Orkambi for those with cystic fibrosis in Ireland). Issues of organ transplantation, shortage, procurement, and distribution of organs, or who should receive access to the limited number of ventilators available when demand may greatly outstrip availability, as in the recent COVID-19 pandemic, are also common topics. Less frequently issues of access to healthcare for particular groups in society also hit the headlines (McCarthy 2017).

To date, the topic of resource allocation in nursing has not generated extensive public discussion. However, over the past decade or so inquiries such as that of

Francis (2013) and Ockenden (2022) in England, the Vale of Leven Inquiry in Scotland (Vale of Leven 2014), and the Tallaght Hospital, Halappanavar and Portlaoise Hospital inquiries in Ireland (HIQA 2012, 2013, 2015) all have important things to say about the nursing (and midwifery) resource and its impact on patient care.

In addition, but separately, over the past two decades a concept variously called 'missed nursing care' (MNC), 'covert rationing of nursing care', 'unfinished care', or 'nursing care left undone' has become a topic of growing research interest internationally (Willis et al. 2021; Gurková et al. 2022). Recent studies persistently demonstrate a weak to moderate (statistical) effect of this covert rationing of nursing care[1] on patient adverse events and on nursing outcomes such as job satisfaction, intention to leave, and so forth (Mandal et al. 2019).

All of the above would seem to suggest that it is timely to explore issues of resource allocation and rationing and their relevance for nursing and the provision of nursing care. This is particularly the case as we know that in a number of countries, including Ireland, the impact of the 2008 financial crisis and subsequent recession, followed by the imposition of austerity measures across the public sector, has had a direct impact on front line staffing in the health service. For example, the Irish health system experienced the loss of 5000 nursing and midwifery posts from the sector between the years 2009 and 2014. This reduction in staffing in Ireland happened at a time when the general population continued to increase and to age, with significant pressures emerging across both acute hospital and community services. As Burke et al. (2014, p. 3) indicate:

> *Approximately €4 billion has been cut from the Irish health system since 2008 and there are over 12,000 fewer Health Service Executive (HSE) staff in December 2013 than there were at the height of public health sector employment in 2007. ... Simultaneously, Ireland's unemployment rate grew from 4% in 2008 to 12.3% in January 2014. .. Reflecting lower incomes and higher levels of unemployment by December 2014. ... These figures combined with a growing, ageing population demonstrate increased demand on a health system which has fewer resources.*

Although in the post-austerity period, there have been concerted attempts by the Irish government to work to ameliorate the drastic impact of austerity on the Irish health system, by increasing the health budget and investing in increasing numbers of staff, among other measures, this is a slow process that has not yet realised significant positive impacts (Cullinan et al. 2020). Thus in the Irish health system, as in many others, already serious resource issues have been compounded by the COVID-19 pandemic, and the consequent pressures imposed on health systems and healthcare staff, particularly nursing staff (Buchan et al. 2022; Gurková et al. 2022; Fino et al. 2023).

---

[1] The term 'covert rationing of nursing care' is being used here to include 'missed/unfinished care' and 'nursing care left undone'.

Resource Allocation and Rationing: Some Definitions

To begin to explore issues of resource allocation and rationing in nursing, it is important to consider what we mean by the relevant terms. Resource allocation refers to the allocation of resources to a service, department, or project. It is important, at the outset, to differentiate between resource allocation and rationing. These are related but nonetheless distinct notions. In allocating resources we are making decisions regarding how to distribute the available resources. There is an implicit assumption that, broadly speaking, there is enough of the resources in question to go around. In situations of rationing, by definition, we are starting from a position that there is not enough of the particular resource to satisfy the needs of all those requiring it. While on occasion in both the economics and ethics literature the concept of rationing may be used to cover any allocation decision, Caplan (1992 p. 322), referring to the medical context, argues for a narrower, more focused definition of rationing:

> ... in health care, rationing refers to a very well-defined subset of allocation policies—those which require a conscious decision or the adoption of an explicit policy wherein certain persons of known medical need are excluded from treatment that might save, prolong, or significantly enhance the quality of their lives.
>
> The stakes are high where rationing in health care is concerned. Thus the overriding moral imperative with respect to rationing in the health care system is not to determine what criteria or rules are fair. It is to make sure that, in the face of apparent scarcity, there is no distributional policy which is a viable alternative to rationing.

The point being made here is that although rationing may occur at the level of both general and specific allocation decisions, not all allocation decisions are rationing decisions. That is, not all allocation decisions contain the conscious choice to give some patients significantly less than optimal care and/or let some patients die, while other patients will receive optimal care/the care that they need to continue living.

Caplan goes on to suggest that in most cases of scarcity, healthcare resources are rationed at the micro allocation level—direct access for specific patients to specific resources, while allocated at the macro level—e.g. funding programme X of healthcare versus funding programme Y.

In a somewhat similar view to that expressed by Caplan in the quote above, Harris (2009) cautions on assuming that healthcare resources are finite, scarce, and therefore must be rationed. He suggests that while such resources are not infinite, they are in fact not finite either—'they are indefinite and can be expanded' (Harris 2009, p. 335). Harris's position was exemplified, for example, in recent hugely increased government investments in public health, healthcare, and social welfare across the Western world, in response to the COVID-19 pandemic (Global Burden of Disease 2021 Health Financing Collaborative Network 2023). Therefore, before rushing to assume rationing is required and trying to grapple with all the attendant difficulties of coming up with a fair, transparent, and acceptable way to ration, Harris suggests that: '... the option of finding a higher level of resource for healthcare might not seem so unattractive or so onerous.' (Harris 2009, p. 349).

To consider resource allocation in the first instance, we can conceive of allocation of resources at a number of different levels. Commonly three levels are used to help frame various types of allocation discussions and decisions—macro-level allocation, meso-level allocation, and micro-level allocation (Tønnessen et al. 2020). The most general level of decision-making in resource allocation is at the macro level. This is the level at which the government, through the Ministry of Finance (or equivalent) or other authorised body, decides the size of the health budget compared, for example, with the budget for education, social welfare, or defence. From this macro decision-making level, the extent of the resources budgeted for healthcare, relative to other social needs such as education, becomes clear. There may be disagreement, among various government departments and/or vested interests, regarding the proportion of funds allocated to health as against education, for example. However, regardless of such concerns and disagreements, the purse available to healthcare will, inevitably, be limited by allocation decisions involving other competing calls on the public purse.

The influence that the individual practitioner in a democratic country can have at this level is as a voting citizen (though there are examples of practising clinicians sitting as elected/appointed members of parliament, as was until recently the case with Dr. Daniel Poulter, in England for example). Pressure groups from within the healthcare professions, patient advocacy groups, or commercial entities[2] may also have an influence at this level. If sufficiently well-organised, there is potential to be much more effective as a collective, as opposed to an individual voter or advocate. It is at this level also that the public discussion of healthcare costs, the resources available, and the potential criteria for explicit rationing of some elements of healthcare, when deemed necessary, can help inform government policy and decision-makers.

The next level of decreasing generality is the meso-economic level; however, many authors include this tier under the heading of macro-economic decision-making (Caplan 1992). It is at this level that decisions regarding allocation of resources among the various healthcare sectors (primary care versus secondary or tertiary care, for example, or women's health versus mental health and so on), are reached. In the normal course of events, there is lobbying, trade-off, and cost benefit-driven decision-making regarding the budget allocation between, for example, primary and acute care sectors.

Again contributions from professional bodies, as well as professional, patient, and commercial pressure groups, may impact on discussions and negotiations during meso-allocation decision-making. Recognition of the importance of negotiation at this level, in terms of the resources for nursing care, may lead one to suggest the need for nurses to develop specific skills, in order to enable them to articulate, more effectively, not only the health but also the economic impact of nursing care. In order to be equipped to participate in these debates, it would benefit nurses to be educated in the concepts, ideas, and approaches to resource allocation and rationing.

---

[2] For example, insurance companies, pharma, and medical devices companies, among others, have very significant lobbying power in this arena particularly in the USA.

This middle level of resource allocation decision-making seems particularly important. It is the potential meeting ground for negotiation between those who come from a top-down (government) and bottom-up (grassroots practitioners) approach to resource allocation.

The micro economic level deals with allocation of resources at the day-to-day operational level. An example of this level of allocation is the posting of the three agency staff available to a hospital to the acute units instead of the emergency department (ED), on the basis of explicit, urgent need. Nurses tend to be acutely aware of the stresses and demands on resources at this level because it affects their everyday clinical practice. For example, if there is a linen shortage, micro allocation decisions concern which patient gets the fresh linen and why. If two patients are demanding the attention of the only nurse on duty, micro allocation decisions, implicitly or explicitly, determine how the needs of these patients, balanced against each other and against the needs of the other patients on that particular unit, will be met.

This is where resource allocation and rationing are directly linked and directly impact on the provision of care. Rationing is also about the distribution of available resources. However, deciding to ration X is based on acceptance that X is scarce—i.e. there is not enough of the particular resource X to go around. Given conditions of scarcity, and with a view to distributive justice, how does one distribute that which is available? The underlying principle here is normally assumed to be that of ensuring the best outcomes for the greatest number. This is known as the Utility Principle.[3] The egalitarian principle of equality of opportunity and the principle of greatest need are also influential in healthcare allocation and rationing decisions (Kuhse and Singer 2009).

Maria Schubert, a Swiss scholar who has published some of the first work in Europe exploring rationing in nursing, defines rationing of nursing care as:

> ... the withholding or failure to carry out necessary nursing tasks due to inadequate time, staffing level and skill mix. (Schubert et al. (2008), p. 228)

In a development of Schubert's position, a recent successful COST Action[4] grant application defined rationing in nursing care as follows:

> Rationing of nursing care occurs when resources are not sufficient to provide necessary care to all patients. The reason for this phenomenon include staff reductions, increased demands for care due to the technological advancements, more treatment options, more informed service users, all requiring more time and attention from care professionals. Rationing of nursing care may also occur due to particular approaches of nurses' clinical judgement and knowledge in allocating the resources and the wider value basis of society on care. As a result, fundamental patient needs may not be fulfilled and human rights linked

---

[3] Please see Chap. 8 of this text for an introduction to Utilitarianism. Utilitarianism is a single-principle theory. That single principle is the Utility Principle.

[4] COST Action grants are research and innovation networking grants funded by the European Commission to enable transnational co-operation. For further information please visit the COST website: http://www.cost.eu/about_cost.

to discrimination may be affected. (RANCARE 2016, Technical Annex, Overview Summary p. 3)

It is important to note that the Schubert definition in particular focuses attention on rationing of nursing care at the bedside —i.e. the micro allocation level.

Consideration of the different positions, presented in the above definitions, seems important for a number of reasons. For example, it does seem that Caplan is correct to draw a distinction between resource allocation and rationing. In resource allocation we allocate the resources we have, one's salary for example, to do particular things—pay our mortgage, buy food, clothes, entertainment, and so forth. In an ideal world, we may wish we had slightly more resource to allocate. However, generally, most people try to work within their means (where this becomes increasingly impossible, for groups or populations, social unrest becomes an increasing risk). Allocating family budget for a holiday might be an example here. If Family A had €10,000 to spend, they might choose to go on a 10-day cruise on the Mediterranean. However, because they actually only have €5,000 to allocate towards a holiday, they choose a 2-week holiday on Lake Garda. While a cruise on the Mediterranean is still a dream to be worked towards, the family are happy with their choice of holiday.

In the nursing context, let us imagine that there are normally 12 staff on the day shift on Medical Ward B. This is, in general, an adequate number of nurses to provide the required patient care, assuming staff work at a reasonable pace, and there are no more than the normal admissions, discharges, and activity demands. Staff are allocated according to the model of care being used, and the normal patient care is given during the nursing shift. However, if one morning the nurse in charge comes on duty and the normal 12 members of staff is reduced to 8, as a result of illness or other reasons, then she may well have to consider how to ration care, including nursing time, to some patients in order to ensure that others get the care they require. This should involve explicit discussion, agreement, and direction at the nursing hand-over and reporting period at the commencement of and throughout the particular shift—in order to try to ensure some degree of transparency, fairness, and peer review of the rationing decisions. The lack of this kind of discussion, transparency, and explicit planning for changing circumstances has led to many recent examples of nurses, for example, during the COVID-19 pandemic, reporting feeling overwhelmed, isolated, unsupported, and incapable of providing adequate care for their patients (Hillestad et al. 2023; Peter et al. 2022; Sperling 2021).

The nurse in charge of Medical Ward B will normally also alert the central nursing office in order to try to get additional help for this particular shift, so that the depleted nursing resource can be augmented, by agency nurses or nurses "on loan" from a quieter part of the hospital—to try to maintain the normal, good standard of care provided to the patients on Ward B. In addition she will alert senior staff of the potential problems that may arise because of the staff shortage. This is akin to acting on Caplan's stricture above that we should ensure that there is no other distributional (allocation) approach available, that will help avoid rationing, and Harris's suggestion that increasing the available resource may be better and less onerous than rationing.

Rationing in Nursing: Design or Default?

As Caplan (1992) points out (see p. 322), rationing decisions exclude certain persons of known need from treatment, or in this case from nursing care. In exploring what such exclusions might look like in terms of nursing care, it is important to take account of three distinctions (Scott et al. 2018, p. 3):

1. The distinction between rationing as implemented by an institution (through their policies or operational practices) and rationing as implemented by individuals (through their actions in their context of practice).
2. The distinction between rationing as based on explicit principles or policies and rationing as based on implicit practices, which may be shared in particular practice contexts or performed by a single individual without making explicit its normative basis.
3. The distinction between rationing of the nursing resource per se (i.e. rationing the number of nurses available to provide the required care) and rationing of actual nursing care at the bedside.

It appears that Caplan's reflections on rationing, referred to above, assumes institutional level rationing based on explicit principles and policy, with doctors and/or other actors involved exercising a gatekeeping role in terms of access to medical care. Frequently these rationing decisions were based on cost-effectiveness or other such assessments and follow largely utilitarian approaches.

However, there is evidence that doctors also engage in additional, covert rationing of medical care at the bedside, based not only on utilitarianism but also, for example, on implicit principles of need and egalitarianism (Scott et al. 2018), or even on administrative burden and/or disengagement, for whatever reason (Ockenden 2022; HIQA 2015).

At the same time, while staff shortages in medicine due to recruitment pressures are a matter of concern internationally, deliberate rationing of medical staff resource does not appear to be a prominent topic of the discussion of rationing medical care.

In contrast, in terms of nursing, there is little if any discussion regarding explicit exclusion either of types of nursing care interventions or of particular patients, in a context of nursing shortages—though shortage of nursing staff is a well-recognised, international problem (Buchan et al. 2022). Even in the face of severe staff reductions and/or increased demands by the institution, the individual nurse's role is still understood to include the provision of the full range of nursing care activities. This simply becomes less possible/impossible as demands increase on the individual nurse or nursing team. Healthcare organisations expect nurses to continue to meet patients' needs fully, while in fact nurses frequently have to miss out/ration nursing care to patients due to lack of time to provide the needed care (Gurková et al. 2022; Witczak et al. 2021):

> *Rationing decisions with regard to the allocation of nursing care, accordingly, appear to be primarily left to practitioners; without explicit normative frameworks, rationing principles*

or specific instructions provided by institutions to guide individual practitioners' decision-making.[5] *The very fact that substantive ethical decision-making regarding rationing is required from nursing staff becomes obscured by this lack of explicitness. It is telling that in the nursing literature on the issue, it is the outcome of 'missed care' or 'care left undone' that provides the impetus to work back to rationing as an underlying ethical problem, rather than beginning with an acknowledgement that constraints regarding availability of resources (in this case nursing staff time) might at times imply the provision of less than optimal care for patients, as is generally the case in the discussion on rationing in medicine.* (Scott et al. 2018, p. 4)

The exclusive focus on rationing care at the bedside (as in missed care/care left undone/unfinished care), in the to date limited discussion of rationing in nursing, is problematic for a number of reasons. This "bedside" focus contributes to obscuring the nature of the ethical problem of rationing in nursing, insofar as it does not appear to (a) recognise a reduced allocation of nursing staff as itself being rationing of a crucial resource and (b) understand that with such a focus, any discussion taking place is kept entirely within the context of the responsibility (and potential culpability) of the individual nurse or nursing team.

Reducing the nursing resource, without a reduction of need, demand, population reduction, and so forth, must be recognised as rationing of nursing care—rather than simply 'cutting staff numbers' or 'reducing the number of training places available':

An ethical justification of rationing the resource of nursing staff, in light of its likely consequences, needs to be provided, rather than effectively rationing the staff resource, but passing on the responsibility for specific rationing decisions in care to individual nurses. Both problems of rationing, the institutional and the individual, need to be recognised as such, and ethical reflection needs to be applied to both. (Scott et al. 2018, p. 4)

Passing on rationing decisions to individual practitioners places onerous ethical demands on individual nurses: ethical demands which often may not be recognised as such. It also risks leading to largely covert rationing of nursing care, akin to that described by Schubert et al. (2008) and RANCRE (2016) Consortium.

Numerous reports (Francis 2013; Vale of Leven 2014; DoH 2014; HIQA 2015; Ockenden 2022) and empirical studies (Ausserhofer et al. 2014; Ball et al. 2013; Witczak et al. 2021) all suggest significant restriction, in fact covert rationing of the nursing resource. Ausserhofer et al. (2014) and Ball et al. (2013) among others report that the nurses they surveyed, in acute medical and surgical units in hospitals across Europe, reported leaving care undone at the end of a shift, as a result of not having enough time to carry out all the patient care required.

Decisions regarding what care to carry out and what care to leave undone due to time or other constraints, unless explicitly discussed and agreed upon at a unit or ward management level, are covert rationing decisions, made by individual practitioners. Covert rationing of nursing care in this way is potentially detrimental to the

---

[5] A stark example of such unsupported rationing decision-making is seen in the case of Ms. Trink, described in the case study in Chap. 4.

care and experience of patients who are not receiving the amount of nursing care required. It is also potentially dangerous as it is not open to peer review or scrutiny. The fact that such covert rationing is not open to peer review and scrutiny and is not openly discussed with either patients or the general public also suggests that there are significant risks of unfairness—covert rationing of this type is based on the judgements and biases of the individual nurse. Much of this covert rationing of care may go unnoticed by nurse managers and unreported by either nursing staff or patients—the latter may feel too vulnerable to do so or may not realise they have a right of fair access to nursing care and a right to complain when this is not provided to them.

If decisions to ration nursing care are not made explicit a number of important questions arise, for example, the following:

- How is the rationing of care monitored?
- Who maintains oversight of care rationing, and who is accountable for the impact on patient care?
- Are there any other factors that can help with more effective allocation of the nursing resource available and thus potentially reduce or remove the need to ration nursing care in certain contexts and circumstances? And how does this question emerge as an issue for discussion?

It seems that implicit/covert rationing decisions are particularly problematic as, by definition, these decisions are unlikely to be transparent, or open to review or challenge. Implicit rationing decisions therefore also do not provide the stimulus or opportunity to consider alternative ways of allocating the available nursing resource, which may remove the need to ration nursing care in the first place.

Cases to Consider

Alice

Let us return briefly to Alice whom we met in Chap. 2 (please see p. 23 above). Alice seems to have very little nursing resource allocated to her. In Alice's case it seems pertinent to ask 'who determined that Alice should receive such limited attention from nursing staff?' Is the decision related to limited nursing resource or to other factors? If due to limited resource, who is responsible and who is accountable for the decision to ration nursing care to Alice and on what criteria? Who knows about the decision? Are the nurses on Alice's ward aware, as a collective staff group, that Alice is receiving little or no nursing care—or has Alice somehow become 'invisible' to nursing staff; is she being actively discriminated against (Bandola and Dobrowolska 2023) for whatever reason? Is the decision to ration nursing care explicit or implicit—and does this matter?

As indicated above, explicit decisions are transparent, thus potentially open to review and challenge, and may be modified in light of further consideration. Implicit decisions are by definition covert, hidden from view. Implicit decisions are therefore not open to review or scrutiny by the team. Because such decisions are covert, and not open to review, they are more likely to suffer from biases and prejudiced decision-making. Implicit decisions carry greater risk of bias, prejudice, and lack of fairness.

Ms. P

A second case study involves a 59-year-old woman, herself a nurse, admitted to an acute surgical unit with a perforation of the large bowel, diagnosed in the emergency department (ED) and confirmed later by CT scan. Ms. P was seriously ill, and initially the surgical team were of the view that resection of her bowel was likely to be required. However, conservative treatment, including intravenous (IV) antibiotics and pain relief, was commenced in the ED and maintained on transfer of Ms. P to an acute surgical ward in a public hospital.

Ms. P (based on her own observation records) received a total of 4–7 min direct nursing contact per 12-h day shift, and between 7 and 15 min per 12-h shift during her first 5 days in the surgical unit. During the final 4 days of her 9-day hospitalisation, 4 of the minutes on day shift were linked with peripherally inserted central catheter (PICC) line care and administration of IV antibiotics; on the night shift, this accounted for approximately 8 min of direct nursing contact (two different 8 hourly administration of drugs). The remainder of nursing time which Ms. P received was taken up with 4-hourly temperature, pulse, and blood pressure monitoring, and the final 2/3 min on day shift occurred if and when Ms. P's bed was made by nursing staff.

For the entire 9-day hospitalisation Ms. P received no nursing input that attempted to explore if Ms. P understood her condition/predicament. She received no advice regarding the importance of trying to sit out of bed, even for short periods, no help or advice regarding general mobilisation, or assistance to go for short walks—though within 24 h of admission she walked across the two-bedded unit, pushing her drip stand, to use the toilet herself. There was no monitoring of fluid intake (despite being 'nil orally' for the first 48-h and then on 'sips' for 3 further days. Prior to commencing 'low residue' diet. Ms. P was 'chased' to the bathroom by a well-meaning student nurse, for a wash on the first 2 days following admission, when she could barely stand—but there was no offer of help or assistance. By day 3 Ms. P knew she should be sitting out of bed for as long as she could cope with it, and she asked her husband and daughter to take her for short walks along and out of the ward, as she was still too unsteady on her feet to go by herself.

The clinical nurse manager (CNM) walked by the foot of Ms. P's bed, on her way to the second patient in the two-bedded room, at least four to five times during Ms. P's hospital stay, without once acknowledging Ms. P in any way. Ms. P was very distressed by this and began to question if she was somehow in the wrong ward, was some kind of 'lodger' who did not deserve to be in hospital, and who did not warrant the care and attention that the other patient ('a proper, deserving patient' with cancer in the bed beside her) in her room was receiving.

From Ms. P's perspective, she was quite ill, undemanding, and mostly continent and as such was largely ignored by nursing staff—including the CNM—and left to her own devices. Ms. P feels that she was neglected as a patient in terms of lack of reasonable, acceptable access to nursing time. She also indicated that she was potentially discriminated against because she did not 'fit' some unarticulated version of 'a deserving patient'.[6]

The cases of Alice (Chap. 2) and Ms. P provide important insights into some of the significant issues with covert rationing of nursing care, regardless of the perceived reasons for such rationing. If nurses ration their care without an explicit, fair, and agreed set of criteria, we face three significant risks:

1. There is a significant risk of unnecessary patient neglect and possible death (Francis 2013; HIQA 2013, 2015; Ockenden 2022).
2. We risk eroding a model of good care as the norm for nursing provision and nursing staffs' expectation that this is the model of care they can and should provide (Mandal et al. 2019).
3. We risk undermining the trust and respect the general public have for nurses and the nursing profession.

In the studies by Auserhoffer et al. (2014), Ball et al. (2013), and Gurková et al. (2022) a consistent pattern of nursing care left undone emerges across Europe. While physical care activities such as patient observations and medication were consistently carried out patient hygiene, comfort care, patient education, and discharge planning, as well as documentation of care, were frequently and consistently among the care activities left undone. Such a pattern portrays a 'hollowed out' notion of nursing care that is extraordinarily limited in its conception of such care (Mandal et al. 2019).

This largely invisible, unaccounted for rationing of nursing care is likely to undermine the core of nursing and those elements of nursing care that patients place much value on—a supportive presence, comfort care, patient education, information about their condition and medication, and what to do when the patient goes home. There is an individual and a collective responsibility to challenge the provision of a reduced, rationed version of nursing care, in the name of good nursing, of patient safety, and of humane, ethically appropriate patient care (Tønnessen et al. 2020).

There is growing evidence indicating a need to recognise the impact of factors such as registered nurse-to-patient ratios, the work environment, nurse characteristics, and leadership on the quality of nursing care provided to patients. A number of studies also indicate that some of the more detrimental effects of nurse staffing shortages can be ameliorated, to some extent, by a positive work environment and inclusive supportive nursing leadership (Aiken et al. 2011; Mandal et al. 2019;

---

[6]The source of this case: direct contact between Ms. P and the author.

Gurková et al. 2022). Aiken et al. (2014) suggest that staffing wards with nurses who have degree-level education, or above, can have an impact on 30-day mortality rates in surgical patients. Papastravrou et al. (2012) argue that both team working and nursing leadership impacts on the covert/implicit rationing of nursing care; increasing the effectiveness of team working reduces implicit rationing of nursing care, as does supportive nursing leadership. This has been confirmed in more recent work in this area (Gurková et al. 2022; Mandal et al. 2019).

These studies appear to provide support for Caplan's demand that instead of focusing on devising fair rules for rationing as our starting point, we should begin by identifying when we are making implicit or explicit decisions to ration and make sure that there is no alternative—no better way of distributing our limited resources—that would avoid or minimise rationing. The potential impact of enhanced team working, nurse education levels, and nursing leadership on the effective use of the nursing resource seem important issues to explore in deciding the overall nursing resource requirements at macro, meso, and micro allocation levels. These also seem important impacts to explore in working towards enhancing patient care and avoiding what may be unrecognised, unmonitored, implicit rationing of nursing care at micro allocation levels in particular. The results of these studies also provide an important reason to argue for explicit rather than implicit rationing of nursing care.

Conclusion

The COVID-19 pandemic highlighted to the public the vital necessity of a functioning healthcare system and the importance of adequate healthcare resources, in a way unprecedented in recent history. The pandemic thus assisted the recognition of nursing, globally, as a valuable healthcare resource, essential to patient care. A corollary of this recognition is the fact that valuable nursing resource should be treated with care and consideration at macro, meso, and micro allocation levels. Nurses should explicitly and consistently discuss the perceived need to make rationing of care decisions with their managers and patients, in order that such decisions are scrutinised, challenged, and, where necessary, explicitly articulated to the Director of Nursing, the hospital CEO, the hospital Board of Directors, and regional and national healthcare managers.

Allocation of the nursing resource is overseen by ward managers/charge nurses on a daily basis across nursing shifts. Nurses then have considerable discretion regarding how their time is allocated to the care activities they engage in with the patients under their care. It seems important, on the basis of the evidence and arguments offered in this chapter, that explicit discussion around this allocation of the care time of the individual nurse, to their patients, be encouraged. In order to do so more effectively and to identify and discuss actual conditions of scarcity and the consequent need to ration nursing care, nurses and their managers need to be educated in the principles and concepts of resource allocation and rationing. They also need to be educated to observe for, and monitor the effects of, both implicit and explicit rationing of nursing care.

Key Learning Points
- Resource allocation refers to the distribution of available resources.
- Rationing assumes that one is existing in conditions of scarcity and thus there is not enough of the required resource to meet existing needs.
- Rationing decisions should be explicit and open to scrutiny, review, and challenge.
- Implicit (covert) rationing of nursing care is detrimental to good patient care. It potentially normalises suboptimal approaches to nursing care and erodes public trust in the nursing profession.
- Health service and nursing leadership, as well as nurses themselves, should treat nursing time as an important healthcare resource to be allocated with careful consideration.

References

Aiken LH, Cimiotti J, Sloane DM, Smith HL, Flynn L, Neff D (2011) The effects of nurse staffing and nurse education on patient deaths in hospitals with different nurse work environments. Med Care 49:1047–1053

Aiken LH, Sloan DM, Bruyneel L, Van de Heede K, Griffith P, Busse R, Diomidous M, Kinnunen J, Koska M, Lesaffre E, McHugh MD, Moreno Casbes MT, Rafferty AM, Schwedimann R, Scott PA, Tichelman C, van Achterberg T, Sermeus W (2014) Association of nurse staffing and education with hospital mortality in 9 European countries. Lancet 2014. https://doi.org/10.1016/S0140-6736(13)62631-8

Ausserhofer D, Zander B, Busse R, Schubert M, De Geest S, Rafferty AM, Ball J, Scott PA, Kinnunen J, Heinen M, Strømseng Sjetne I, Moreno-Casbas T, Kózka M, Lindqvist R, Diomidous M, Bruyneel L, Sermeus W, Aiken L, Schwendimann R (2014) Prevalence, patterns and predictors of nursing care left undone in European hospitals: results from the multicountry cross-sectional RN4CAST study. BMJ Qual Saf 2(23):126–135. Available online 11th Nov 2013. http://qualitysafety.bmj.com/cgi/content/full/bmjqs2013-002318

Ball JE, Murrells T, Rafferty AM, Morrow E, Griffiths P (2013) 'Care left undone' during nursing shifts: associations with workload and perceived quality of care. BMJ Qual Saf. Available at: http://qualitysafety.bmj.com/content/early/2013/07/08/bmjqs-2012-001767.full.pdf+html. Accessed 12th Sept 2023

Bandoła K, Dobrowolska B (2023) Determinants of the rationing of nursing care provided to older patients. Medycyna Ogólna i Nauki o Zdrowiu. https://doi.org/10.26444/monz/171757

Buchan J, Catton H, Shaffer FA (2022) Sustain and retain in 2022 and beyond: the global nursing workforce and the COVID-19 pandemic. International Centre for Nurse Migration, Philadelphia

Burke S, Thomas S, Barry S, Keegan C (2014) Measuring, mapping and making sense of Irish health sector performance in the recession. A working paper for the Resilience project. The Centre for Health Policy and Management, School of Medicine Trinity College, Dublin. https://www.tcd.ie/medicine/health_policy_management/assets/pdf/Resilience-working-paper-March-2014.pdf. Accessed 8 July 2023

Caplan AL (1992) If I were a rich man could I buy a pancreas? And other essays in the ethics of health care. Indiana University Press, Indiana

Cullinan J, Connolly S, Whyte R (2020) The sustainability of Ireland's health care system. Centre for Economic Research on Inclusivity and sustainability (CERIS) Working Paper Series, 2020/02. https://www.universityofgalway.ie/media/research/ceris/files/WP-2020-02.pdf. Accessed 25 August 2023

DoH (2014) HSE midland regional hospital, portlaoise perinatal deaths (2006-to date). Stationary Office, Dublin

European Council, Council of the European Union (2021) COVID-19: the EU's response in the field of public health. https://www.consilium.europa.eu/en/policies/coronavirus/covid-19-public-health/. Accessed 24 July 2023

Fino E, Daniels JK, Micheli G, Gazineo D, Godino L, Imbriaco G, Antognoli M, Sist L, Regnano D, Decaro R, Guberti M, Mazzetti M (2023) Moral injury in a global health emergency: a validation study of the Italian version of the Moral Injury Events Scale adjusted to the healthcare setting. Eur J Psychotraumatol 14(2):2263316. https://doi.org/10.1080/20008066.2023.2263316

Francis R (2013) Report of the Mid Staffordshire NHS Foundation Trust Public Inquiry. Chaired by Robert Francis QC. Stationary Office, London

Global Burden of Disease 2021 Health financing Collaborative Network (2023) Global investments in pandemic preparedness and COVID-19: development assistance and spending on health between 1990 and 2026. Lancet Glob Health 2023(11):e385–e413. https://doi.org/10.1016/S2214-109X(23)00007-4

Gurková E, Mikšová Z, Šáteková L (2022) Missed nursing care in hospital environments during the COVID-19 pandemic. Int Nurs Rev 69(2):175–184. https://doi.org/10.1111/inr.12710

Harris J (2009) Deciding between patients. In: Singer P, Kushe H (eds) A companion to bioethics, 2nd edn. Wiley-Blackwell, Chichester, UK, pp 335–350. (chapter 29)

Hillestad AH, Rokstad AMM, Tretteteig S, Julnes SG, Lichtwarck B, Eriksen S (2023) Nurses' ethical challenges when providing care in nursing homes during the COVID-19 pandemic. Nurs Ethics 30(1):32–45

HIQA (2012) Report of the investigation into the quality, safety and governance of the care provided by the Adelaide and Meath Hospital, Dublin incorporating the National Children's Hospital (AMNCH) for patients who require acute admission. https://www.hiqa.ie/publications/report-investigation-quality-safety-and-governance-care-provided-adelaide-and-meath-hos. Accessed 12 September 2023

HIQA (2013) Patient Safety Investigation Report published by Health Information and Quality Authority. Health Information and Quality Authority. 9 Oct 2013. Archived from the original on 30 Nov 2013. Available at: file:///C:/Users/0119275s/Downloads/Patient-Safety-Investigation-UHG.pdf. Accessed 12th Sept 2016 https://www.hiqa.ie/press-release/2013-10-09-patient-safety-investigation-report-published-health-information-and-qualit. Accessed 12 September 2023

HIQA (2015) Report of the investigation into the safety, quality and standards of services provided by the Health Service Executive to patients in the Midland Regional Hospital, Portlaoise. Available at: https://www.hiqa.ie/publications/report-investigation-safety-quality-and-standards-services-provided-health-service-exec. Accessed 12 September 2023

Kuhse H, Singer P (eds) (2009) A companion to bioethics, 2nd edn. Wiley-blackwell, Chichester, UK

Mandal L, Seethalakshmi A, Rajendrababu A (2019) Rationing of nursing care a deviation from holistic nursing: a systematic review. Nurs Philos 21(1):10.1111/nup.12257

McCarthy J (2017) Americans back higher insurance rates for smokers, not for obese. Gallup: https://nws.gallup.com/poll/214244/americans-back-higher-insurance-rates-smokers-not-obese.aspx. Accessed 19 July 2023

Ockenden D (2022) Ockenden report—final: findings, conclusions and essential actions from the independent review of maternity services at the Shrewsbury and Telford trust hospital NHS trust. Her Majesty's Stationary Office, London. https://www.ockendenmaternityreview.org.uk/wp-content/uploads/2022/03/FINAL.INDEPENDENT_MATERNITY_REVIEW_OF_MATERNITY_SERVICES_REPORT.pdf. Accessed 5 July 2023

Papastravrou E, Andreou P, Schubert M, De Geest S (2012) Rationing of nursing care within professional, environmental constraints: a correlational study. Clin Nurs Res 20(10):1–22. https://doi.org/10.1177/1054773812469543

Peter E, Mohammed S, Killackey T, MacInver J, Variath C (2022) Nurses experience of ethical responsibilities of care during the COVID-19 pandemic. Nurs Ethics 29(4):844–857

RANCARE COST Action (2016) Rationing—missed nursing care: an international and multidimensional problem. CA15208. COST is supported by the EU Framework Programm Horizon 2020, Brussels, COST Association

Savulescu J, Cameron J, Wilkinson D (2020) Equality of utility? Ethics and law of rationing ventilators. Br J Anaesth 125(1):10–15

Schubert M, Glass T, Clarke SP, Aiken LH, Schaffert-Witvlet B, Sloane DM, De Geest S (2008) Rationing of nursing care and its relationship to patient outcomes: the Swiss extension of the International hospital study. Int J Qual Health Care 20(4):227–237

Scott PA, Harvey C, Felzmann H, Suhonen R, Habermann M, Halvorsen K, Christiansen K, Toffoli L, Papastavrou E (2018) Resource allocation and rationing in nursing care: a discussion paper. Nurs Ethics 26(5):1528–1539. https://doi.org/10.1177/0969733018759831

Shanahan C (2017) Meet the brave people who fought to give cystic fibrosis sufferers a new lease of life. Irish Examiner April 15th 2017: https://irishexaminer.com/business/arid-20447866.html . Accessed 19 July 2023

Sperling D (2021) Ethical dilemmas, perceived risk, and motivation among nurses during the COVID-19 pandemic. Nurs Ethics 28(1):9–22

Tønnessen S, Scott PA, Nortvedt P (2020) Safe and competent nursing care: an argument for a minimum standard? Nurs Ethics 27(6):1396–1407. https://doi.org/10.1177/0969733020919137

Turale S, Meechammaan C, Kunaviktikul W (2020) Challenging times: ethics, nursing and the COVID-19 pandemic. Int Nurs Rev 67(2):164–167. https://pubmed.ncbi.nlm.nih.gov/32578249/. Accessed 19 July 2023

Vale of Leven Hospital Inquiry Report (2014) Chaired by Rt Hon Lord MacLean. Published on behalf of The Vale of Leven Hospital Inquiry by APS Group An online version of the Report is available at www.valeoflevenhospitalinquiry.org. Accessed 12 September 2023

Willis E, Zelenikova R, Bail K, Papastavrou E (2021) The globalization of missed nursing care terminology. Int J Nurs Pract 27(1):10.1111/ijn.12859

Witczak I, Rypicz Ł, Karniej P, Młynarska A, Kubielas G, Uchmanowicz I (2021) Rationing of nursing care and patient safety. Front Psychol 12:676970. https://doi.org/10.3389/fpsyg.2021.676970

Yip YC, Yip KH, Tsui WK (2022) When rationing becomes inevitable in a pandemic: a discussion on the ethical considerations from a public health perspective. Public Health Pract 4:100294

Moral Injury and Nursing Practice

4

Anto Čartolovni, Minna Stolt, Riitta Suhonen, and P. Anne Scott

Abstract

The idea of moral injury in healthcare attracted much public attention during the recent COVID-19 pandemic. Duty to care, particularly in circumstances such as the pandemic, raised the awareness of the phenomenon of moral injury in nursing among practising nurse and nurse leaders and managers. The concept of moral injury was introduced originally from a military context, mostly identified, and observed among veterans. Some evidence from the early literature on the concept suggests that moral injury, as an experience, was conceptually confused with other existing experiences conceptualised as burnout and/or moral distress. This may have led to an under recognition and lack of awareness of moral injury as a discreet experience.

Although the experiences conceptualised as moral injury, moral distress, and burnout have some commonalities in symptoms and outcomes, it is argued that as individual experiences these three differ in humanly and ethically important

---

A. Čartolovni (✉)
School of Medicine, Catholic University of Croatia, Zagreb, Croatia
e-mail: anto.cartolovni@unicath.hr

M. Stolt
Department of Nursing Science, University of Turku, Turku, Finland

Wellbeing Services County of Satakunta, Pori, Finland
e-mail: Minna.stolt@utu.fi

R. Suhonen
Department of Nursing Science, University of Turku, Turku, Finland

Turku University Hospital, Wellbeing Services County of Southwest Finland, Turku, Finland
e-mail: riisuh@utu.fi

P. A. Scott
University of Galway, Galway, Co Galway, Ireland
e-mail: Anne.scott@universityofgalway.ie

ways. It is further argued that these different experiences need to be recognised and addressed appropriately. Failing to do so may add to the rising number of nursing professionals leaving their profession.

This reality raises significant challenges for both nurse leaders and managers and for healthcare organisations. It is incumbent on leaders and managers in healthcare organisations to be sensitive to the development of moral distress, moral injury, and burnout in staff members and colleagues, and to work to find ways to support the well-being of nurses and other healthcare practitioners, thus enabling them to flourish as persons and as healthcare professionals.

In this chapter we will consider the evolving use of the concept of moral injury in the healthcare literature, including attempts to differentiate it from concepts of moral distress and burnout. We will also consider some of the factors identified as contributing to the experience of moral injury in individual practitioners. The chapter will conclude by suggesting some measures that can be taken to help ameliorate and or mitigate the experience of moral injury.

Keywords

Moral injury · Moral integrity · Nursing practice · Moral dissonance · Burnout · Moral distress

Case Study

The narrative quoted below is indicative of the experiences of many frontline nurses during the COVID-19 pandemic:

> Tassia Trink, a registered nurse in southern California, says pandemic numbers rose so rapidly that emergency room patients would be waiting up to 18 hours for a bed. Consequently, nurses were forced to make decisions about which patient was moved into an ER bed first. As a seriously ill couple waited for care, Trink was forced to pick which spouse should be moved first. Although both spouses were eventually seen, Trink selected the partner with the lowest oxygen saturation (70%) …
>
> Nurses may have been unfamiliar with the process of rationing care, but the pandemic has changed that perspective. Nurses are now dealing with a form of rationing that leaves them miserable, in tears, and in persistent distress. Providing care for 10 patients as opposed to a maximum of five forces nurses to make appalling decisions. Which patient needs my attention now? Will another patient die while I am in this room? How can I choose, without suffering lasting trauma from my decisions?
>
> Nurses have repeatedly been placed in impossible situations throughout the pandemic." (Goodman, Diane M. 2022)

The enormous uncertainly, conflict, and distress experienced by nurses such as Ms. Trink during the pandemic crisis is difficult to articulate. In the case above, decisions had to be made about which acutely ill patients to treat when all could not be treated. The lack of reference in the case to ethical decision-making frameworks or protocols suggests that no such frameworks or protocols existed to assist Ms. Trink or her colleagues make rationing decisions fairly, transparently and with support. Ms. Trink was on her own – desperately trying to cope with overwhelmingly ill people, with severely limited resources, knowing that some of her patients would die, often alone and in distress, and there was nothing she could do about it. As a once off scenario this would have been distressing and painful. As an ongoing reality, over days and weeks and month, the experience is so traumatising that it is very difficult to describe it either accurately or sensitively.

Introduction

The experiences of nurses such as Ms. Trink have brought to attention, within the healthcare domain, the recently recognised phenomenon of moral injury. There is no doubt that Ms. Trink faced a moral dilemma during the triage process, followed by the emotional aftermath of her decision based on prioritisation. The inability to provide the required care to both husband and wife, due to the acute shortage of resources resulting from the exponential demand during the pandemic, caused Ms. Trink acute distress, uncertainty, and conflict regarding the right thing to do, in addition to the exhaustion that comes with working under such sustained pressure. In this scenario Ms. Trink is forced to choose between two people, both of whom requires urgent, lifesaving care, in a context where resources dictate that only one person can receive the required emergency room (ER) bed. This scenario may seem like a scenario that would create a form of moral distress in a committed, conscientious practitioner. However, the circumstances raised by the pandemic, linked with Ms. Trink's personal characteristics (such as depth of experience as a nurse, moral resilience,[1] religious beliefs and so forth), may lead to the experience of moral injury by Ms. Trink.

Moral distress and moral injury are two distinguishable, individual responses of practitioners. These practitioners are involved in situations in which the individual is exposed to incidents, interventions, or situations that give rise to perceived clashes of moral principles and/or deeply held moral values (personal and/or professional), in decision-making about patient care.

The individual personal responses to a situation are based on the personal perceptions, cognitions, and appraisals of the situation understood as inducing a moral issue/problem/conflict/ dilemma. Such individual cognitions may be influenced by both internal and external factors—personal, interpersonal, institutional, and societal (Griffin et al. 2023).

> Gibbons et al. (2013, p. 248) *makes a clear distinction between moral distress and moral injury .. stating that 'moral distress among military health professionals occurs when an*

---

[1] Moral resilience refers to one's ability to sustain or restore a sense of moral integrity in the face of moral confusion, complexity distress, or setback.

individual makes a moral judgment about a patient situation but does not act accordingly. This occurs when actions are obstructed by an organisation or by a more powerful individual'. On the contrary, in defining 'moral injury', Gibbons et al. (2013) refers to the work of Litz et al. (2009) stating that 'Moral injury involves a deeper emotional wound and is unique to those who bear witness to intense human suffering and cruelty'. ...

The main difference between moral distress and moral injury is that moral distress represents a form of situational problem (due to the external or internal constraints), while moral injury represents an experience of the problem that results in a long-lasting change to an individual's sense of losing hope, trust, integrity and so on. In fact, moral distress represents a challenge which may be relatively easy to prevent, if the external constraints are removed and the internal constraints mitigated by reinforcing and increasing moral resilience. .. On the contrary, moral injury results in long-term emotional scarring or damage contributing to permanent numbness, malfunctioning and social isolation, which may on the other hand result, if treated in time, in a posttraumatic growth.

However, we would also not exclude the possibility that some cases of moral distress may turn into moral injury with time, and in certain circumstances and contexts. The relationship between these two concepts needs further investigation and confirmation through empirical studies, particularly in terms of where to draw the line as to when significant moral distress turns into moral injury leading to severe consequences. (Čartolovni et al. 2021, pp. 5–8)

Moral problems, issues, and dilemmas are labels applied to situations, perceived as involving a combination of moral elements such as important moral values, duties, and principles. In the case of moral dilemmas, these values, principles, or duties are in direct conflict, such that choosing to be guided by value A violates value B. For example, an individual witnesses the mugging of an old women and recognises this as a bad act (a moral issue) for a variety of reasons, e.g. the mugger has hurt the old woman by knocking her to the ground, has stolen her bag and has left the old woman shaken, angry, and frightened. Moral distress or moral injury are labels applied to individual personal responses in those individuals who are engaged with or involved in such situations. For example, our witness may feel moral distress at the mugging, which caused trauma and damage to an innocent old woman, because they were unable to intervene through fear for their own safety, or because having intervened ineffectively the mugger still got away with the old woman's property and left the old woman distraught, because the only photo she had of her dead husband was in the bag.

Persistent exposure to feelings of moral distress, i.e. chronic moral distress, may result ultimately in moral injury (a long-term emotional scarring or damage inflicted on one's sense of moral integrity) (Litz et al. 2009; Mewborn et al. 2023; Griffin et al. 2023).

Profound, inescapable moral trauma caused by cruel, devastating situations or incidents such as those experienced by both civilians and healthcare workers (HCWs) in the war in Syria, Ukraine, and Gaza can also cause moral injury in an individual (Cuadra 2023; Abbara et al. 2023; BBC 2023). Whether the individual experience is one of moral distress or moral injury is down to the response of the individual—a response that is driven by internal individual factors (e.g. moral resilience, personal history, self-confidence, feeling of self-worth and being supported, etc.). These individual factors are, however, heavily influenced by interpersonal, institutional, and societal factors—leadership support, etc. (Griffin et al. 2023).

Some evidence suggested that the risk of functionally impairing moral injury was higher among women (versus men), younger (versus older) HCWs, nurses (versus physicians), those who worked more versus fewer hours, and providers with less experience (Akhtar et al. 2022). Also, the risk of severe moral injury symptoms was lower among individuals who identified as religious/spiritual versus those who did not (Mantri et al. 2021; Griffin et al. 2023).

Conceptualisation of the experience now called 'moral injury' stems from the work of psychiatrist Shay, who first observed it as an internal wound among Vietnam veterans (Shay 1995). Moral injury for Shay was not only related to exposure to trauma but also to the moral dilemma in specific actions, defining it as present *'when (i) there has been a betrayal of what is morally right, (ii) by someone who holds the legitimate authority and (iii) in a high stakes situation'* (Shay 1995). However, Shay's definition is focused only on the power relations between the superior and the soldier, presenting a reduced understanding of moral injury concentrating only on external aspects and negating the internal aspects of disappointment with the moral actions taken and their accompanying negative feelings. Furthermore, this has motivated researchers to change focus to the personal perspective and potentially morally injurious events (PMIEs). PMIEs are defined as *'perpetrating, failing to prevent, or bearing witness to acts that transgress deeply held moral beliefs and expectations'* (Litz et al. 2009), to which longer severe/repeated exposure might lead to moral injury. In short, PMIEs might violate deeply held moral beliefs through acts of perpetration, omission, or bearing witness to suffering, mistakes or accidents causing them.

Ms. Trink's testimony, articulated in the case study above, is like that of many of the healthcare workers, especially nurses, who actively contributed during the COVID-19 pandemic. During the pandemic, many studies reported moral injury levels among healthcare professionals (HCPs) due to the pandemic's extreme circumstances. This included morally challenging or relatively unfamiliar situations to the HCPs involved, such as overcrowded hospitals, patient overload, lack of beds, respirators, personal protective equipment (PPE), and exhausted healthcare professionals (Thibodeau et al. 2023).

The pandemic has demonstrated that occupational factors can play a detrimental role in the development of moral injury. Factors such as lack of PPE for nurses and patients, uncertainty of the transmissibility of COVID-19, high patient mortality, triage with scarce resources, lack of support from management and colleagues, and incongruent remuneration for the required sacrifice and work, all contribute to the sense that top-level management, organisations, government, and broader society, do not take the safety and needs of HCPs into account. This leads to feelings of anger, betrayal, resentment, powerlessness, and inability to forgive. Considering Shay's definitions, these high-stakes situations during the pandemic led to hard choices in which HCPs needed to make morally problematic and/or distressing decisions. It may have led to a sense of betrayal by their leaders, organisation, and system afterwards. Furthermore, HCPs were frequently labelled as 'angels' or 'heroes' by the media, creating a false image of invincibility and lack of vulnerability, and thus no need to provide any special care or concern for HCPs during the pandemic; this may have created a barrier for care, making it more difficult for HCPs to seek help for their state or condition (Rabin et al. 2023).

The pandemic placed unprecedented pressure on healthcare organisational structures internationally, and nurses needed to work longer hours and care for more patients with fewer resources (Hegarty et al. 2022). Furthermore, due to the reallocation of resources to the frontlines to combat the pandemic, patients' health deteriorated (due partially to diverting of resources to the front line and to the fact that many people did not present to the health services for required screening, assessment, and treatment), and eventually, some patients died, creating a more significant risk of moral injury for the nurses responsible for their care. In addition, this was often followed by a system-wide lack of response to nurses' feedback, leading to a feeling that their organisations did not look out for their well-being (Rabin et al. 2023). In addition, a recent study (Fitzpatrick et al. 2022) among nurses and nursing leaders demonstrated a significant association between moral injury and negative well-being and a negative association between moral injury and resilience, with no significant differences observed between nurses and nursing leaders.

Nurses experience difficult and stressful ethical challenges in their everyday work, which, in significant part, they can handle. Still, in such exceptional circumstances as those which existed during the COVID-19 pandemic, the primary moral priorities needed clarification; for example, those between nurses preserving their own life and health by not getting infected and nurses fulfilling the ethical and professional responsibility of providing good care to (all) those who required it. These morally conflicting situations create internal dissonance by impacting biological, psychological/emotional, social/familial, and spiritual dimensions (Carey and Hodgson 2018). This internal dissonance is followed by feelings of guilt or shame, a sense of betrayal, anger, disgust, anxiety, helplessness, cynicism, loss of confidence, isolation, sadness, negative thoughts about oneself, about others, and about the world (Rabin et al. 2023).

Conceptual and Terminological Conundrums

Despite its roots in the military/war context, moral injury has also been observed among other professionals such as firefighters, police, and paramedics (Lentz et al. 2021) or even civilians (Morriss and Berle 2023). Regarding nurses, the first empirical study on moral injury among healthcare professionals, at the beginning of the pandemic, reported that nurses had the highest moral injury functional impairment symptoms among all respondents (Mantri et al. 2021). However, a much deeper discussion about moral injury in healthcare started within the medical burnout literature. A key theme emerging in this literature argues that physicians are not suffering from burnout but from moral injury, emphasising that moral injury has its roots in a broken system that uses a reductionist business model, which prioritises profit over healing (Dean et al. 2019).

Nevertheless, it is important to point out that there is likely to be a connection between both phenomena, i.e. burnout and moral injury. The World Health Organisation (WHO) has recently recognised burnout as an occupational phenomenon *'resulting from chronic workplace stress that has not been successfully managed'* (World Health Organisation 2019). Moreover, burnout *'is characterised by three dimensions: (a) feelings of energy depletion or exhaustion; (b) increased mental distance from one's job, or feelings of negativism or cynicism related to one's job; and (c) reduced professional efficacy'* (World Health Organisation 2019).

It is important to emphasise that moral injury can contribute to the core burnout symptoms, particularly distressing situations where nurses cannot practise in a way that coheres with their moral/ethical expectations. Consequently, doubts about their ability to provide good nursing care can lead to ineffectiveness and a reduced sense of personal accomplishment, leading to cynicism, depersonalisation, and disengagement (Rosen et al. 2022). Furthermore, this relatedness is perceived in a recent study conducted by Zahiriharsini et al. (2022) during the third wave of the COVID-19 pandemic in Quebec. This study demonstrated that HCPs exposed to psychosocial stressors at work (PSW) were two to five times more likely to experience moral injury. The strongest association was seen in situations identified as having a poor ethical culture.

Therefore, it is important to emphasise that occupational stress can be related to moral injury, and moral injury may be related to burnout (Rosen et al. 2022). However to frame the entire discussion, placing a discussion and analysis of 'moral injury' within a discussion on 'burnout' might lead to an underestimation of the moral aspects of 'moral injury' and may also result in 'moral injury' being treated as a mental disorder or issue (Čartolovni et al. 2021), versus a mental disorder that has institutional roots that the institution/service needs to address.

Despite being interrelated and existing on a continuum, there are differences which distinguish moral distress, moral injury, and burnout in relation to focus. Burnout relates to the mental health aspects of occupational stress, and moral distress and moral injury focus on the moral aspects of certain actions and situations. However, the clear distinction between moral injury and moral distress is hard to draw because both relate to the individual's moral integrity and the inner feelings they share.

Andrew Jameton first defined moral distress as a phenomenon *'when one knows the right thing to do, but institutional constraints make it nearly impossible to pursue the right course of action'* (Jameton 1984). In other words, moral distress appears when the HCP is clear on what is ethical but something or someone is preventing it from happening (omission). Moral injury appears when the HCP is required to do something (or observe something) that he/she believes is wrong (commission of or observation of wrongdoing). Therefore, based on the definitions of moral injury and moral distress, it seems that moral distress relates to the more situational problem (due to external or internal constraints) (Čartolovni et al. 2021) in which an individual is unable to act according to their moral judgement, while moral injury has a psychological impact in a more long standing and severe experience of suffering, occurring as a result of hyper acute or chronic moral adversity or moral distress (generated via acts of commission or omission), which results in long-lasting change such as a deep emotional wound (Gibbons et al. 2013). A recent study (Stanojević and Čartolovni 2022) among oncology and palliative nurses demonstrated a correlation between moral distress and moral injury, which also correlated with the decision to leave or consider leaving their positions.

Therefore, it is important to acknowledge that all three experiences described by the concepts moral distress, moral injury, and burnout might have some overlaps in symptoms or outcomes or are correlated with each other, existing on a spectrum with a movement back and forth along the continuum (Rosen et al. 2022). However, this overlap does not mean that one approach/solution can be applied to resolve and deal with them all. It is likely that each of the experiences (moral distress, moral injury, burnout) requires different interventions to help resolve each set of symptoms. The current global situation of nursing professionals' understaffing, where the number of nurses who left or are planning to leave the profession increased by up to one-third in 2022 (Mandowara and Leo 2023), raises a concern that some of these decisions to exit nursing might be due to unrecognised moral injury or misplaced and misdiagnosed moral distress or burnout (Rosen et al. 2022).

Contributing Factors to the Occurrence of Moral Injury

Most of the situations in which moral injury or moral distress emerge appear to be situations that are ethically problematical, situations of ethical conflict, ethical uncertainty, and/or situations giving rise to ethical dilemmas. The latter are situations where different options can be supported by various ethical concepts/principles, but none of the solutions are ethically satisfactory. Such an outcome might result in the violations of one or more ethical values, concepts, or principles leading to emotions such as guilt, disappointment, frustration, etc. The case Ms. Trink faced, with the triage process and emotional aftermath of the decision taken, appeared to be one such ethical dilemma. These situations create moral dissonance in an individual between performed behaviour and morally more desirable behaviour. Furthermore, the theoretical explanations have tried to explain moral injury emerging through the Moral Dissonance Model (MDM) (Te Brake and Nauta 2022) as providing an explanation of the continuous interplay between individual experience and contextual aspects. This might be more pressing by changing moral contexts as Te Brake and Nauta (2022) argue, *'there is a continuous change between displayed behaviour and a present, ever-changing sense of how the individual should have acted differently'*. The MDM model relates not only to exceptional circumstances but also to everyday situations that can be distressing, but not all ending in moral injury.

However, besides moral dissonance within the inner self, some of the factors outlined in the existing literature, that have been observed in moral distress and burnout phenomena, are recognised as contributing factors of moral injury as well. Rabin et al. (2023) distinguish these factors at three different levels: macro (systematic factors), micro (team) factors, and individual ones. They do not exist independently, but they are intertwined, impacting each other, i.e. individuals making an impact on team and system level and vice versa. Furthermore, all these factors need to be understood as contributing and not causative factors that could potentially lead to moral injury by creating ethical dilemmas and moral dissonance in the HCP's inner self. This is important to emphasise because only in situations where these factors lead towards acts of commission or witnessing of wrongdoing may moral injury result.

Such contributing factors may be present in everyday practice, such as chronic understaffing or lack of resources. This can be seen nowadays when healthcare organisations view patient care through the lens of business and financial interest, particularly when this business model comes into conflict with healthcare delivery, resulting in situations where nurses need to care for more patients than they are able, with an inadequate level of resources. This often emerges in health system cultures, which discourage caring relationships, by limiting time with patients to focus nurses' attention on administrative tasks, electronic health records, or paperwork for insurance companies (Pittman 2021).

After the pandemic, the reality for nurses in many health systems became very difficult: working long hours and being under-resourced put greater pressure on nursing professionals. This type of situation may lead to the need to make decisions that are not in accordance with nurses' moral beliefs or values. Moreover, some of a nurse's everyday practice can involve trying to balance allocating nursing resources (time for example) as effectively as possible, given all the demands on the nursing resource in a particular patient care context. All these difficult situations with patients are sometimes followed by challenging situations with third parties, such as experiencing violence (physical or verbal from the patient's relatives), or nurses being required to be actively involved in emotionally charged conversations with grieving or angry family members (Rabin et al. 2023).

The contributing factors at the micro (team) level, such as lack of preparedness and perceived lack of empathy and respect from supervisors (Riedel et al. 2022), are potential risk factors for developing moral injury. These factors create a sense that nurses are providing lower-quality patient care and lacking adequate support—from organisations, units, superiors, and colleagues—to help them identify, manage/specify, and deal with ethical issues. Such circumstances may lead to nurses leaving the profession entirely, further exacerbating the issue of understaffing for those who stay, thus creating even more adverse working environments, reducing their workplace effectiveness, and exposing nurses to a much higher risk of moral injury (Rabin et al. 2023).

Ultimately, the determining factors can be present at the individual level, depending on the nurses' life and work experience, where junior and less experienced nurses are at elevated risk for higher levels of moral injury. Nurses with frequent and prolonged contact with patients, and lacking decision-making power, are more likely to experience PMIEs. Nurses who report mental health problems are prone to moral injury. Nurses who experience stressful life events, such as the death of their loved ones, may also be at higher risk of experiencing PMIEs and suffering from moral injury (Rabin et al. 2023).

How to Prevent, Reduce, and Recover from Moral Injury

The first step in dealing with moral injury is identifying and recognising the causes of moral injury such as we have seen in Ms. Trink's case, followed by a willingness to support the individual in confronting them. After a recognition of the issue, we need to help ameliorate the situation and support a person experiencing moral injury to recovery, by addressing systemic, team, and personal/individual factors in an effective way. One of the common systemic problems is understaffing, which can be solved by equipping the teams with enough personnel. Besides understaffing, another hot issue is appropriate remuneration for the challenging work nurses perform. Remunerating nurses appropriately will help attract and retain more nurses in the health service and may also improve the perceived status of the profession with the public. At the team/individual level, exhaustion and work saturation can be resolved by allowing and implementing adequate meal and rest breaks for nurses during their working shift and ensuring they can take their annual leave entitlement. Finding a good balance between the business model in use and humane, competent, high-quality healthcare delivery is essential to protect the well-being of healthcare personnel and enable healthcare workers to flourish in their professions (Williamson et al. 2023).

The second step would be to reframe moral injury into predictable occupational exposure that could alleviate the management of PMIEs with other occupational hazards, keeping in mind the potential occurrence of moral injury during the assessment and prevention of other occupational hazards. This would be possible if nursing professionals were adequately prepared, including psychological preparation, for their roles through preparatory briefings about the nature of PMIEs' and where they might encounter them, ensuring they can speak freely to their supervisors without fear of retribution or ridicule. Nursing leaders and managers need to be empowered to lead psychologically informed conversations with their team members about any concerns, identify solutions, and provide encouragement; this might contribute to fostering a supportive work environment. Nurses are less likely to suffer from moral injury if they are more prepared for their roles, including recognising potential challenges and consequences, and ways of coping—thus assisting the development of moral resilience (Fitzpatrick et al. 2022).

However, preparation is also needed for nursing leaders and managers to improve their active listening skills and feelings of confidence in supporting their staff (Rabin et al. 2023), leading towards an increase of psychological capital and strengthening of organisational justice (Flinkman et al. 2023). Leadership support is important, particularly in recognising and assessing moral injury, in a timely manner. In order to achieve this, there are a couple of instruments that might be helpful in the identification and evaluation of moral injury symptoms, such as the Moral Injury Symptom Scale-Health Professional (MISS-HP) (Mantri et al. 2020) developed during the COVID-19 pandemic or the more recent Occupational Moral Injury Scale (OMIS) (Thomas et al. 2023). Other instruments facilitating the assessment and recognition of emotions, such as the Moral Injury Experience Wheel (Fleming 2023), might also be helpful. However, such instruments should only be used (and such data only be collected) if the nurses being assessed have given their fully informed consent for assessment and data collection, including being made fully aware of the purposes for which the data is being collected, and the consequences for the nurse participants themselves. This should include assurances on how the nurse's personal data will be stored, who will have access to the data and for what purposes. It is also important to emphasise that in cases where there is no willingness, or little or no ability/capacity to address causative factors, assessing/diagnosing an individual as 'suffering from' moral injury may be stigmatising and harmful.

So far there is no agreed method on retroactively mitigating moral injury because it is classified as experiencing moral adversity rather than a diagnosed psychological illness (Rabin et al. 2023). However, if moral injury occurs, one of the important aspects to start dealing with is self-forgiveness and self-compassion (Buhagar 2021). Furthermore, a combination of different approaches, such as mindfulness and compassion-based approaches in combination with cognitive behavioural therapy, might help manage stress and increase productivity to facilitate the processing of anger, shame, and guilt through cultivating compassion towards self, others, and the world (Rabin et al. 2023). However, these approaches alone, aimed at the individual, cannot provide the complete answer to fix/resolve moral injury. This is because moral injury is a context-driven, often systemic, and multifactor-induced problem. Therefore it is a problem that requires context, system, and/or community-based solutions (Rosen et al. 2022; Cahill et al. 2023), in addition to those solutions aimed at the individual.

Such system and/or community-based solutions might start with nursing leaders regularly discussing ethical issues with nurses. This could form a part of annual development discussions. Leadership support could be better planned and executed at several levels: primary level (dissemination of information about moral injury, encouraging informal seeking of help, proactive check-ins), secondary level (reducing stigma and training staff to identify symptoms of moral injury), and tertiary level (accessible, confidential and rapid availability of mental health services, ethics support in the form of moral deliberations and ethics rounds) (Tracy et al. 2020; Williamson et al. 2020; Maguen and Griffin 2022; Stanojević and Čartolovni 2022). All these activities lead towards building and developing moral resilience among nurses. A recent study conducted by Berdida and Grande (2023), among nurses from the Philippines demonstrates that moral resilience and moral courage negatively impact—i.e. mitigates or reduces—moral injury and distress, implying that healthcare organisations and nurse managers should endorse morally resilient and courageous therapeutic practices.

Other approaches aiming for moral recovery, in which individuals recover their sense of well-being and moral integrity by engaging in restorative communal actions (by addressing the social causes of unethical practices), take the shape of practical ethical leadership (Cullen 2022; Stanojević and Čartolovni 2022). The existing interventions that encompass the above-mentioned approaches and focus on the healthcare practitioners' informative qualities of moral pain and facilitate moral healing are acceptance and commitment therapy (ACT), relational dynamic group therapy, a meaning-oriented collaborative care model (Reclaiming Experiences and

Loss [REAL]), and a communal intervention model (moral engagement group [MEG] (Evans et al. 2023).

Conclusion

Recognition of moral injury has entered the healthcare domain and discussion, attracted attention during the COVID-19 pandemic, and continues to be important in everyday healthcare situations.

Moral injury represents an internal dissonance between the actions being taken or witnessed and what is perceived as being good to do. It represents an internal reaction to moral adversity by having a deep impact in the form of an emotional wound. We may distinguish different factors that might lead to moral injury; they are present at different levels: systemic, team, and individual.

We acknowledge that many of these factors have been seen in the discussion about the experiences labelled with the concepts of moral distress and burnout, but this should not lead us to conclude that the experiences of moral injury, moral distress, and burnout are the same. It also does not mean that these experiences are not correlated with each other. We share the view of early studies that moral distress, moral injury, and burnout exist on a continuum and are correlated in some way. Moreover, the interplay between these three phenomena may impact some nurses leaving their profession.

It is incumbent on nurse leaders and nurse educators to support practicing nurses in identifying and articulating feelings of moral distress, moral injury, and burnout and in seeking assistance and support in managing, coping with, and mitigating such experiences—which are detrimental to both nurses' and patients' outcomes.

> **Key Learning Points**
> - Moral injury is a recently identified phenomenon in nursing practice that has attracted professional attention during the pandemic.
> - Moral injury is a phenomenon occurring due to accumulation of moral stressors affecting healthcare workers differently.
> - Moral injury differs from moral distress and burnout despite overlaps in symptoms and outcomes.
> - Moral injury is a permanent and severe experience of suffering resulting from hyper acute and/or chronic moral adversity or moral distress, resulting in long-lasting change such as deep emotional wounds.
> - Moral injury deserves more attention from organisations, institutions, nursing leaders, and educators to identify and implement preventative measures against its occurrence.

References

Abbara A, Rayes D, Tappis H, Hamze M, Wais R, Alahmad H, Amharic N, Rubenstein L, Haar R (2023) "Actually, the psychological wounds are more difficult than physical injuries:" a qualitative analysis of the impacts of attacks on health on the personal and professional lives of health workers in the Syrian conflict. Confl Heal 17(1):48. https://doi.org/10.1186/s13031-023-00546-5

Akhtar M, Faize FA, Malik RZ, Tabusam A (2022) Moral injury and psychological resilience among healthcare professionals amid COVID-19 pandemic. Pak J Med Sci 38(5). https://doi.org/10.12669/pjms.38.5.5122

BBC (2023) Gaza: surgeon ready to help says moral duty trumps fear. In: BBC News. https://www.bbc.com/news/uk-england-67334666. Accessed 15 Nov 2023

Berdida DJE, Grande RAN (2023) Moral distress, moral resilience, moral courage, and moral injury among nurses in the Philippines during the COVID-19 pandemic: a mediation analysis. J Relig Health. https://doi.org/10.1007/s10943-023-01873-w

Buhagar DC (2021) The forgiveness interview protocol: a narrative therapy writing-process model for the treatment of moral injury. J Relig Health 60(5):3100–3129. https://doi.org/10.1007/s10943-021-01395-3

Cahill JM, Kinghorn W, Dugdale L (2023) Repairing moral injury takes a team: what clinicians can learn from combat veterans. J Med Ethics 49(5):361. https://doi.org/10.1136/medethics-2022-108163

Carey LB, Hodgson TJ (2018) Chaplaincy, spiritual care and moral injury: considerations regarding screening and treatment. Front Psych 9. https://doi.org/10.3389/fpsyt.2018.00619

Čartolovni A, Stolt M, Scott PA, Suhonen R (2021) Moral injury in healthcare professionals: a scoping review and discussion. Nurs Ethics 28(5):590–602. https://doi.org/10.1177/0969733020966776

Cuadra D (2023) What Ukrainian healthcare workers can teach employers about burnout. In: Empl. Benefit News. https://www.benefitnews.com/news/what-ukrainian-healthcare-workers-can-teach-employers-about-burnout. Accessed 21 Nov 2023

Cullen JG (2022) Moral recovery and ethical leadership. J Bus Ethics 175(3):485–497. https://doi.org/10.1007/s10551-020-04658-3

Dean W, Talbot S, Dean A (2019) Reframing clinician distress: moral injury not burnout. Fed Pract 36(9):400–402

Evans WR, Smigelsky MA, Frankfurt SB, Antal CJ, Yeomans PD, Check C, Bhatt-Mackin SM (2023) Emerging interventions for moral injury: expanding pathways to moral healing. Curr Treat Options Psychiatry. https://doi.org/10.1007/s40501-023-00303-8

Fitzpatrick JJ, Pignatiello G, Kim M, Jun J, O'Mathúna DP, Duah HO, Taibl J, Tucker S (2022) Moral injury, nurse well-being, and resilience among nurses practicing during the COVID-19 pandemic. JONA J Nurs Adm 52(7/8):392–398

Fleming WH (2023) The moral injury experience wheel: an instrument for identifying moral emotions and conceptualizing the mechanisms of moral injury. J Relig Health 62(1):194–227. https://doi.org/10.1007/s10943-022-01676-5

Flinkman M, Rudman A, Pasanen M, Leino-Kilpi H (2023) Psychological capital, grit and organizational justice as positive strengths and resources among registered nurses: a path analysis. Nurs Open 10(8):5314–5327. https://doi.org/10.1002/nop2.1769

Gibbons S, Shafer M, Hickling EJ, Ramsey G (2013) How do deployed health care providers experience moral injury? Narrat Inq Bioeth 3:247–259

Goodman, Diane M. (2022) The moral injury of COVID: how will nurses survive? In: Medscape. https://www.medscape.com/viewarticle/968051. Accessed 28 Aug 2023

Griffin BJ, Weber MC, Hinkson KD, Jendro AM, Pyne JM, Smith AJ, Usset T, Cucciare MA, Norman SB, Khan A, Purcell N, Maguen S (2023) Toward a dimensional contextual model of moral injury: A scoping review on healthcare workers. Curr Treat Options Psychiatry 10(3):199–216. https://doi.org/10.1007/s40501-023-00296-4

Hegarty S, Lamb D, Stevelink SAM, Bhundia R, Raine R, Doherty MJ, Scott HR, Marie Rafferty A, Williamson V, Dorrington S, Hotopf M, Razavi R, Greenberg N, Wessely S (2022) "It hurts your heart": frontline healthcare worker experiences of moral injury during the COVID-19 pandemic. Eur J Psychotraumatol 13(2):2128028–2128028. https://doi.org/10.1080/20008066.2022.2128028

Jameton A (1984) Nursing practice: the ethical issues. Prentice-Hall Englewood Cliffs, NJ, Englewood Cliffs, N.J

Lentz LM, Smith-MacDonald L, Malloy D, Carleton RN, Brémault-Phillips S (2021) Compromised conscience: a scoping review of moral injury among firefighters, paramedics, and police officers. Front Psychol 12. https://doi.org/10.3389/fpsyg.2021.639781

Litz BT, Stein N, Delaney E, Lebowitz L, Nash WP, Silva C, Maguen S (2009) Moral injury and moral repair in war veterans: a preliminary model and intervention strategy. Posttraumatic Stress Disord Wars Afghan Iraq 29(8):695–706. https://doi.org/10.1016/j.cpr.2009.07.003

Maguen S, Griffin BJ (2022) Research gaps and recommendations to guide research on assessment, prevention, and treatment of moral injury among healthcare workers. Front Psych 13. https://doi.org/10.3389/fpsyt.2022.874729. eCollection 2022

Mandowara K, Leo L (2023) One-third of US nurses plan to quit profession, survey shows. Reuters. https://www.reuters.com/world/us/one-third-us-nurses-plan-quit-profession-report-2023-05-01/. Accessed 19 Sep 2023

Mantri S, Lawson JM, Wang Z, Koenig HG (2020) Identifying moral injury in healthcare professionals: the moral injury symptom scale-hp. J Relig Health 59(5):2323–2340. https://doi.org/10.1007/s10943-020-01065-w

Mantri S, Lawson JM, Wang Z, Koenig HG (2021) Prevalence and predictors of moral injury symptoms in health care professionals. J Nerv Ment Dis 209(3):174–180

Mewborn EK, Fingerhood ML, Johanson L, Hughes V (2023) Examining moral injury in clinical practice: a narrative literature review. Nurs Ethics 30(7–8):960–974. https://doi.org/10.1177/09697330231164762

Morriss M, Berle D (2023) Measuring moral injury: further validation of the MIES-C and EMIS-C in a civilian population. J Psychopathol Behav Assess. https://doi.org/10.1007/s10862-023-10071-7

Pittman, P (2021) Moral injury-from understanding to action. In: Am. Fed. Teach. https://www.aft.org/hc/spring2021/pittman. Accessed 30 Aug 2023

Rabin S, Kika N, Lamb D, Murphy D, Stevelink SA, Williamson V, Wessely S, Greenberg N (2023) Moral injuries in healthcare workers: what causes them and what to do about them? J Healthc Leadersh 15:153–160. https://doi.org/10.2147/JHL.S396659

Riedel P-L, Kreh A, Kulcar V, Lieber A, Juen B (2022) A scoping review of moral stressors, moral distress and moral injury in healthcare workers during COVID-19. Int J Environ Res Public Health 19(3). https://doi.org/10.3390/ijerph19031666

Rosen A, Cahill JM, Dugdale LS (2022) Moral Injury in Health Care: Identification and Repair in the COVID-19 Era. J Gen Intern Med 37(14):3739–3743. https://doi.org/10.1007/s11606-022-07761-5

Shay J (1995) Achilles in Vietnam: combat trauma and the undoing of character, 1st Scribner ed. Scribner New York, New York

Stanojević S, Čartolovni A (2022) Moral distress and moral injury and their interplay as a challenge for leadership and management: the case of Croatia. J Nurs Manag 30(7):2335–2345. https://doi.org/10.1111/jonm.13835

Te Brake H, Nauta B (2022) Caught between is and ought: the moral dissonance model. Front Psych 13:906231. https://doi.org/10.3389/fpsyt.2022.906231

Thibodeau PS, Nash A, Greenfield JC, Bellamy JL (2023) The association of moral injury and healthcare clinicians' wellbeing: a systematic review. Int J Environ Res Public Health 20(13). https://doi.org/10.3390/ijerph20136300

Thomas V, Bizumic B, Quinn S (2023) The occupational moral injury scale (OMIS)—development and validation in frontline health and first responder workers. https://osf.io/ht7ne/. Accessed 19 Sep 2023

Tracy DK, Tarn M, Eldridge R, Cooke J, Calder JDF, Greenberg N (2020) What should be done to support the mental health of healthcare staff treating COVID-19 patients? Br J Psychiatry 217(4):537–539. https://doi.org/10.1192/bjp.2020.109

Williamson V, Murphy D, Greenberg N (2020) COVID-19 and experiences of moral injury in front-line key workers. Occup Med 70(5):317–319. https://doi.org/10.1093/occmed/kqaa052

Williamson V, Lamb D, Hotopf M, Raine R, Stevelink S, Wessely S, Docherty M, Madan I, Murphy D, Greenberg N (2023) Moral injury and psychological wellbeing in UK healthcare staff. J Ment Health 1–9. https://doi.org/10.1080/09638237.2023.2182414

World Health Organisation (2019) Burn-out an "occupational phenomenon": International Classification of Diseases. https://www.who.int/news/item/28-05-2019-burn-out-an-occupational-phenomenon-international-classification-of-diseases. Accessed 19 Sep 2023

Zahiriharsini A, Gilbert-Ouimet M, Langlois L, Biron C, Pelletier J, Beaulieu M, Truchon M (2022) Associations between psychosocial stressors at work and moral injury in frontline healthcare workers and leaders facing the COVID-19 pandemic in Quebec, Canada: a cross-sectional study. J Psychiatr Res 155:269–278. https://doi.org/10.1016/j.jpsychires.2022.09.006

Values-Based Nursing and Fitness to Practice Issues

5

Julie-Ann Hayes

Abstract

Values are often viewed as a reflection of moral, personal and cultural beliefs. Yet nurses are challenged with the additional consideration of professional values. In the United Kingdom (UK), the values that underpin the profession are articulated within the regulatory guidance from the Nursing and Midwifery Council (NMC). This guidance is a measurable tool of both practice and behaviour, and falling short of this standard raises the question of fitness to practise.

This chapter explores the importance of values and how these values not only underpin practice but determine fitness to Practise.

Keywords

Values · Morals · Professionalism · Fitness to practise · Standards; Trust

Introduction (Including Case Study)

This chapter will explore the personal and professional values that we utilise within nursing practice. The chapter will draw upon healthcare values applied across healthcare practice and not only within nursing. A case study will allow us to explore these values in a nursing context.

J.-A. Hayes (✉)
School of Nursing and Allied Health, Liverpool John Moores University, Liverpool, UK
e-mail: J.Nicholson@ljmu.ac.uk

© The Author(s), under exclusive license to Springer Nature Switzerland AG 2024
P. A. Scott, S. M. Scott (eds.), *Key Concepts and Issues in Nursing Ethics*,
https://doi.org/10.1007/978-3-031-54108-7_5

Case Study

Kate is in the 3rd year of her nursing programme of study. She is finding it difficult to balance her current workload and is struggling to complete her academic assessments within the deadlines. However, she is flourishing within the clinical environment and has received positive verbal feedback regarding her performance.

Kate has an assignment to complete in the next 48 hours but has limited time to work on this and is still unsure on how to tackle the assignment. She discusses this with the fellow student, Lucy, who is working on the same shift. Lucy offers to let Kate use her assignment so she can submit on time. Kate is relived. Once she reads the assignment, she makes some slight amendments to the assignment and then submits the assignment on time.

What Is Value-Based Nursing?

Values are an important aspect of nursing and have received a huge amount of attention and emphasis in recent debate and discussion regarding healthcare and the drive to ensure that nurses possess the 'right' values. It is crucial to ensure that we understand what values are before we begin to attempt to 'measure' their existence in a workforce such as nursing. Developing a successful workforce depends on providing the necessary skills, behaviours and values, as set out in the 2015 review by Lord Willis, *Raising the bar—Shape of caring; a review of the future education and training of registered nurses and care assistants* (Health Education England 2015). Skills are measureable activities through competences and agreed frameworks; however, behaviour and values are less tangible in their scope to be benchmarked.

Understanding the concept of values is an important starting point. Horton et al. (2007, p. 722) suggested that 'Values are what are important, worthwhile and worth striving for'. Horton et al. place 'worth' at the centre of their definition of values and indicate that values have both importance and an aspirational quality. Horton et al. (2007, p. 722) provide further, more detailed, understanding of the concept by highlighting that 'Values determine a person's beliefs and actions… values direct the priorities we live by and shape our being in the world'. However, we can explore this concept further by considering terms that are used in relation to values in nursing. Table 5.1, adapted from Horton et al. (2007), lists terms that are frequently used when discussing values in nursing and illustrates that values are often assumed to be the origins of social behaviour.

These values are reflective of the six fundamental virtues necessary in nursing as asserted by Beauchamp and Childress (2013, p. 33–44) who suggested the following:

- Care
- Compassion
- Discernment
- Trustiness
- Integrity
- Conscientiousness

Table 5.1 Frequently used terms relating to values

Responsibility	Compassion
Honesty/truth	Caring
Dignity	Altruism
Autonomy	Competence
Nurturing	Trust/trustworthy
Integrity	Empowering
Privacy	Morals
Courage	Judgement

Adapted from Horton et al. (2007)

The terms that emerge through the work of Beauchamp and Childress (2013) and Horton et al. (2007) are mirrored within other literature (Hawley 2007; Baillie and Black 2015).

Moral and Personal Values

Moral values have an important influence on the approach that nurses adopt, the way in which they think and act and consequently the care they deliver. Jormsri et al. (2005, p. 586) suggest 'Morals are an individual's application of values'. However, Horton et al. (2007) defines morals as the distinction between good and bad or right and wrong and highlights that the terms morals and values are frequently used in conjunction with each other. If moral behaviour (i.e. acting on the distinction between good and bad, right and wrong, for example) is reflective of our values, then consideration of our values is crucially important.

If our personal values and beliefs influence our thinking, attitudes to people, and situations and thus also influence our behaviours, this is a significant issue when we consider our professional roles as nurses. Of course it is essential to recognise that we are human beings first and foremost, and secondly we are professionals. However, one of our aims as professional nurses is to enhance the nurse-patient caring relationship, as the important means through which we deliver good quality care, while respecting patient's ethical values and beliefs.[1] Developing an understanding of the values and moral behaviour that influences and shapes their practice is central to a nurse's role. Haighighat et al. (2020) explore the concept of moral competency and the relationship between moral competencies and the formation of professional identity and suggest that professional identity is a continuous process and that this is critical to effective and safe practice. This premise that professional identify is a process is linked to the work of Buzgova and Sikorova (2013) who suggest that moral development is defined as the change in moral behaviour over time. Both sets of authors propose fluidity in the development of both identity and moral development.

---

[1] For further description and discussion of the nurse patient relationship, please see Chap. 1.

Conflicting Values

Values can influence our ethical decision-making, and for nurses values influence our perspectives on the delivery of patient care. However, conflict may occur between professional and personal values and present the nurse with complex challenges. For example, we may personally feel it is acceptable to tell a lie in certain circumstances, and yet in our professional roles, honesty is viewed as paramount and the cornerstone of trust in the nurse-patient relationship. Understanding professional values is crucial to equipping nurses with the skills and knowledge in dealing with these conflicting values.

Professional Values

Professional values can be viewed as the tools which enable you to become a morally sensitive practitioner. The values of the profession are captured not only in codes of practice such as within the Nursing and Midwifery Council (NMC) code of conduct (2018) but are also articulated within the English healthcare context, through the Department of Health publication 'Compassion in Practice: Nursing, Midwifery and Care Staff: Our Vision and Strategy (Department of Health 2012)'. This work outlines what is believed to be the six core values that underpin health and social care. These values are branded as the 6Cs of caring:

- Care
- Compassion
- Competence
- Communication
- Courage
- Commitment

These values are not dissimilar to those personal virtues articulated by Beauchamp and Childress (2013, p. 33–44).

Three of the core values identified within the DoH (2012) guidance are relevant when we consider the case of Kate. The values that raise some concerns are competence, courage and communication. If communication is central to a trusting and caring relationship with our patients and an effective and successful relationship with our colleagues, then the cornerstone to all communication needs to that of honesty and integrity. Kate is presented with the challenge of communicating her situation to staff in both the university and the clinical setting or plagiarising her colleague's work. Honesty and integrity in this situation would require Kate to openly acknowledge her failure to complete the assignment which may result in a failure of the assessment. This acknowledgement of her failure also indicates a requirement for Kate to show courage, as being late with her assignment will have potentially serious implication for her ability to progress through her programme successfully and within the required time frame. Kate makes the decision to plagiarise her colleagues work—indicating a lack of courage, honesty and integrity. Having integrity is an essential aspect of good character and is considered to be a desirable quality in members of the nursing profession. Laabs (2011) describes integrity in terms of being a certain kind of person who is honest and trustworthy, consistently does the right thing and is able to stand up for what is right despite the consequences.

Values of the NHS

Following the Francis Inquiry (Francis 2013), there has been an increased emphasis on values within the NHS. The NHS Constitution (Department of Health 2015) clearly outlines the rights and responsibilities for patients and staff. It identifies its core values as respect and dignity, quality of care, compassion, improving lives and working together.

The Francis Inquiry (Francis 2013, p. 1399) suggested that the NHS Constitution was a source of values and principles and stated 'All staff should be required to commit to abiding by its values and principles'. This suggests that NHS staff should have an understanding of the values and principles required for caring for patients. The NMC (2018) also stipulates the standards (values) required of registered and student practitioners.

When we consider an individual case such as Kate's, it is important to remember that the broad ideas of the NHS Constitution (Department of Health 2015) are reflective of the 6Cs (Department of Health 2012). Care, compassion, competence, communication, courage and commitment are relevant to every individual case and nurse. Kate is required to deliver a high quality of nursing care and to demonstrate this through her assessed competence, compassion and commitment. The latter, i.e. commitment, may, on occasion, also demand the personal characteristic of courage—for example, in advocating for a patient[2] or reporting inappropriate or inadequate care. Demonstration of competence to practice underlies the notion of being fit to practice, that is, being deemed worthy of a licence to practice as a nurse that is enshrined in the nurse's registration, with the national body responsible for nurse registration—in the United Kingdom this is the NMC.

Professionalism

Professionalism is the term most frequently used in relation to aspects of behaviour that relate to fitness to practise (FtP). Professionalism is defined in a variety of ways and could include aspects of character and ethical behaviour, as well as skill and competence (Boak et al. 2). The NMC (2018) advises that standards of professional behaviour are based on the code of conduct. This informs the practitioner and the student that good character forms the foundation of professionalism. The structures

---

[2] For a discussion of the nurse's role in advocating for patients please see Chap. 2.

in place to measure the professional standards of nurses are that of 'fitness to practise'. We therefore may find ourselves asking the question 'Is professionalism and fitness to practise the same thing'?

Arguably professionalism is concerned with high standards and the best aspired to behaviour. In contrast fitness to practise is concerned with maintaining the minimum standards required for safe practice. Understanding the concept of fitness to practise as well as the relevant processes, however, may inform our understanding of how the regulatory body, in England this is the NMC, view and consider professional conduct and professionalism. In the context of the case study, does the measure of professional standards 'fitness to practise' extend to academic conduct or indeed misconduct?

Understanding Fitness to Practise

Health and social care professionals are often subject to scrutiny regarding their practice and their professional conduct. The lens of that scrutiny is not only fellow professionals but also public concern. This is reflected in investigations of high-profile incidents of patient harm, which involve health and social care professionals, such as the Clothier (Beverley Allit) Report (Clothier 1994) and more recently the Francis Inquiry (Francis 2013). The resultant inquiries have recommended the need for effective professional regulation of health and social care professionals and reform across healthcare professions. Such inquiries have also formed the basis for changes in the regulation and the concept of fitness to practise (FtP).

In the United Kingdom, the nursing profession is regulated by the Nursing and Midwifery Council (NMC). This body has both regulatory and statutory powers and came into force in 2002. One of its key functions is regulation. Professional regulation is achieved through a process of fitness to practise (FtP) which is defined by the Nursing and Midwifery Council (NMC) as:

> *Being fit to practice requires a nurse or midwife to have the skills, knowledge, good health and good character to do their job safely and effectively* (NMC 2021).

The Nursing and Midwifery Council (NMC) came into force following the introduction of Project 2000 and the significant educational changes within the nursing profession which led to the replacement of its predecessor the United Kingdom Central Council for Nursing, Midwifery and Health Visiting (UKCC). The UKCC was set up in 1983 and had the function of maintaining a register of nurses, midwives and health visitors in the United Kingdom in addition to management of professional misconduct. The NMC continues with this structure for regulation and provides clear guidance regarding best practice for nurses and midwives. The most recent advice is via the NMC (2018) Code of Conduct. This guidance includes defining professional standards and what constitutes 'fit for practice'. A referral to the NMC is a concern or complaint that is reported to the NMC. The concerns can be raised against the registered practitioner, by an employer, a colleague or a member of the public. During 2022–2023 the Nursing and Midwifery Council received a total of 5068 new referrals (0.64% of the register) in comparison to 5291 new referrals (0.70% of the register) during 2021–2022. This illustrates a drop in 4% of concerns raised.

The top three types of categories of allegations found proved have remained the same each year since 2020. In 2022–2023 patient care was the most common category (22% of allegations), followed by prescribing and medicines management (16% of allegations) and finally record-keeping (13% of allegations). These are illustrated in the Table 5.2 below

These figures indicate a decrease in the number of FtP cases since 2021–2022 by 4%; however, the areas of concerns have remained consistent since 2020.

Determination of fitness to practise for registered practitioners is agreed by the NMC.

The NMC fitness to practise panel hears evidence regarding alleged poor practice of both midwives and nurses, but they do not regulate preregistration student nurses or student midwives (i.e. those undertaking their training). The responsibility regarding regulation of students lies with the Higher Education Institution (HEI). As part of a contractual agreement with professional bodies, Higher Education Institutions (HEIs) are required to monitor good health, character, discipline, standards of conduct and performance throughout all preregistration/qualification programmes and other programmes leading to professional qualifications. This includes monitoring such issues as occupational health checks and criminal record disclosure and self-declaration of good health and character.

Several other functional aspects of the NMC include:

- Maintaining a register- this includes a register, which can be accessed by the profession and by the public, of all registered practitioners.
- Setting standards for practice - this involves a series of guidance documents appraising students and registered nurses of expected standards
- Setting standards for education - this involves agreeing and setting standards for education programmes
- Conducting research

Table 5.2 Categories of allegations found proven NMC (2023)

Type of allegations	Percentage of allegations 2022–2023	Nature of allegations
Patient care	22%	Diagnosis, observations, assessment
		Inappropriate or delayed response to negative signs, deterioration or incidents
Prescribing and medicines Management	16%	Not administering or refusing to administer medication
		Inappropriate storage, transportation, preparation and disposal
Record-keeping	13%	Patient or clinical records
		Drugs or medication records

Data from NMC (2022–2023) Fitness to Practise Annual Report (2023)

- Advising the government on aspects of nursing and midwifery
- Determining fitness to practise of registered practitioners - this involves conducting investigations into FtP

A number of the above functional aspects of the NMC are self-explanatory; however the concept of FtP requires some consideration.

What Does Fitness to Practise Actually Mean?

There is an expectation from the public that registered practitioners are fit to practice throughout their careers. The NMC suggests that being fit means that nurses have the skills, knowledge, good health and good character to do their jobs safely and effectively by adhering to principles of good practice set out by the NMC.

The NMC (2021) outlines two clear aims for fitness to practise: firstly, a professional culture that values equality, diversity and inclusion and prioritises openness and learning in the interests of patient safety, and, secondly, nurses, midwives and nursing associates who are fit to practise safely and professionally. The NMC provides a set of 12 principles to help deliver these aims.

1. A person-centred approach to fitness to practise.
2. Fitness to practise is about managing the risk that a nurse, midwife or nursing associate poses to patients or members of the public in the future. It is not about punishing people for past events.
3. We can best protect patients and members of the public by making final fitness to practise decisions swiftly and publishing the reasons openly.
4. Employers should act first to deal with concerns about a nurse, midwife or nursing associate's practice, unless the risk to patients or the public is so serious that we need to take immediate action.
5. We always take regulatory action when there is a risk to patient safety that is not being effectively managed by an employer.
6. We take account of the context in which the nurse, midwife or nursing associate was practising when deciding whether there is a risk to patient safety that requires us to take regulatory action.
7. We may not need to take regulatory action for a clinical mistake, even where there has been serious harm to a patient or servicer-user, if there is no longer a risk to patient safety and the nurse, midwife or nursing associate has been open about what went wrong and can demonstrate that they have learned from it.
8. Deliberately covering up when things go wrong seriously undermines patient safety and damages public trust in the professions. Restrictive regulatory action is likely to be required in such cases.
9. In cases about clinical practice, taking action solely to maintain public confidence or uphold standards is only likely to be needed if the regulatory concern cannot be addressed.

5 Values-Based Nursing and Fitness to Practice Issues   77

10. In cases that are not about clinical practice, taking action to maintain public confidence or uphold standards is only likely to be needed if the concerns raise fundamental questions about the trustworthiness of a nurse, midwife or nursing associate as a professional.
11. Some regulatory concerns, particularly if they raise fundamental concerns about the nurse, midwife or nursing associate's professionalism, cannot be addressed and require restrictive regulatory action.
12. Hearings best protect patients and members of the public by resolving central aspects of a case that we and the nurse, midwife or nursing associate do not agree on.

The NMC indicates however that it is not only our professional performance that is at issue in terms of fitness to practise. The NMC also suggests that anything that we do that might have an impact on public safety or confidence in the profession may be subject to challenge. This suggests to the registered practitioner and the student practitioner that the expectations of conduct and behaviour apply not only to professional life but also personal life.

The NMC (2021) outlines what allegations of fitness to practise can be based on:

- **Misconduct**—This considers behaviour that falls short of what is expected of a registered nurse.
- **Lack of competence**—This considers lack of knowledge, skill, performance or judgement.
- **Criminal convictions and cautions**
- **Health**—This relates to long-term serious physical and mental health conditions.
- **Determinations by other health or social care organisations**
- **Not having the necessary knowledge of English**

Even with a definition of the concept of 'fitness to practise' from the NMC, there are still aspects of FtP that leave the registered practitioner and student practitioner alike unsure of what is expected from the professional body, in terms of their conduct and performance. The Professional Standards Authority (PSA, previously Council for Healthcare Regulatory Excellence CHRE) is the independent body accountable to parliament that oversees the work of the regulators of healthcare, including the NMC. The CHRE (2008) recognised this cloudy uncertainty surrounding FtP and provided the 'statement explaining the purpose of FtP'.

In order to ensure public confidence, the process of dealing with fitness to practise needs to be transparent and open to ongoing audit and review. It could be argued that this is achieved through regulation of the regulators by the Professional Standards Authority. The NMC reports all of its decisions to the Professional Standards Authority for Health and Social Care, and they provide feedback on the decisions made by the various panels.

The NMC requires that registered and student nurses have 'character and health'. What equates to 'character and health' is derived from the two key documents: 'Character and health decision-making guidance' (Nursing and Midwifery Council

2016) and 'The Code- Professional Standards of Practice and Behaviour for Nurses and Midwives' (Nursing and Midwifery Council (NMC) 2018). Public trust in nurses, as well as in the regulation and accountability of the profession, is vital for an effective nurse-patient relationship. Core professional values must be upheld not only by those who are qualified but also by student nurses. The previous NMC (2010) guidance on professional conduct for nursing and midwifery, for students, stated 'Your personal life counts too!'. It further outlines how personal life counts by stipulating that behaviour and conduct, both during the programme of study and in personal life, may impact on fitness to practise and ability to complete the programme, in addition to the willingness of the university to declare good health and good character for its students to become registered nurses. This guidance was replaced by the NMC (2015) 'The Code- Professional standards of practice and behaviour for nurses and midwives' which is a set of standards for all nurses—both registered and student and then further in the NMC (2018). When we consider the case of Kate, is her willingness to plagiarise a reflection of character?

'Good' Character and Integrity

'Good' Character

The NMC (2010) defined good character 'is such that you are capable of safe and effective practice as a nurse, midwife or nursing associate'. The assessment of good character also took into consideration criminal convictions. This guidance alongside the NMC (2018) code: Professional standards of practice and behaviour for nurses, midwives and nursing associates, must be adhered to by HEIs. HEIs are required to carry out a disclosure check on all applicants. Once on a course of study, students must inform the HEI of any changes in their status. Sellman (2007) suggests that verifying the good character of the student is problematic for the HEI to do and that the 'assessment' of good character itself is too simplistic, is not actually reflective of good character and is arguably based on assumptions regarding traits that are neither fixed nor static. Sellman's philosophical consideration of this concept of 'character' and indeed 'good' is a challenge to organisations such as the NMC (and other regulatory bodies) that attempt to assess these traits without providing guidance or instruction to HEIs on this moral assessment.

The Council for Health Regulatory Excellence (CHRE) (2008) recommended that there should be a common approach to the understanding of 'good' character across healthcare professions. The CHRE (2008) argued that this would ensure that students aspiring to join a healthcare profession would clearly understand what was required of them in order to demonstrate 'good' character. The CHRE (2008) does not formally define the concept of good character, but they do seek instead to provide underlying principles. The concept of 'good character' is a dynamic concept: it is enacted in relation to other people, it is located in the context of changing social norms and it takes account of the ability to reflect on past actions and the development of insight into past conduct (CHRE 2008, p. 3). The CHRE advises that the assessment of good character be in line with the core principles of protection of the public, maintaining public confidence in a profession, 'acting in accordance with the standards of the profession' and 'honesty and trustworthiness'.

Assessment of 'good' character can be based on negative or positive features. For example, 'good' character can be the assessment that a candidate will not and has not acted in ways which will risk harm to the public, 'undermine public confidence', show an 'unwillingness to act in accordance with the standards of the profession' or 'act dishonesty' (CHRE 2008). Alternatively 'good' character can be assessed positively, as the possession of qualities such as commitment to the well-being of others, justifying public confidence, acting according to professional standards and being honest and trustworthy (CHRE 2008). However, the CHRE (2008) argues that it is important for regulators to be realistic about their ability to determine a person's 'good' character and states 'The regulators cannot assure that an individual possesses (positive character traits) only that given the evidence available it is not reasonable to believe the individual lacks them'. The CHRE (2008, p. 2–3).

Good character when contextualised to the case study of Kate is central to principles of honesty and trustworthiness even though the conduct under examination is outside of clinical practice. This leads us to pose the question 'Is plagiarism an ethical issue?' Carter et al. (2019) highlight that plagiarism is a violation of academic integrity. When we consider the concept of integrity and dishonest acts within nursing, do we locate plagiarism in this definition?

Integrity

Having integrity is an essential aspect of good character and is considered to be a desirable quality in the professional. The concept of trust and integrity underpins the 'code' with the following statement:

> You should uphold the reputation of your profession at all times. You should display a personal commitment to the standard of practice and behaviour set out in the code. You should be a model of integrity and leadership for others to aspire to. This should lead to trust and confidence in the professions from patients, people receiving care, other health and care professionals and the public. NMC (2018, p. 21).

It further instructs how that trust and confidence will be achieved with a number of directives such as upholding the reputation of the profession, upholding your position as a registered nurse, co-operating with investigations and audits, responding to complaints and providing leadership to ensure people's well-being is protected.

These instructions are an attempt to outline to the practitioner how trust and confidence are achieved, rather than working on an assumption that a practitioner simply knows how to gain trust. We often transfer societal norms to our professional behaviour and integrity, and trust may be one such example of this. The reality is that trust is a necessary condition of healthcare. The willingness of one party to rely on another to act in a certain way is gained through the practitioners' actions, but also to some degree, society expects that practitioners will act in a certain way (this is a condition of their licence to practice as a nurse). By fulfilling their role, as expected, the practitioner gains pubic trust and is seen as trustworthy. An example of this is veracity or truth-telling which is often used as a measure within the trust debate. Veracity is crucial to the trusting relationship between practitioners and their patients. Although traditionally professional 'codes' (such as the Hippocratic oath) have not explicitly referred to veracity, the more recent NMC code (2018) has made reference to the approach advocated by Beauchamp and Childress (2013) of health practitioners dealing with patients openly and honestly, suggesting that adhering to these principles facilitates the development of a trusting relationship between the patient and practitioner. It is important to be aware of the differences between trust and trustworthiness. Being trustworthy provides no guarantee that the patient's trust is apportioned in a sound manner. Therefore even though systems of accountability and aims towards transparency (e.g. the NMC (2022) Duty of Candour guidance) are in place, if patients have a distrust of these systems, then trust itself may be hard to establish. Providing detailed instructions of 'actions' or 'behaviour' that will move towards gaining trust is a massive step for the NMC (2019) and reflects insight into the consideration of what society wants and expects from its nurses (and student nurses). It is also an acknowledgement that trust is no longer assumed but needs to be gained.

The NMC (2010) student guidance, which defines 'good' character, also provides detailed guidance on behaviour and conduct. This includes guidance on issues such as aggressive, violent or threatening behaviour, cheating or plagiarising, criminal conviction or cautions, dishonesty, drug or alcohol misuse, health concerns and persistent inappropriate attitude or behaviour. It clearly outlines to students what it considers unprofessional behaviour and defines this as:

> Breach of confidentiality, misuse of the internet and social networking sites, failure to keep appropriate professional or sexual boundaries, persistent rudeness to people, colleagues or others and finally unlawful discrimination NMC (2010, p. 3).

This guidance by the NMC has been replaced in 2018 by the revised NMC code NMC (2018). Following this shift, each HEI is required to provide a code of conduct and a fitness to practise policy. Arguably with such explicit guidance, it would be reasonable to suggest that there is no doubt on what is viewed as unprofessional behaviour. Yet David and Lee-Wolf (2010) suggest that uncertainty does exist. They highlight that new students often do not appreciate that 'misbehaviour' in their spare time can undermine public confidence in them and their profession and may endanger their career. David and Lee-Wolf (2010) also highlighted that one of the major perils appears to surround the use of social networking in the context of patients and colleagues contrary to explicit guidance by the NMC. It is clear that students cannot be held to the same standard as registered professionals, simply by the nature of their developmental 'learning' role, and that feedback on their performance should not be isolated simply to their clinical and academic progression but also refer to their professional performance. David and Lee-Wolf (2010) assert that developing professional behaviour occurs through a combination of information, education, role modelling and reflective practice. They further suggest that managing that development requires an acknowledgement that students are colleagues who are novices.

In the case of Kate, the student nurse we met earlier in this chapter, the issue of professionalism is a developing rather than a fully formed concept. However, it is important to note that as a 3rd year student, there would be an expectation of a greater understanding and application of the principles of professionalism. This lack of insight from a more senior learner would raise concerns of fitness to practise.

David and Lee-Wolf (2010) highlighted that there should be clear guidance of what is expected in terms of behaviour at each stage of the programme of study and that it is vital that the level of expectation reflects the student's progress on the course and also the level at which the student is called to account. When considering professional behaviour, this is approached in a developmental manner. David and Lee-Wolf (2010) provide an example of this approach suggesting that a first year student called in to account for their actions would be reminded of the requirements of professional behaviour and the significance of their actions. Should the activity continue, a further discussion would follow, with a further reminder of why these actions would be considered unprofessional, and the student would be asked to reflect on their behaviour and possibly a warning issued. If the student repeats the activity in the second or third year, then such actions would become less understandable and acceptable, and this may proceed to a fitness to practise panel.

In the case of Kate, a 3rd year student nurse, this is the first issue raised, and we can identify external pressures that could be seen as mitigation. However, it is important to consider that although this is the first issue raised, the serious nature of the concern warrants consideration with the student and the potential escalation to an FtP investigation. A lack of previous concerns should not automatically abolish the need for an investigation. The nature of the concerns should be the deciding factor.

These developmental concerns that are raised regarding student understanding of unprofessional conduct clearly do not exist for the registered practitioner. The NMC would consider that every registered practitioner has a fully formed understanding of the concept of professional conduct and the code of conduct outlines the requirements in practice. The NMC has a number of options at their disposal to deal with any falling short of the expected standards. These are:

1. Close case with no further action
2. Refer case for an interim order hearing
3. Refer case to an investigating committee panel
4. Refer case to a conduct and competence committee
5. Refer case to the health committee

As stated above within the NMC (2023) annual fitness report, a total of 5068 new referrals were received in 2022–2023 in comparison to 5291 new referrals during 2021–2022. These figures, illustrated in Table 5.2 above signify a decrease in cases. This decrease could be attributed to a raised awareness of the expected standard of conduct for nurses.

Conclusion

This chapter examines values, both moral and professional, for nursing practice. There are a number of expectations on nurses, both registered and student. The way in which nurses conduct themselves is what constitutes fitness to practise, and this is a reflection of knowledge, skill, performance, and judgement. This is also a reflection of nurses' professionalism which is built on agreed and shared values.

Through the consideration of the case of Kate, we can see a challenging situation. The values we hold as human beings may sometimes conflict with that of our professional bodies. Being part of a profession requires an acceptance of certain standards. Such standards not only reflect professional competency but, importantly, also reflect the professional values that underpin the profession. Kate as a student nurse has agreed to abide by the standards determined by the NMC (2018) code of conduct. The code clearly demands that practitioners 'act with honesty and integrity at all times', and this clearly applies to the context outlined within the case study. Therefore there is a reasonable challenge to the student's fitness to practise.

Having clearly defined professional values has a number of potential positive impacts, such as strengthening the nurse-patient relationship and gaining trust in the profession. If we are prepared to put aside these agreed standards that capture the values of our profession, the result can only lead to the erosion of the trust that is central to the nurse-patient relationship.

Key Learning Points
- Value-based nursing is ensuring that values underpin care delivery.
- Our professional and personal values can differ; however, there are common values that are transferable across both our personal and professional conduct.
- The NMC code of conduct (Nursing and Midwifery Council (NMC) 2018) outlines values that underpin our practice and promote safe and effective care.
- Guidance from the Department of Health (2012) 'Compassion in Practice: Nursing, Midwifery and Care Staff: Our Vision and Strategy' provides more detailed guidance for practitioners in recognising values that underpin practice.
- Fitness to practise simply means that nurses have the skills, knowledge, good health and good character to do their jobs safely and effectively, by adhering to the principles of good practice set out by the NMC, and this includes academic misconduct.
- Failure to adhere to the guidance, maintain the good character and values that underpin our practice and promote safe and effective care can bring your fitness to practise into question.

References

Beauchamp TL, Childress JF (2013) Principles of biomedical ethics, 7th edn. Oxford University Press, New York

Buzgova R, Sikorova L (2013) Moral judgement competence of nursing students in the Czech Republic. Nurse Educ Today 33(10):1201–1206

Carter H, Hussey J, Forehand JW (2019) Plagiarism in nursing education and the ethical implications in practice. Heliyon 5(3):e01350. https://doi.org/10.1016/j.heliyon.2019.e01350

Clothier (1994) Allitt Independent Inquiry relating to deaths and injuries on the children's ward at Grantham and Kesteven General Hospital. HMSO, London

Council for Healthcare Regulatory Excellence (2008) A common approach to good character across the health professions regulators. CHRE, London

David TJ, Lee-Wolf E (2010) Fitness to Practice for student nurses: principles, standards and procedures. Nurs Times 106(39):23–26

Department of Health (2012) Compassion in Practice. https://www.england.nhs.uk/wp-content/uploads/2012/12/compassion-in-practice.pdf. Accessed 13th Sept 2016

Department of Health (updated, 2015) The NHS constitution. https://www.gov.uk/government/uploads/system/uploads/attachment_data/file/170656/NHS_Constitution.pdf

Francis, R (2013) Report of the Mid Staffordshire NHS Foundation trust public inquiry. Executive Summary. http://www.midstaffspublicinquiry.com/sites/default/files/report/Executive%20summary.pdf. Accessed 13th Sept 2016

Haighighat S, Borhani F, Ranjbar H (2020) Is there a relationship between moral competencies and the formation of professional identity among nursing students? BMC Nursing 19:49. https://doi.org/10.1186/s12912-020-00440-y

Hawley G (ed) (2007) Ethics in clinical practice: an interprofessional approach. Pearson Education, Harlow

Health Education England (2015) Raising the bar—shape of caring: a review of the future education and training of registered nurses and care assistants. Health Education, England

Horton K, Tschudin V, Forget A (2007) The value of nursing: a literature review. Nurs Ethics 14(6):716–740

Jormsri P, Kunaviktikul W, Ketefian S, Chaowalit D (2005) A moral competence in nursing practice. Nurs Ethics 12:582–594

Laabs C (2011) Perceptions of moral integrity: contradictions in need of explanation. Nurs Ethics 18(3):431–440

Nursing and Midwifery Council (2010) Good Health and Good character: guidance for approved Education Institutions. NMC, London

Nursing and Midwifery Council (2015) The code—professional standards of practice and behaviour for nurses and midwives. NMC, London

Nursing and Midwifery Council (2016) Health and character guidance for AEI's. NMC, London

Nursing and Midwifery Council (2022) Duty of candour. NMC, London. https://www.nmc.org.uk/globalassets/sitedocuments/nmc-publications/openness-and-honesty-professional-duty-of-candout.pdf. Accessed 21 Nov 2023

Nursing and Midwifery Council (NMC) (2018) The code: professional standards of practice and behaviour for nurse and midwives. NMC, London

Nursing and Midwifery Council (NMC) (2021) Our fitness to practise aims and objectives. https://www.nmc.org.uk/ftp-library/understanding-fitness-to-practise/using-fitness-to-practise/. Accessed 21 Nov 2023

Nursing and Midwifery Council (NMC) (2023) Annual report and accounts 2022–2023 and strategic plan 2023–2025. NMC, London

Sellman D (2007) Trusting patients, trusting nurses. Nurs Philos 8(1):28–36

Patient Autonomy in Nursing and Healthcare Contexts

6

Anna-Marie Greaney and Dónal P. O'Mathúna

Abstract

Respect for patient autonomy continues to gain momentum in nursing and healthcare practice. The general public is more aware of the right to self-determination and choice regarding the care, support, and treatment they can receive. This right is supported by healthcare policy, enshrined in professional codes, mandated by legislation, and underpinned by a human rights-based care agenda. While respect for patient autonomy, as well as associated patient choice, is accepted in professional practice, supporting autonomy can create tensions for nurses and healthcare professionals. Such tensions arise when patient choice conflicts with professional care obligations and available clinical evidence, raising concerns about professional accountability for patient welfare. This chapter explores the complexities of respecting patient autonomy in 'real-world' nursing and healthcare contexts. We argue that equating autonomy with independence is unrealistic in the lives we live. A case study highlights practical concerns. We propose ways of reconciling professional accountability with respect for patient autonomy. We draw on recent research, a more relational understanding of autonomy and contemporary health and social care guidance. We conclude that *Autonomy by Negotiation* represents a more accurate account of our autonomy as social beings.

A.-M. Greaney (✉)
Department of Nursing and Healthcare Sciences, Munster Technological University, Tralee, Co. Kerry, Ireland
e-mail: anna.marie.greaney@mtu.ie

D. P. O'Mathúna
College of Nursing, The Ohio State University, Columbus, OH, USA
e-mail: omathuna.6@osu.edu

© The Author(s), under exclusive license to Springer Nature Switzerland AG 2024
P. A. Scott, S. M. Scott (eds.), *Key Concepts and Issues in Nursing Ethics*,
https://doi.org/10.1007/978-3-031-54108-7_6

Keywords

Autonomy · Choice · Professional accountability · Care · Vulnerability · Human rights · Relational autonomy · Autonomy by negotiation

Autonomy is most useful as an ethical norm when we recognise that it does not mean simply being left alone to decide (Dove et al. 2017, p. 13).

Introduction: Autonomy and the 'Patient'

This chapter presents an overview of autonomy as a concept and explores the practical realities of respecting autonomy within nursing and healthcare. We begin with a working explanation of autonomy, providing further analysis as the chapter proceeds. Autonomy denotes an understanding of human beings as being worthy of respect. Being autonomous means that persons live in accordance with their own values and wishes. We illustrate autonomy's practical dimensions through a case study where Bronagh's expressed preferences conflict with what a nurse and others see as favourable. This case allows us to explore various philosophical accounts of autonomy in the real, 'murky' world of everyday, patient-family-healthcare professional interactions. We also explore the associated concepts of choice, freedom, decision-making, professional accountability, culture, human rights, and legislative guidance. We conclude with suggestions for reconciling professional accountability with respect for autonomy, drawing on empirical and philosophical research. We propose a relational, as opposed to individualistic, and negotiated understanding of autonomy as a more realistic account of our interdependent existence.

We begin by explaining our use of the term 'patient'. As health and social care systems have evolved, the term 'patient' and its associated meanings have also developed. The terms 'person', 'client', and 'service-user' are frequently used for the individual receiving care, support or treatment from health and social care professionals. Some argue that the term 'patient' limits a person's autonomy by confining them to a dependant relationship. This position has merit in certain contexts, but we present briefly three interrelated claims to defend using the term 'patient' here.

Firstly, the word 'patient' denotes a traditional understanding of a person in a professional caregiving relationship, who is *"more-than-ordinarily* vulnerable" (Sellman 2011 p. 51). Sellman elaborates that this vulnerability is an extension of that which every person experiences as a biological entity. The word 'vulnerable' comes from the Latin term *vulnus* meaning 'wound', identifying someone as being capable of being wounded. This does not mean that the person cannot protect themselves but rather acknowledges that patients engage in professional relationships to help overcome impediments to their flourishing.[1] Secondly, the term 'patient' counteracts consumer-orientated terms like 'service-user', 'customer', and 'client'. The business world can view clients as individuals to be satisfied, sometimes no matter what they want (hence the adage 'the customer is always right'). However, clients are also those to be managed and sometimes outsmarted in a market-based, capitalist society. A business model of the person-carer relationship may hide the threat of power imbalances, yet also undermine professional ideals of care, compassion, advocacy, and professional accountability. Finally, describing those we care for as patients need not create a power imbalance but instead remind everyone of the potential for power imbalances. Misuse of power arises when those involved intend to use their power inappropriately or fail to recognise the power inherent in their roles. In highlighting the vulnerability of the 'patient', we do not subscribe to a form of 'othering', or an observance of paternalistic practices, as some suggest (Condon 2021). Rather, we remind ourselves of the care and due diligence required in our relationships as responsible professionals engaged with 'autonomous' patients. This perception of patients in nursing and healthcare underpins the understanding of autonomy presented throughout the chapter. Respecting autonomy must involve an appreciation of vulnerability, care, humanity, and associated accountability if healthcare professionals are to care responsibly. Framing autonomy this way helps to avoid an unscrupulous application of a rights-based agenda, a focus on blind consumerism and misinterpretation of legislative reform.

Defining Autonomy in Nursing and Healthcare Contexts

The term 'autonomy' derives from the Greek *autos*, meaning self, and *nomos*, meaning law. Ancient Greek cities had *autonomia* when the people established their own laws (Dworkin 1988). The emergence of individual autonomy is more recent, often attributed to Kantian philosophy. For Kant, autonomy is associated with notions of free will and reason that characterise humanity (1998). However, a Kantian understanding of autonomy is not a defence of individualistic free choice, as is often assumed, but rather a way of living underpinned by duty and reason as opposed to individual desire. In contrast, Mill's (1859) account of autonomy suggests that people's liberty, or freedom of choice, remains paramount unless their autonomous choices harm others. According to Mill, we should not interfere with others' choices just because we feel those choices are unwise.

> *The only purpose for which power can be rightfully exercised over any member of a civilized community, against his will, is to prevent harm to others. His own good, either physical or moral, is not a sufficient warrant.* (Mill 1859, p. 22)

---

[1] Our use of the term vulnerable here should not be confused with the concept of 'vulnerable persons' as outlined in safeguarding legislation and policy. Rather we refer to a more generalised vulnerability associated with the human condition that is more apparent in healthcare contexts.

Philosophical accounts of autonomy present different perspectives, but the general understanding of 'autonomy' is concerned with 'self-governance', 'self-rule', 'self-determination', and 'independence'. In short: 'I decide what happens to me'.

Autonomy in nursing and healthcare is largely associated with free choice. The Code of Professional Conduct and Ethics for Registered Nurses and Registered Midwives in Ireland outline autonomy as 'self-determination; a person's ability to make choices on the basis of their own values' (Nursing and Midwifery Board of Ireland (NMBI) 2021, p. 4). This is consistent with the 'right' to choose outlined by the International Council of Nurses Code of Ethics (ICN 2021) and views of autonomy in other nursing ethics codes. For example, the American Nurses Association (ANA) Code of Ethics for Nurses aligns autonomy with respect for human dignity and self-determination (ANA 2015). The Code of Professional Standards of Practice and Behaviour for Nurses in the UK (Nursing and Midwifery Council (NMC) 2018) does not use 'autonomy' in a patient context but associates human dignity with respect for personal preference, human rights, and individual choice. The UK code suggests a more shared approach to decision-making, but generally, registered nurses internationally are duty-bound to respect patients' right to self-determination and their healthcare choices.

This emphasis on patient autonomy reflects a global shift away from traditional, paternalistic healthcare models often characterised as 'doctor knows best'. We welcome the replacing of medical dominance with a greater focus on patient autonomy. The National Consent Policy in Ireland (Health Service Executive (HSE) 2022) outlines the significance of autonomy and personal will and preference, including respect for what others may consider 'unwise' decisions. Decisions 'perceived as being ill-advised or risky' (p. 96) by healthcare professionals must be respected in patients with decision-making capacity. The 2019 version of this consent policy referred to the significance of other ethical principles and underlined healthcare professionals' 'responsibility to try and maximise the health and well-being of, and to minimise harm to, service users and others' (p. 21). However, this caveat, and accompanying ethics section, is not found in the 2022 version which places greater emphasis on human rights within healthcare.[2]

Complex social and legal changes have contributed to the growth of this view of autonomy, but it also owes much to the four-principle approach to medical ethics (Beauchamp and Childress 2019). The four principles are autonomy, beneficence (to do good), non-maleficence (to do no harm) and justice (to treat people fairly). These collectively represent a middle-range theory of ethical decision-making which suggests that actions are ethical if they accord with the principles. Debate continues over the merits of this approach, especially how priority is often given to autonomy, but it has endured as a core foundation of bioethics, particularly in American contexts.[3]

---

[2] The FREDA principles (fairness, respect, equality, dignity, and autonomy) are applied in health and social care contexts to ensure the individual's human rights are protected, promoted, and supported (Health Information and Quality Authority (HIQA) 2019).

[3] For an in depth discussion of these principles in the context of nursing ethics please see Chap. 7.

In their eighth edition, Beauchamp and Childress (2019, p. 101) define autonomy as:

> At a minimum, personal autonomy encompasses self-rule that is free from both controlling interference by others and limitations that prevent meaningful choice, such as adequate understanding.

Adopting this view of autonomy would require that patients' choices should be respected so long as a person is competent. However, they, along with Kant (1998) and Mill (1859), suggest alternative, somewhat conflicting, understandings of respecting autonomy. Should we respect all choices based on free will and reasoned understandings, as Kant suggests? Should we respect any choice that does not harm others regardless of how unwise it seems, in accordance with Mill? What about choices that result in harm to one's self? Should healthcare professionals abstain from interference with patients' choices, as Beauchamp and Childress seem to suggest? Answering such questions also requires careful consideration of the meaning of 'controlling' and 'interreference' and whether degrees of these are acceptable in healthcare.

The significance of other ethical principles in patient choice became evident in COVID-19 pandemic policy and legislation. This period clearly revealed the difficulties with viewing autonomy as freedom from controlling influences and preventing meaningful choice. Public health restrictions deemed necessary to protect others' health, such as mask mandates and restricted visitation policies, limited people's autonomy, and free choices. Yet many held them to be ethically justified, if not ethically required, for the good of others and to prevent harm (Kopar et al. 2021). During this global crisis, public health ethics replaced individualism, and personal autonomy had to be balanced against beneficence and non-maleficence. Various reasons were raised against such policies, with personal autonomy used to argue against restrictions (Rubin 2020). Overall, the view that autonomy is respected only when a person's free choices are fully supported was seen to be untenable during a crisis like a pandemic (for a detailed ethics case analysis, see Kopar et al. 2021).

Such complex ethical issues cannot be understood in isolation from the healthcare environments and personal narratives where questions of autonomy and choice arise. Bronagh's story presents a 'real-world' example of patient choice.

Autonomy in Context: Bronagh's Story

Bronagh is an 82-year-old retired teacher living at home with her husband Ray. Bronagh was diagnosed with dementia but lives well at home with Ray's assistance. Their adult children live significantly faraway. Bronagh enjoys gardening, reading, and their local musical society. Previously, Bronagh had leading roles and sometimes was its director. Recently, Bronagh becomes agitated at night, sleeping less and raising concerns about intruders when none are found. She expresses frustration with her reading ability and capacity to complete ordinary tasks. One evening, thinking she was in bed, Ray found her in the garden looking lost and unaware of how she got there. Ray very recently told their son Matt about this. He is becoming exhausted as he sleeps poorly, worrying about Bronagh's deteriorating condition and their shared future. He is staunchly protective of his beloved wife and dismisses any question of residential care, even for a respite period.

Matt and his siblings are concerned for both parents. Matt visits frequently to help out and was there when the Public Health Nurse, Margot, visits. Margot suggests various supports including home help, the local voluntary dementia association, and respite care. Bronagh is fully engaged with the conversation and becomes upset at the mention of residential care and refuses professional carers. Margot is aware of the Assisted Decision-Making (Capacity) Act 2015[4] and what it means for people with impaired decision-making capacity. She recently attended training which emphasised the importance of the individual's will and preferences, despite their diagnosis. Margot understands how much Bronagh and Ray want to be together but is concerned about Bronagh's deteriorating condition, Ray's health and the impacts on the wider family.

- How can we understand autonomy within the context of this complex range of factors?
- Is there a workable solution that aligns Bronagh's preferences, the law, and Margot's professional accountability?
- What is Margot to do?

Autonomy and Interference: Are they Compatible for Professional Carers?

We begin by questioning the assumption that respect for Bronagh's autonomy requires healthcare professionals to abstain from interfering with her wishes. This depends on our understanding of 'interference'. Does interference allow for questioning choices, assessing understanding, and convincing or persuading? Alternatively, is 'interference' confined to situations involving coercion? What do Beauchamp and Childress (2019) mean by 'controlling interference'? Empirical research suggests that patients value their autonomy in decision-making and also prefer more shared approaches to decision-making within trust-based relationships (Schildmann et al. 2013). A rights-based approach to autonomy where liberty and independence always take precedence has been questioned also (Mol 2008; Greaney et al. 2012; Dove et al. 2017; Heidenreich et al. 2018; McCarthy 2021). Margot is concerned that accepting Bronagh's refusal of additional support without further

---

[4] The Assisted-Decision Making (Capacity) Act 2015 (Government of Ireland 2015) was fully commenced in Ireland in April 2023. This act enables individuals to exercise their legal capacity and provides a range of supports to facilitate people to make their own decisions. We will provide a more detailed outline of the legislation and its impact in a later section.

interaction might respect her autonomy but also violate other professional obligations such as accountability, responsibility, and quality practice.

A libertarian understanding of autonomy, rooted in individualism, is predominantly a Westernised phenomenon. Different cultures include others in their decision-making processes, both in healthcare and wider contexts. This can create ethical challenges when different cultures interact, such as when husbands want to make healthcare decisions for females in Western contexts. In other situations, benefits arise when patients' family members participate actively in decision-making. Even within one culture, subgroups may prefer different levels of engagement with others. For example, younger adults may value more active interactions with healthcare professionals, while older adults may defer more to professionals. An individualistic view of autonomy easily becomes one where patients are left alone and isolated in making what can be difficult decisions.

Returning to interference, Fleisje (2023) refers to a continuum of controlling/non-controlling terms that denote types of communication that doctors[5] can use when presenting their preferred courses of action. Doctors may approach patients in ways that seek to inform, recommend, convince, persuade, manipulate, or coerce. One end of the spectrum is non-paternalistic (inform and recommend) and the other, paternalistic (manipulate and coerce), with the middle (convince and persuade) eliciting most debate. If we relate the more polarised terms to Bronagh's situation, 'informing' and 'recommending' would involve outlining the benefits of additional home supports and awaiting Bronagh's decision in a non-paternalistic approach. Bronagh would make her decision independently. Conversely, if Bronagh's son Matt threatened to remove his support, or Margot indicated that residential care was inevitable if Bronagh refused professional home carers, this could be construed as paternalistic acts of 'manipulation' and 'coercion'.

In regard to the more central point of the continuum, Fleisje contends that while 'convincing' is acceptable, 'persuasion' is paternalistic. Conversely, Dooley and McCarthy (2012) contend that persuading patients to change their minds based on reasoned arguments is legitimate but that coercion and manipulation are not. While we have some discomfort with 'persuasion', our 2017 chapter argued that when individuals concede to a course of action they previously refused, some degree of persuasion has occurred. This need not be coercion or manipulation, but a change of mind supported by information and engagement with others. Fleisje argues that 'persuasion' involves the patient agreeing to something because they feel pressurised to do so. He suggests that 'convincing' is more appropriate as the patient changes her mind based on information and understanding gleaned through engagement. In this sense, Fleisje's 'convincing' accords with Dooley and McCarthy's 'persuading'. They recommend a dialogical approach based on shared communication and professional engagement. More recently, McCarthy (2021 p. 62) affirms the significance of autonomy as 'an antidote to the paternalism of the past', but cautions against an over individualistic approach that fails to recognise the social

---

[5] While Fleisje related his work to medical doctors, we argue that this continuum can apply to the communication styles of all health and social care professionals and nonprofessional carers.

embeddedness of our lives. A relational understanding of autonomy captures this social dimension. We will return to this point. Arguably, as responsible and accountable healthcare professionals, nurses engage in some form of 'interference' every day. For example, health promotion involves activities that seek to educate, empower, encourage, and 'convince' or 'persuade' people to alter their behaviour. Perhaps 'convince' is preferable because the term suggests an active cognitive process as with Fleisje's position. What is important is not the word chosen but the description of what actually happens. Nurses do not ask patients if they may convince or persuade them. However, they will engage in some verbal exchange with the patient. We believe that nurses should do what Fleisje describes as convince and avoid what he describes as persuasion.

In seeking to 'convince' Bronagh to agree to additional supports, Margot and her family would engage with her and explain the reality of long-term caring commitments on her husband and wider family, and the benefits that additional home care or the involvement of the local dementia association could provide. The local dementia association may have a performing arts group or a gardening class which would appeal specifically to Bronagh. Ray may explain that he wants them to stay living together as a couple in their home but that he worries about how long this can continue without additional support. This process of dialogue may lead Bronagh to appreciate the needs of others to a greater extent and understand the value of an alternative perspective. She may decide to accept additional professional care through this more interdependent approach. Bronagh may be open to this engagement (arguably interference) from Margot, Ray, and her son, Matt. Bronagh may be glad that Margot and others interfered with her initial choices through engagement, explanation, and deliberation. Conversely, Bronagh may not be open to further engagement, dialogue, or being convinced. A refusal to engage, or agree with proposals, cannot be construed as a lack of capacity. Bronagh has a right to make decisions that others may consider unwise (Government of Ireland 2015; HSE 2022). However, Bronagh should understand the associated implications for herself, her husband, and others. Once dialogue has occurred and everyone assured that Bronagh understands the consequences of her decision, she cannot be forced to do something against her will. Regardless, Margot and other healthcare professionals should continue to engage with Bronagh and evaluate her care needs and the support in place. A subsequent deterioration in Bronagh's condition may necessitate further engagement and, should certain triggers suggest, possible assessment of her capacity (to be explored later).

We propose this more nuanced or 'middle-ground' approach legitimises some interference with personal choices but avoids coercion. The middle-ground respects autonomy and individual choice but recognises that other moral principles, such as beneficence, non-maleficence, and associated obligations, are at play. The choices of others are also significant. A middle-ground perspective can provide solutions that respect autonomy, demonstrate care, and uphold professional accountability. In this sense, respect for Bronagh as a person precedes respect for her autonomy.

McCarthy (2021) further notes that respect for autonomy does not mean that those using health services are permitted to have everything they want. Resource constraints, treatment efficacy, and public health factors must be considered. The moral obligations of healthcare professionals extend beyond an absolute adherence to patient autonomy where personal choices remain unchallenged. Nurses' professional codes of conduct accept that obligations to respect autonomous choices coexist with requirements to deliver safe, compassionate, evidence-based care. Empirical evidence supports such tensions. Heidenreich et al. (2018) explored the reasoning of interprofessional teams in Sweden during moral case deliberations. Central to their considerations were ways of reconciling their perspectives on good care when patients expressed alterative preferences. The authors concluded that autonomy can only be 'achieved by interaction and engagement, rather than abandoning the patient to decide for themselves' (Heidenreich et al. 2018, p. 475).

Earlier work used the concepts of 'protective responsibility' (Holm 1997) and 'protective empowering' (Chiovitti 2008) to describe this middle ground. This 'protective' sense underpins Margot's indecision over Bronagh's care. Knowing Bronagh and her significant relationships leads her to wonder about Bronagh's initial position which prompts further reflection and engagement. Margot respects Bronagh's autonomy but first and foremost respects her as a person. This requires considering the principles of beneficence and non-maleficence also. Fuelled by a sense of moral obligation and protective responsibility, Margot 'interferes' with Bronagh's choices by suggesting and promoting alternatives.

This approach is congruent with the philosophical foundations of nursing whereby the concept of care remains the most dominant characteristic of the nurse-patient relationship.[6] Nurse regulators, while emphasising self-determination, also suggest certain caveats that require nurses to move beyond blind adherence to personal choice (ANA 2015; NMC 2018; NMBI 2021). From a moral theory perspective, the ethics of care as expressed by Gilligan (1982) and others[7] echoes the need to move beyond impartial moral rules related to duty and consequences and understand the nuances of the human condition. In comparison to rule-based moral theories, an ethics of care is rooted in relatedness and connectivity. Mol (2008, p. 43) articulates the difficulties that can exist in healthcare when a pronounced focus on personal autonomy and choice exist. Mol's central thesis is that a 'logic of choice' is not consistent with a 'logic of care' and may lead to 'poor' care. Mol sees the logic of choice being concerned with patients as customers and autonomous, independent individuals, while the 'logic of care' suggests a far messier landscape. For her, 'the logic of care is attuned to people who are first and foremost related' (p. 62). More recent discussion supports this analysis and shows how to reconcile respect for persons and their well-being *with* respect for their autonomy (Dove et al. 2017; McCarthy 2021; O'Keefe 2023). We have previously articulated the significance of care, relationality, and responsibility as an alternative to a libertarian focus on personal choice and independent decision-making (Greaney et al. 2012; Greaney 2014). We do not support a return to paternalism by another name. Dove et al. (2017 p. 162) caution that a 'mere extension of personal autonomy to the familial' creates

---

[6] See Chap. 1 for further discussion of the nurse-patient relationship.
[7] For an introduction to the ethics of care, please see Chap. 10.

an opportunity for power imbalances. Rather, healthcare ethics should not be reduced to an unquestioning adherence to autonomy and independent decision-making, to the detriment of other moral principles, human caring, and wider professional considerations.

Autonomy, Capacity, and the Law

International law mostly respects an individual's right to autonomy in healthcare decisions. Exceptions exist, for example, as with public health regulations during the COVID-19 pandemic referred to earlier. In general, the overriding legal position is that competent individuals have the right to consent to, and refuse, treatment even if such refusal results in death. This right is enshrined in both constitutional and case law in many jurisdictions and has a distinct human rights dimension. The United Nations Convention on the Rights of Persons with Disabilities (UNCRPD 2006) asserts the specific rights of people with disabilities to have legal capacity on an equal basis with others and an associated right to make decisions that reflect their personal will and preference. Member states are obliged to provide the supports necessary to enable people with disabilities to make their own decisions. One cannot be presumed to lack capacity on the basis of their diagnosis. The Convention also replaces a previously established approach of substituted decision-making, based on the perceived best interests of the person, with an appeal to personal will and preference. In essence, the paternalistic approach of *deciding for* is no longer fully supported by international law.

In Ireland, the Assisted Decision-Making (Capacity) Act (Government of Ireland 2015), and later amendments (Government of Ireland 2022), facilitates the formal ratification of UNCRPD and provides practical steps towards its implementation. The act was fully commenced on April 26 2023. This Act reforms the law for people who require assistance, or may require assistance, in decision-making. It upholds the rights of people to make decisions that others may consider unwise. It provides for a range of supportive measures to assist individuals to make their own decisions and applies a functional assessment of capacity. In accordance with this legislation, Bronagh has a right to legal capacity (the right to make legal decisions) and a presumption of mental capacity (the ability to make a decision), irrespective of her diagnosis of dementia. Margot and other healthcare team members must understand this as they interact with Bronagh. She cannot be deemed unable to make her own decisions unless all necessary efforts have been made to facilitate her understanding. To 'jump to' capacity assessments to ensure certain healthcare outcomes is unethical and incompatible with legal principles. Bronagh's refusal to accept additional supports should not prompt a capacity assessment without additional triggers. In accordance with the law and codes of practice, Bronagh may appoint somebody to assist her with decision-making or nominate an enduring power of attorney. This support person may be her husband, her son, another relative, or another individual of her choosing. Margot's concerns for Bronagh's well-being cannot be resolved by a rush to capacity assessment. However, nothing in the legislation or codes preclude Margot from questioning Bronagh's decision and proposing alternatives.

Bronagh's cognitive ability *could* decline further. If she demonstrated a lack of understanding or unusual behaviour, a capacity assessment may be required. This would determine her mental capacity to refuse professional care and supportive measures. The functional assessment of capacity is time and decision-specific. Bronagh has the necessary capacity to refuse, if she understands information relating to the decision, is capable of retaining this information, can weigh up the associated issues (including the risks), and can communicate her decision.[8]

The UNCRPD (2006) attaches significant weight to Bronagh's personal will and preference, even if the healthcare team believes her decision is unwise and may lead to harm. If Bronagh is deemed to lack mental capacity, the least restrictive possible measures could be legally applied to maintain her safety. If Bronagh is determined to have mental capacity, her decision to stay at home cannot be contested legally but may be questioned by those who care for, and about, her. However, in keeping with the UNCRPD (2006), healthcare professionals should work with people, understand their preferences, and support their decision-making, even if those decisions cause some unease. A genuine respect for the choices of others is important, and energies should be invested in realising those choices in creative, sometimes safer, ways as opposed to challenging them.

Ideally, a form of advance care planning would be in existence, which could have evidence of Bronagh's preferences with regard to living arrangements. This approach is particularly relevant in the context of individuals with dementia whose mental capacity will deteriorate over time. Commencement of the Assisted Decision-Making (Capacity) Act (2015) establishes a legal framework for Advance Care Directives in Ireland. Despite agreements that are in accordance with the law, Margot may still be left with various reactions to Bronagh's decision ranging from unease to moral distress. In keeping with the middle-ground approach, we propose below that both Bronagh's preference to stay at home and her safety can be realised through a process of engagement, dialogue, and negotiation. We suggest this is more ethical than 'abandoning' people to the hazards of their own choices under the guise of autonomy, or alternatively applying restrictive practices, even if supported by the law.

---

[8] O'Keefe (2023) raises some concerns about a functional approach to capacity which emphasises individual autonomy and independent decision-making. Reflecting concerns about isolated decision-making raised earlier in this chapter, O'Keefe (p.79) refers to people as 'socially embedded' and the significance of relationships and obligation within the decision-making process. In a detailed analysis, beyond the scope of this chapter, O'Keefe outlines a number of problems with the functional approach and sets out a series of mitigating strategies. These include fairness and consistency in capacity assessments, the involvement of independent advocates and moving beyond an exclusively rational approach to capacity to allow due recognition to non-cognitive factors. If armed with this level of understanding, healthcare professionals like Margot will find it easier to respect personal will and preference in tandem with a more situated appreciation of people, their environment, and social connections.

Autonomy and Others: Relational Autonomy

Another understanding of autonomy embodies the concepts of care, relationality, and responsibility articulated above: relational autonomy. This is an umbrella term for approaches that value the 'role social relations play in the development and exercise of autonomy' (Ashley 2012, p. 19). Relational autonomy acknowledges that we do not live in isolation and that our decisions reflect our interactions with, and obligations towards, others. It reflects a socially embedded autonomy outlined in our earlier discussions. Relational autonomy is 'interdependent', as opposed to 'independent', and offers an alternative to an isolated individualistic perspective (Heidenreich et al. 2018; McCarthy 2021; O'Keefe 2023). As we plan our weekend, our autonomous choice, our will, and preference may be to stay at home by the fire watching our favourite television series. But how often does this materialise? We have numerous other activities and obligations that require our attention. In reality, we meet the obligations of our busy lives and negotiate a pathway between what we want to do, what we feel we should do, the needs of others, and what we actually do. Does this mean we are not autonomous? This example raises questions about what we mean by autonomy. We propose that exercising our autonomy encompasses more than fulfilling our basic desires to do what we want (stay home and hibernate perhaps). Autonomy includes being congruent with the type of person we want to be (an individual committed to helping others). We negotiate with ourselves and others over our desires and our final choices.

Dworkin (1988) makes this distinction and explains that autonomy is sometimes misunderstood as synonymous with freedom. For Dworkin, 'autonomy is a richer notion than liberty' and relates to being 'more than a passive spectator of one's desires and feelings' (p. 107). This supports Fleisje's (2023) analysis that it is morally acceptable to 'convince' an individual to pursue a different course of action than they initially suggested. If Bronagh decides to accept additional home supports, she may have abandoned her initial desire to refuse professional carers, in favour of her greater desires to ensure her husband's well-being and increase the likelihood of living at home long term. Autonomy is not about freedom to act independently in ways that fulfil our own desires. Relational autonomy reflects the fact that we live in a world with others and make decisions in this context. An isolated, independent understanding of autonomy 'makes autonomy inconsistent with loyalty, objectivity, commitment, benevolence and love' (Dworkin, p. 21). Relational autonomy acknowledges that individual autonomy fails to capture the interdependent nature of our lives. Dove et al. (2017) use case studies to explore the extent to which relational autonomy is workable in practice. They conclude that relational autonomy provides a practical alternative that is more consistent with the interdependent ways in which we make choices. They promote a form of relational autonomy that embodies self-rule that is informed by relationships, responsibilities, and care for others. For Dove et al. (2017, p. 161) 'relational autonomy offers greater analytic and normative value than individualistic autonomy by encouraging wider appreciation of the socially situated person, whose decisions are shaped by and consequential for society, and whose interests are rarely purely self-interested'.

This understanding of relational autonomy embodies Margot's unease with adhering to Bronagh's choices without interference. Relational autonomy underpins her concern for Bronagh and her attempt to influence her to review her decision. Margot is concerned that a lack of community supports may eventually mean residential care is the only option. Relational autonomy also suggests that Bronagh be encouraged to consider the impact of her decision on Ray and her family. If Bronagh endures an injury, Ray is called upon to help. Ray lies awake at night wondering if Bronagh will fall and whether he will be able to respond adequately. Margot could bring Ray's perspective into her interactions with Bronagh. In addition, Margot needs to consider Bronagh's request from a broad range of perspectives, not just safety. Margot could also engage with Bronagh to understand her reasons for refusing professional home care. There may be issues in her past experiences that have influenced this decision. A true relational approach involves negotiation on all sides.

Autonomy Solutions in Contemporary Healthcare Practice

We need to move towards a practical resolution of Bronagh's story. Is there a workable solution that respects autonomy and aligns well with Bronagh's preferences, the law and Margot's professional accountability? The answer to this question lies in a relational, interdependent understanding of autonomy that goes beyond capacity assessments when people disagree. Contemporary healthcare practice is increasingly aware of the complexities of respecting autonomy in the real world (Dove et al. 2017; Heidenreich et al. 2018; O'Keefe 2023). The nuances of practice reflect a more complex reality of autonomy. Autonomy, as explained earlier, goes beyond *I decide what happens to me* and involves our relationships with, and obligations towards, other people. We advocate this 'middle-ground' approach as an alternative to more libertarian perspectives on autonomy. Some contemporary examples explain what this approach means in practice.

In a previous phenomenological study, we explored the meaning of autonomy in people who use self-testing devices to measure their blood glucose levels (Greaney 2014). The participants' experiences revealed an understanding of autonomy as an interdependent and context-dependent process—*Autonomy as Lived*. This 'process' involved mutual respect and understanding between patients and professionals and was not confined to discrete moments of choice. Participants reported that autonomy in their everyday lives was contingent on personal issues related to the overall stage in their illness trajectory, their experiences of chronic illness, their willingness to take an active role in managing their own health, and their ability to understand and master a technological device. Phenomenological analysis revealed the sub-theme, *Autonomy within constraints*, to signify the somewhat diminished sense of autonomy experienced by people when living with a long-term illness. Interdependence is evident in the participants' accounts of living with diabetes and the self-testing process. Engagement, interference, and influence from others were seen not only as permissible but necessary to enable more autonomous living. *Autonomy as Lived* reflected a relational understanding of autonomy and is congruent with Sellman's (2011) understanding of patients as people who are 'more-than-ordinarily vulnerable'. This contextualised, interdependent understanding of autonomy has previously been articulated in phenomenological accounts of older adult care settings (Agich 2003) and in more contemporary work (Dove et al. 2017).

Greaney (2014) proposed *Negotiated Autonomy* as a process to address the tensions experienced in healthcare when an individual's choices conflict with healthcare professionals' moral intuition and professional obligation to provide safe, evidence-based care. We articulated this understanding in the first edition of this chapter. Upon further reflection, we propose here that *Autonomy by Negotiation* provides a better account of our position. We previously asserted that 'while an individual retains his or her autonomy, it is in exercising that autonomy that negotiation occurs; in the decision-making process' (Greaney and O'Mathúna 2017, p. 95). *Autonomy by Negotiation* more clearly captures our meaning. One's autonomy endures but is 'shaped' by negotiation. We negotiate our choices, not our autonomy, by choosing between our initial desires and higher-order preferences in accordance with Dworkin's (1988) analysis, yet also between our preferences and our concern for and obligations towards others as relational beings. *Autonomy by Negotiation* understands autonomy as relational. It recognises that while patient decisions may be rational, this does not mean they cannot be questioned. It supports a 'logic of care' as opposed to blind adherence to a 'logic of choice' (Mol 2008). *Autonomy by Negotiation* does not condone coercion but is underpinned by mutual respect and understanding. *Autonomy by Negotiation* allows the concepts of care, responsibility, and relationality to be realised. Figure 6.1 presents the elements of *Autonomy as Lived* and associated *Autonomy by Negotiation*. Moving clockwise, these are Respect for Persons, Respect for Autonomy, Openness to Negotiation, Acceptance of Personal Responsibility, Dialogical Practice, and Outcome and Review. This model is adapted from that presented in our earlier edition of this chapter.

Our model begins with *Respect for Persons* which involves respecting the dignity of autonomous and nonautonomous persons that is not dependent on a rational expression of capacity. *Respect for Persons* appreciates an individual's whole life story. It is congruent with a relational understanding of autonomy whereby decision-making is guided by an ethic of care and moral responsibility (Gilligan 1982; Dove et al. 2017; Heidenreich et al. 2018). *Respect for Persons* encourages all involved to seek solutions that move beyond Bronagh's initial desires, to consider how she can best continue to flourish. As previously noted, activities within the local dementia centre that reflect Bronagh's specific interests may assist in this regard. *Respect for Persons* involves both patients and healthcare professionals appreciating the others' perspective. In Bronagh's story, Margot and family members should respect the significance of Bronagh's preference to remain in her own home. *Respect for Persons* also involves Bronagh understanding her husband's predicament. This is congruent with an understanding of autonomy whereby the impact of our decisions on others is not merely considered but valued (Dove et al. 2017).

Respect for Autonomy ensures that engagement with Bronagh places her will and preference centre stage in negotiations. It requires a presumption of capacity and

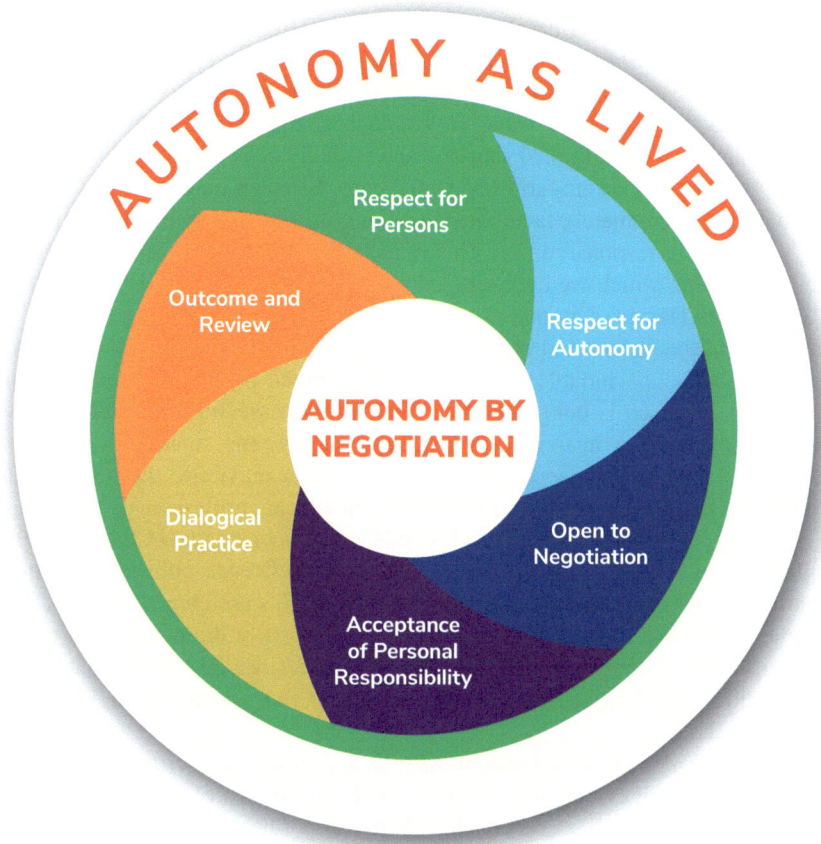

Fig. 6.1 Autonomy by Negotiation (adapted from Greaney and O'Mathúna 2017)

involves respecting the rights of others to make decisions that may be considered unwise. This respect for autonomy may involve what Olsen (2003) refers to as the 'ethical use of influence' to encourage people to make healthier, safer choices. This reflects the special relationship that exists between patients and healthcare professionals whereby a sense of 'protective responsibility' (Holm 1997) or protective empowering (Chiovitti 2008) prevails. For Olsen, influence is an ongoing feature of patient-healthcare professional interactions. It involves a relational approach whereby every action of influence, despite its magnitude, is assessed for its ethical suitability. This assessment occurs through self-reflection where healthcare professionals explore their actions and underlying motivations. Margot can respect Bronagh's autonomy but also seek to influence her, possibly 'convince' her, to reconsider her initial decision to reject additional supports, and understand the risks involved and the consequences for her, her husband and wider family. *Respect for Autonomy* ensures that Autonomy by Negotiation is congruent with legal frameworks (Government of Ireland 2015), professional codes of practice (NMBI 2021), and a human rights-based approach to care (HIQA 2019).

Open to Negotiation means that all stakeholders are amenable to this negotiation. If not, the process becomes a covert means to 'force' patients to conform or 'get' professionals to do what I want. In Bronagh's story, negotiation may involve Bronagh agreeing to additional supports and possibly considering a short period of respite, thus avoiding long-term residential care. Bronagh may be happy with this negotiation as it ultimately facilitates remaining in her own home but also reduces Ray's caregiving responsibilities. This reflects the more interdependent nature of decision-making which we have alluded to earlier (Dove et al. 2017; Heidenreich et al. 2018). During negotiation, Margot, others in the healthcare team, and Bronagh's husband Ray and son Matt may accept the degree of risk this entails. Risk of harm is unavoidable unless Bronagh's human rights are extensively violated. This approach is congruent with positive risk assessment, which acknowledges the role of risk in living fulfilled lives. Positive risk management seeks to identify risks and minimise those risks in ways that maximise the potential and priorities of the person involved. In this sense, healthcare professionals are engaged in risk management as opposed to risk avoidance. Beauchamp and Childress (2019) explore the concept of harm and note that non-maleficence obliges us to justify harmful actions. In this scenario, appealing to Bronagh's preference to stay at home and the associated impact on quality of life could justify the possible harms that may arise in the absence of further supervision in a residential context. Harm could be reduced by use of a sensor mat that would alert Ray should Bronagh leave her bed during the night.

Acceptance of Personal Responsibility is a feature of interdependent living. Margot acknowledges her responsibility for Bronagh's care and the support she requires, while Bronagh accepts responsibility for her health and well-being, as far as her fluctuating capacity allows. In understanding Bronagh's story, alternative services may be considered. This may involve linking with her musical society who have previously asked to assist. Time with a like-minded friend at rehearsals could mean more to Bronagh than other activities at a local dementia support group that Bronagh finds less meaningful. This would also provide some welcome respite for Ray. *Dialogical practice* involves moving beyond a contractual account of the caring relationship, to working in ways that engage with personal narrative (Brody 2002). In this sense, Margot would engage with Bronagh to understand her choices and associated motivations and seek ways in which they could be realised without compromising her well-being.

The final stage, *Outcome and Review*, signifies that *Autonomy as Lived* is an ongoing cyclical process and not a moment of discrete choice, or abandonment to isolated decision-making. Supports agreed are put in place. Bronagh's refusal of a wider range of possible services should not result in a withdrawal of nursing services. Margot and the healthcare team should continue to engage with Bronagh and her family to review her progress. Further negotiation may be required in time.

Conclusion: Autonomy, Accountability, and Bronagh

Bronagh's story may reach a favourable conclusion through realising *Autonomy by Negotiation* that reflects the interconnected, contextual nature of our daily lives. This approach values personal autonomy, person-centred communication, and supportive practices to achieve a balance between Bronagh's expressed preferences, Margot's professional accountability for her care, and the needs of family members. A process of dialogue and negotiation could result in Bronagh agreeing to accept some services. Dialogue and negotiation should not assign lower priority to her personal will and preference but facilitate exploration of her personal choices with her in light of the risks they pose and their impact on others. The introduction of additional supports will not eliminate risks entirely. We recognise the importance of risk in human flourishing and appreciate that quality of life involves more than keeping people safe. A range of person-centred supports can minimise the risk of harm occurring. This approach may avoid the need for capacity assessments, which provide a legal basis for action, but may also instil fear and mistrust if people '*more-than-ordinarily* vulnerable' (Sellman 2011) are legally bound to submit to restrictive practices. We suggest that the approach presented here is more compatible with a human rights agenda and the ethos of the UN Convention as it seeks to engage with people in less restrictive ways. Through real engagement, Margot can act as an advocate for Bronagh and comply with her professional obligations as a registered nurse. Respect for Bronagh as a person and respect for her autonomy can mutually exist though a relational understanding of *Autonomy by Negotiation*.

> **Key Learning Points**
> - Autonomy is concerned with respect for persons, their values, preferences, and choices.
> - In nursing and healthcare contexts, patients have a right to autonomy and the associated right to make choices that accord with their personal values, even if others consider them unwise.
> - Respecting autonomy can create challenges for healthcare professionals when patient choices conflict with best available evidence and promotion of health, safety, and well-being.
> - A middle-ground approach that values care, relationality, and responsibility, in addition to autonomy, can provide some solutions.
> - This chapter outlines some contemporary perspectives on autonomy that reconcile the principle of autonomy with other moral and professional principles through a process of engagement and negotiation. This middle-ground approach values autonomy yet also recognises the vulnerability of patients in the care setting.
> - *Autonomy by Negotiation* is introduced as a relational understanding of how we exercise autonomy and choice as social beings.

Acknowledgements 1. The authors would like to acknowledge the contribution of Professor P. Anne Scott as co-supervisor on the referenced PhD work. The PhD study was partly funded by the School of Nursing and Human Sciences, Dublin City University and Science Foundation Ireland (SFI) (SFI 05/CE3/B754 and SFI 10/CE/B1821). We thank the many patients, service users, health and social care professionals, and academic colleagues whose comments and experiences have contributed to the ideas presented.

2. We also thank Brooke Sheridan and Troy Huffman from the Marketing and Communications team at The Ohio State University College of Nursing for creating Fig. 6.1.

References

Agich GJ (2003) Dependency and autonomy in old age. Cambridge University Press, Cambridge

American Nurses Association (ANA) (2015) Code of ethics for nurses. ANA, Silver Springs, MD

Ashley V (2012) Philosophical models of autonomy. Essex Autonomy Project, Essex. Available via http://autonomy.essex.ac.uk/philosophical-models-of-autonomy. Accessed 14 June 2016

Beauchamp T, Childress J (2019) Principles of biomedical ethics, 8th edn. Oxford University Press, New York

Brody H (2002) My story is broken; can you help me fix it. In: Fulford KWM, Dickenson DL, Murray TH (eds) Healthcare ethics and human values: an introductory text with readings and values. Blackwell publishers, Oxford, pp 133–140

Chiovitti RF (2008) Nurses' meaning of caring with patients in acute psychiatric hospital settings: a grounded theory study. Int J Nurs Stud 45(2):203–223

Condon J (2021) Advocacy and the assisted decision-making (capacity) Act 2015. In: Donnelly M, Gleeson C (eds) The assisted decision-making (capacity) Act 2015: personal and professional reflections. Dublin, Health Service Executive, pp 151–156

Dooley D, McCarthy J (2012) Nursing ethics: Irish cases and concerns, 2nd edn. Gill and Macmillan, Dublin

Dove ES, Kelly SE, Lucivero F, Machirori M, Dheensa S, Prainsack B (2017) Beyond individualism: is there a place for relational autonomy in clinical practice and research? Clin Ethics 12(3):150–165

Dworkin G (1988) The theory and practice of autonomy. Cambridge University Press, Cambridge

Fleisje A (2023) Paternalistic persuasion: are doctors paternalistic when persuading patients, and how does persuasion differ from convincing and recommending? Med Health Care Philos 26(2):257–269

Gilligan C (1982) In a different voice: psychological theory and women's development. Harvard University Press, Boston

Government of Ireland (2015) Assisted decision-making (capacity) act. The Stationery Office, Dublin

Government of Ireland (2022) Assisted decision-making (capacity) (Amendmet) act. The Stationery Office, Dublin

Greaney AM (2014) Autonomy as lived: an empirical-ethical analysis of patient autonomy in the clinical context of individuals engaged with self-testing technology (PhD Dissertation). Dublin City University. Available via http://doras.dcu.ie/20159. Accessed 8 Nov 2023

Greaney AM, O'Mathúna DP (2017) Patient autonomy in nursing and healthcare contexts. In: Scott PA (ed) Key concepts and issues in nursing ethics. Springer, Cham, Switzerland

Greaney AM, O'Mathúna DP, Scott PA (2012) Patient autonomy and choice in healthcare: self-testing devices as a case in point. Med Health Care Philos 15(4):383–395

Health Information and Quality Authority (Ireland) (2019) Guidance on a human rights-based approach in health and social care services. HIQA, Dublin

Health Service Executive (HSE) (2022) National consent policy. HSE, Dublin

Heidenreich K, Bremer A, Materstvedt LJ, Tidefelt U, Svantesson M (2018) Relational autonomy in the care of the vulnerable: health care professionals' reasoning in moral case deliberation (MCD). Med Health Care Philos 21(4):467–477

Holm S (1997) Ethical problems in clinical practice. Manchester University Press, Manchester

International Council of Nurses (ICN) (2021) The ICN code of ethics. ICN, Geneva

Kant I (1998) Groundwork of the metaphysics of morals. Translation by M. Gregor and Introduction and Commentary by C. Korsgaard. Cambridge University Press, Cambridge

Kopar PK, Kramer JB, Brown DE, Bochicchio GV (2021) Critical ethics: how to balance patient autonomy with fairness when patients refuse coronavirus disease 2019 testing. Crit Care Explor 3(1):e0326. https://doi.org/10.1097/CCE.0000000000000326

McCarthy J (2021) The assisted decision-making (capacity) act 2015: the ethical relevance of the relevant person in healthcare decision-making. In: Donnelly M, Gleeson C (eds) The Assisted decision-making (capacity) act 2015: personal and professional reflections. Health Service Executive, Dublin, pp 61–65

Mill JS (1859) On liberty. J.W. Parker and Son, London

Mol AM (2008) The logic of care: health and the problem of patient choice. Routledge, London

Nursing and Midwifery Board of Ireland (NMBI) (2021) Code of professional conduct and ethics for registered nurses and registered midwives. NMBI, Dublin

Nursing and Midwifery Council (UK) (NMC) (2018) The code: professional standards of practice and behaviour for nurses and midwives. NMC, London

O'Keefe S (2023) Functional capacity assessments by healthcare professionals: problems and mitigating strategies. In: Briggs J, Donnelly M, Harding R, Taşcıoğlu E (eds) Supporting legal capacity in socio-legal context. Bloomsbury Publishing, London

Olsen DP (2003) Influence and coercion: relational and rights-based ethical approaches to psychiatric treatment. J Psychiatr Ment Health Nurs 10(6):705–712

Rubin R (2020) First it was masks; now some refuse testing for SARS-CoV-2. JAMA 324(20):2015–2016. https://doi.org/10.1001/jama.2020.22003

Schildmann J, Ritter P, Salloch S, Uhl W, Vollmann J (2013) 'One also needs a bit of trust in the doctor...' a qualitative interview study with pancreatic cancer patients about their perceptions and views on information and treatment decision-making. Ann Oncol 24:2444–2449

Sellman D (2011) What makes a good nurse. Jessica Kingsley Publishers, London

United Nations (UN) Convention on the Rights of Persons with Disabilities (CRPD) (2006) General comment No. 1. Article 12: equal recognition before the law. Committee on the Rights of Persons with Disabilities: Eleventh session

Part II

Theoretical Approaches to Ethical Analysis and Decision-Making

Principles and Nursing Ethics

Alan J. Kearns

Abstract

When engaging in the academic study of ethics, it may quickly become evident that there is a wide range of theoretical resources available that can be drawn from for the purpose of ethical reflection. Included in this range of resources are ethical theories and other frameworks. This chapter examines one seminal resource for nursing, namely, the four principles as articulated by Beauchamp and Childress. First, the chapter presents a brief overview of the consequentialist, deontological, and character-based ethical positions that form the backdrop to the four principles. Second, the principles of beneficence, nonmaleficence, respect for autonomy, and justice are succinctly presented. Third, a hypothetical case study is then examined in the context of the four principles framework. Finally, reference is made to the Irish Assisted Decision-Making (Capacity) Act 2015, and its possible impact on the obligatory standing of the four principles for ethical decision-making.

Keywords

Assisted Decision-Making (Capacity) Act 2015 · Autonomy · Beneficence · Consequentialism · Deontology · Justice · Nonmaleficence · Principles · Virtue

Introduction

Suppose a patient is anxiously waiting for the results of their biopsy. They are clearly worried about receiving a cancer diagnosis. They decide to ask one of the nurses whether there is any news of their tests. Let us suppose that the nurse knows

A. J. Kearns (✉)
School of Theology, Philosophy, and Music, Dublin City University, Dublin, Ireland
e-mail: alan.kearns@dcu.ie

that the results are back and knows that they confirm a cancer diagnosis. They can see that the patient is worried and wanting to help to ease, somewhat, the patient's anxiety, they tell them that the results are not back yet. Would it be morally permissible for the nurse to do this? Would it be morally right or morally wrong? Would this all depend on the consequences of not telling the patient the truth about the results being back? Would there be a moral duty to tell the truth to the patient (i.e. that the results are back)? On what moral principle would either telling the patient the truth or not be based? Could this principle ever be overridden by another moral principle?

Ethical questions about what is morally permissible, what is morally required, and what is morally forbidden (see Timmons 2013, p. 7) inevitably raise their head in the practice of nursing, given its nature as a caring profession and given its focus on patients, who can be very sick and are often vulnerable.

This chapter examines one framework for ethical reflection, namely, the four principles that are articulated by Tom L. Beauchamp and James F. Childress. These four principles have greatly influenced thinking in bioethics and healthcare ethics. Although Beauchamp and Childress' work on principles has sparked much academic literature, challenges, critique, and reflection, it is not possible to capture in one chapter all the various debates that they have prompted, as well as all the aspects of these principles and their accompanying method. This chapter has, therefore, a more modest agenda: first, the chapter will present a brief overview of the consequentialist, deontological, and character-based ethical positions that form the backdrop to the four principles. Second, the principles of beneficence, nonmaleficence, respect for autonomy, and justice will be succinctly presented. Third, a hypothetical case study will then be examined in the context of the four principles framework. Finally, a key aspect to this framework is that none of the principles have a presumptive obligatory priority over one another. Yet, it is well recognised (and widely discussed) that autonomy plays a central role in ethics today. Reference will therefore be made to the significant Irish Assisted Decision-Making (Capacity) Act 2015, and its possible impact on the obligatory standing of the four principles for ethical decision-making.

Ethical Positions of Consequentialism, Deontology, and Virtue

The ethical positions of consequentialism, deontology, and virtue, capture the fact that human acts can do a number of things: they can generate consequences, they can intentionally fulfil obligations, and they can demonstrate virtues (see Briggle and Mitcham 2012, p. 51). In other words, ethical reflection can be outcome-led, duty-led, or character-led.

In the case of an ethical position emphasizing outcomes, or more technically described as consequentialism, the ethical constitution of acts is based on whether their consequences bring about a certain kind of value, such as pleasure or happiness or welfare or preference—utilitarianism would certainly be the leading example of consequentialism (see Kagan 1998, p. 61).[1] Consequentialism is situated in a teleological view of ethics. Coming from the Greek word *telos*, meaning "end", the teleological view understands the object of human acts to be the fulfilment of particular ends (Deigh 2010, pp. 14–15). From an ethics perspective, right and wrong are linked to the achievement of particular ends that are considered to be good (Deigh 2010, pp. 14–15).

In the case of an ethical position emphasizing duty, or more technically described as deontology, the ethical constitution of acts is based on whether they are aligned to a principle (Briggle and Mitcham 2012, p. 51). Like the term teleology, deontology also has its origins in ancient Greek, namely, *deon*, which is translated as duty (Briggle and Mitcham 2012, p. 51). From an ethics perspective, right and wrong are not linked to the achievement of good ends; the fulfilment of duties is linked to what is deemed to be right or wrong (Deigh 2010, pp. 14–15).

In the case of an ethical position emphasizing character, or more technically described as virtue, the ethical constitution of acts is based on their conformity to a certain type of character (see Timmons 2013, pp. 278–281). Virtue ethics is mostly recognised in Aristotle's understanding of the ethical life that combines both intellectual and moral virtues such as prudence and courage (see Timmons 2013, pp. 272–276).[2]

The dominant positions of consequentialism, deontology, and virtue tend to contain a single overarching principle as part of their theoretical architecture, whether it be the principle of utility (as in the case of utilitarianism), the principle of the categorical imperative (as in the case of deontology), or the principle of virtue (as in the case of virtue ethics).[3] An ethical position that is not monist regarding principles but rather pluralistic is the framework articulated by Beauchamp and Childress. These principles have a deontological and a consequentialist backdrop to them and are set in the context of virtuous actions by healthcare workers.[4]

---

[1] For a fuller treatment of the theory of utilitarian ethics, see Chap. 8 of this book.

[2] For a fuller treatment of the theory of virtue ethics, see Chap. 9 of this book.

[3] One version of the principle of utility is "the overall balance of pleasure versus pain that would be produced were the action to be performed"; one version of the principle of the categorical imperative is "act that you use humanity, whether in your own person or in the person of any other, always at the same time as an end, never merely as a means"; one version of the principle of virtue is "An action […] is *obligatory* if and only if […] [it] is an action that a virtuous person […] would not fail to perform in the circumstances in question" (Timmons 2013, p. 117; p. 211; p. 280)

[4] Normally, the ethical theories of deontology and consequentialism are presented as distinctly separate positions. However, the four principles of Beauchamp and Childress can be understood to be framed as both deontological and consequentialist (Chadwick and Schüklenk 2021, p. 31; also see Veatch and Guidry-Grimes 2020, pp. 65–68).

Framework of Principles

The utilisation of a framework of principles has been termed as "principlism" (see Clouser and Gert 1990; Veatch and Guidry-Grimes 2020, pp. 63–64). The principles set out by Beauchamp and Childress (given their association with Georgetown University in the United States) are commonly known, especially among ethicists working in this field, as the "Georgetown Mantra" (Chadwick and Schüklenk 2021, pp. 30–31). Since the original edition of Beauchamp and Childress' *Principles of Biomedical Ethics* back in the 1970s, the four principles have become one of the leading methods for bioethical analysis, with "enduring staying-power" (Chadwick and Schüklenk 2021, p. 33). Yet this does not imply that their work has been, or continues to be, immune from the subject of debate and critique (e.g. Clouser and Gert 1990).

There are a number of premises on which Beauchamp and Childress' (2019) "framework of practical normative principles" (p. vii; also see p. 17) is based: first, the principles find their source in, what Beauchamp and Childress (2019) describe as, "common morality" (p. 3; p. 13)[5]; this is a globally shared catalogue of moral norms recognised and acknowledged across societies and cultures.

Second, the framework of principles has a prima facie obligatory standing, i.e. the principles demand that they be met unless there are other principles which have an overriding obligatory requirement in a specific situation (Beauchamp and Childress 2019, p. 15). For example, a nurse has a prima facie obligation to respect the autonomous choice of patient X. However, should patient X's choice cause harm to patient Y, then the nurse may have an overriding obligatory requirement to prevent harm posed to patient Y rather than to uphold the autonomous choice of patient X. Beauchamp and Childress (2019) are at pains to point out that no principle has an automatic primacy (see p. ix; p. 99; p. 143).

On a surface level, the principles are easy to remember and to understand. The principles can help nurses recognise, identify, and articulate ethical questions or concerns that they have in the care of patients. One advantage of having principles is the possible clarity that can be offered and direction that can be given. However, there is considerable depth and complexity to each principle, and each principle has sparked much analysis and reflection.

Turning now to the particular principles, the prima facie obligation to act for the benefit of patients is articulated in **beneficence**, which can mean positive beneficence (i.e. through furthering welfare) or utility (i.e. through weighing the benefits and risks of healthcare actions for the overall benefit of persons) (Beauchamp and Childress 2019, p. 217). Some authors have derived other principles from beneficence such as compassion, veracity, and fidelity (DeWolf Bosek and Savage 2007, pp. 19–20). Beneficence also underpins the need for evidence-based practice, to ascertain possible benefits and harms (Stanley 1998, p. 47), a key focus in contemporary forms of professional nursing.

---

[5] They originally rooted the principles in a combination of ethical theories but amended that in response to critics (Baker 2022, p. 202).

The prima facie obligation not to do harm, or put others at risk of harm, is articulated in the principle of **nonmaleficence** (Beauchamp and Childress 2019, pp. 155–159). Given that the potential for risk of harm can be part of the very nature of healthcare, it would seem that it is unworkable to demand compliance to the view that the principle of nonmaleficence must always override other prima facie principles (Gillon 1985, pp. 130–131). Following Seay and Nuccetelli (2017), the principle of nonmaleficence should be understood in the sense of avoiding harm that is needless compared to harm that is instrumental, i.e. harm as an instrumental means that is needed to attain a health outcome (p. 59).

The principle of **autonomy**, or the prima facie obligation to respect autonomous choices (Beauchamp and Childress 2019, pp. 99–104), is no doubt a kernel principle in contemporary healthcare and nursing ethics. The historical journey of healthcare professionals, of healthcare institutions and of governments recognising patients as the prime managers of their health, according to their beliefs, values, and preferences—through enactment of codes, protocols, policies—is an extensive one and is still ongoing. The rules regarding consent safeguard the autonomy of the patient (Beauchamp and Childress 2019, pp. 118–119).

For Beauchamp and Childress (2019), an autonomous act is constituted by intention, by substantial (not necessarily complete) understanding and by noncontrolling influences (we are all influenced by many people in our lives, but the issue is whether that influence is in fact of a coercive or manipulative kind) (p. 102).

The prima facie obligation to distribute fairly and equitably to patients, in terms of enjoying the benefits and carrying the burdens of medical treatments and progress, is articulated in the principle of **justice** (Beauchamp and Childress 2019, pp. 267–268). Distributive justice focuses on the allocation of health resources, which tend not to be plentiful in supply (Jecker 1997, p. 30). Whereas the principles of beneficence, nonmaleficence, and autonomy can be primarily focused on the patient, the principle of justice also takes a wider perspective in terms of issues of access to health services and allocation of resources (see DeWolf Bosek and Savage 2007, p. 24).

Case Study

Leonard has made an appointment in the local clinic for a check-up as lately he hasn't been himself and is becoming a bit forgetful. Although he is retired, and his wife passed away a few years ago, Leonard still has a great range of intellectual interests and outdoor hobbies. But the other day, he became very alarmed by not being able to remember how to drive home after playing a round of pitch and putt.

When the day of his appointment arrives, Leonard's condition has already gotten worse, and the clinic's staff are concerned about the anxious behaviour he is displaying in the waiting room. After some initial examinations, they explain to him that more tests need to be carried out. Sometime after he is admitted, Leonard becomes more and more agitated and confused. He accuses the nursing staff of incarcerating him but later apologises and admits that this is nonsense. Yet later he starts shouting again at the staff. Now he is demanding to go home.

Ethical Questions and Discussion

When reflecting on the above hypothetical case study in the context of the framework of the four principles, it is not a matter of simply moving from a principle to a judgment, but rather the principles need to be specified and interpreted in the given situation (Beauchamp 1995, p. 182 and p. 184). Beauchamp and Childress (2019) stress the importance of specifying the four principles into rules to provide directives that are more tangible (p. 17).[6]

What follows below is not an exhaustive specification of the principles in the context of the case study. From the perspective of the four prima facie principles framework, there are a number of initial questions that can emerge, i.e. what is morally permissibly, what is morally required and what is morally forbidden regarding the healthcare team's response to Leonard in the given situation:

1. Should Leonard's present demand to go home be respected? The pinpoint concern here is whether Leonard really wants to go home, i.e. whether it is an autonomous choice to leave. Ethically, we can ask whether Leonard's demand to leave is with intention, with understanding and without undue influence by others? Does Leonard fully appreciate the potential consequences if he leaves the clinic? Can Leonard fully appreciate the potential consequences that his action could bring to himself and to others? Can he make an autonomous choice on this matter at this moment? His illness, at this time, could be having a significant impact on his ability to think things through—but that still needs to be proven.

    A possible specification of the principle of respect for autonomy emerging in such a situation could be *that there is an obligation to respect the autonomous choice of a patient to leave the care of the clinic against the advice of the healthcare team, when they have been fully informed and understand the possible consequences and when they have given valid consent.*
2. Should Leonard be encouraged to stay in the clinic at this time so that he can benefit from a possible programme of care and treatment for his illness? Certainly, the sentiment of beneficence has been the *raison d'être* of healthcare and nursing practice over the years (see DeWolf Bosek and Savage 2007, p. 18). It could be argued that Leonard's welfare can only be properly looked after in the clinic (or in an equivalent setting) in which he has a chance of benefitting from getting a diagnosis and a possible follow-on programme of care and treatment. In terms of weighing up the benefits and harms of a possible treatment and nontreatment, it may seem that there is more benefit for him to stay in the clinic than to leave.

---

[6] See Beauchamp and Childress (2019, pp. 17–19) for more information about the process of specification. Also see Richardson (2000) and Rauprich (2011).

A possible specification of the principle of beneficence in such a situation could be *that there is an obligation to make every reasonable effort to persuade, with reasons, a patient to follow the advice of the healthcare team to remain in the clinic so that they can benefit from a possible programme of treatment and care.*

3. Should Leonard remain in the clinic so that he is not put at risk of harm? The healthcare team will not want to cause Leonard harm by neglecting to provide the treatment and care that he needs, should he decide to remain in the clinic.

    A possible specification of the principle of nonmaleficence in such a situation could be *that there is an obligation not to cause harm to a patient through doing everything possible to ensure that they follow the advice of the healthcare team.*

4. Should Leonard be simply let go home to respect his rights and freedoms and so that resources can be allocated to other patients who wish to remain in the clinic? It may seem that the issue of the fair and equitable distribution of resources is not to the fore in this case study. In analysing cases using the framework of principles, not all principles have to be applied but only the ones that are most pertinent. Yet, we may still want to ensure that the resources of the clinic are allocated to patients in a fair, equitable, and efficient manner so that they are not wasted, especially if they are not wanted or needed by a patient.

A possible specification of the principle of justice in such a situation could be *that there is an obligation to use the resources of the clinic in a fair, equitable, and efficient manner so that they are not wasted, especially if they are not wanted or needed by a patient.*

There may be a feeling of a tug-of-war, as it were, between the obligation to respect Leonard's autonomous choice to leave the care of the clinic and the obligation to make every reasonable effort to persuade (with reasons) him to stay to benefit him and the obligation not to cause him harm. Balancing the "weight" or the "strength" of the principles in conflict is required (Beauchamp and Childress 2020, p. 566). Should the healthcare team come to the view that the obligations arising from the principle of beneficence have more "strength" and "weight" in this situation, this position would need to be justified. For instance, solid reasons would need to be provided for acting according to the principle of beneficence rather than according to another principle: that there is a possibility of benefitting Leonard in the clinic and that although Leonard's demand to leave is not immediately acted on, this doesn't mean that all his other choices (and perhaps future choices to leave) are simply ignored but that he is treated fairly (see Beauchamp and Childress 2019, p. 23). At the conclusion of the deliberation regarding what is morally permissible, what is morally required, and what is morally forbidden regarding the healthcare team's response to Leonard, the ethical decision needs be reflected upon as to whether the stance taken is coherent (see Beauchamp and Childress 2019, pp. 440–441).

There can be no doubt that caring for patients such as Leonard may spark various ethical questions and issues. Some may take the position that obligations arising from the principle of respect for autonomy have more strength and weight. As already said, the journey towards putting, and supporting, patients' autonomous choices regarding their healthcare foremost in decision-making has been a long one (and is perhaps far from over). Significantly, in 2015, the Assisted Decision-Making (Capacity) Act was passed in the Republic of Ireland, and it is seen to have shifted the approach to decision-making for those lacking (or soon will lack) capacity, from a patient's best interest model to a patient's preference and will model (Bury et al. 2019)[7]. The Act contains a range of guiding principles, and structured means, to assist decision-making (Davidson 2022, pp. 2–4): these principles include, for example, the capacity presumption, i.e. except when it is demonstrated not to be the case, the patient is to be presumed to possess capacity to make a decision regarding the particular issue at hand; decisions that are viewed not to be wise, i.e. a decision that is considered not to be wise for a patient is not a decisive confirmation for lack of capacity; interventions are not to take place unless necessary, i.e. interventions need to be necessary for the patient, taking into account their particular situation; and those undertaking the intervention on the patient should, as far as possible, enable the patient's participation and realise the patient's will and preference, both contemporaneous and past (Davidson 2022, pp. 2–4; ADMC 2015, pp. 17–18).

Following some of the principles outlined in Assisted Decision-Making (Capacity) Act, the following could initially be said regarding the situation of Leonard: that he is to be presumed to possess capacity (except when it is demonstrated not to be the case) to make a decision regarding whether to leave the clinic and that should Leonard decide to leave the clinic, although it may be viewed not to be wise, it would not be a decisive confirmation for lack of capacity (see Davidson 2022, pp. 2–3; ADMC 2015, p. 17).

The potential impact of the Assisted Decision-Making (Capacity) Act on healthcare workers is not inconsequential (Usher and Stapleton 2018, p. 130). The effect of the Act on the decision-making in the practice of healthcare in Ireland remains to be seen. In addition, whether, and how, the Act will have a knock-on effect on the prima facie obligatory standing of the four principles is also open to speculation—in terms of respecting the will and preference of patients having a presumptive obligation over other principles in ethical decision-making. On a theoretical level, the four principles have an equal prima facie obligatory standing, but on a practical level, some principles may have been given an automatic precedence over others. Yet, to make any principle overarching would seem not be in line with the thinking behind the framework. At the same time, others warn about the danger of not having some kind of order of principles as it could be left to healthcare workers to arbitrarily adopt one of the principles that supports their way of thinking ethically (Chadwick and Schüklenk 2021, p. 33).

---

[7] Also see Assisted Decision-Making (Capacity) (Amendment) Act 2022.

Conclusion

Nurses face questions about the ethical dimension of nursing practice, i.e. what are their obligations, what is permissible for them to do, and what ought they not do. In facing such questions, there are various ethical resources available to draw from, to provide both theoretical reflection and guidance. Arguably among these resources, the framework of the four principles—doing what is beneficial and not doing needless harm, respecting autonomous choices and distributing fairly—continues to hold a strong position in examining ethical issues in healthcare.

> **Key Learning Points**
> - To identify the key differences in ethical positions that are outcome-led, duty-led, and character-led, which form the backdrop to the framework of the four principles of Beauchamp and Childress.
> - To know some of the kernel aspects of the principles of beneficence, non-maleficence, autonomy, and justice.
> - To reflect on a hypothetical case study in the context of the framework of the four principles.

References

Assisted Decision-Making (Capacity) Act 2015 (ADMC) (2015). https://www.irishstatutebook.ie/eli/2015/act/64/enacted/en/html. Accessed 26 Sept 2023

Baker R (2022) Principles and duties: a critique of common morality theory. Camb Q Healthc Ethics 31(2):199–211. https://doi.org/10.1017/S0963180121000608

Beauchamp TL (1995) Principlism and its alleged competitors. Kennedy Inst Ethics J 5(3):181–198. https://doi.org/10.1353/ken.0.0111

Beauchamp TL, Childress JF (2019) Principles of biomedical ethics, 8th edn. Oxford University Press, New York, Oxford

Beauchamp TL, Childress JF (2020) Response to commentaries. J Med Philos 45(4–5):560–579. https://doi.org/10.1093/jmp/jhaa011

Briggle A, Mitcham C (2012) Ethics and science: an introduction. Cambridge University Press, Cambridge

Bury G, Thompson A, Tobin H, Egan M (2019) Ireland's Assisted Decision Making Capacity Act–the potential for unintended effects in critical emergencies: a cross-sectional study of advanced paramedic decision making. Ir J Med Sci 188(4):1143–1148. https://doi.org/10.1007/s11845-019-01994-w

Chadwick RF, Schüklenk U (2021) This is bioethics: an introduction. Wiley-Blackwell, Hoboken, NJ

Clouser KD, Gert B (1990) A critique of principlism. J Med Philos 15(2):219–236. https://doi.org/10.1093/jmp/15.2.219

Davidson H (2022) The Assisted Decision-Making (Capacity) Act 2015: interrogating the guiding principles for a person with dementia. Int J Law Psychiatry 84:101819. https://doi.org/10.1016/j.ijlp.2022.101819

Deigh J (2010) An introduction to ethics. Cambridge University Press, Cambridge

DeWolf Bosek MS, Savage TA (2007) The ethical component of nursing education: integrating ethics into clinical experience. Lippincott Williams & Wilkins, Philadelphia, London

Gillon R (1985) "Primum non nocere" and the principle of non-maleficence. Br Med J (Clin Res Ed) 291(6488):130–131. https://doi.org/10.1136/bmj.291.6488.130

Jecker NS (1997) Principles and methods of ethical decision making in critical care nursing. Crit Care Nurs Clin North Am 9(1):29–33

Kagan S (1998) Normative ethics. Westview Press, Boulder, Oxford

Rauprich O (2011) Specification and other methods for determining morally relevant facts. J Med Ethics 37(10):592–596

Richardson HS (2000) Specifying, balancing, and interpreting bioethical principles. J Med Philos 25(3):285–307. https://doi.org/10.1076/0360-5310(200006)25:3;1-H;FT285

Seay G, Nuccetelli S (2017) Engaging bioethics: an introduction with case studies. Routledge, London

Stanley R (1998) Applying the four principles of ethics to continence care. Br J Nurs 7(1):44–51. https://doi.org/10.12968/bjon.1998.7.1.5794

Timmons M (2013) Moral theory: an introduction, 2nd edn. Rowman & Littlefield Publishers, Lanham

Usher R, Stapleton T (2018) Overview of the assisted decision-making (capacity) act (2015): implications and opportunities for occupational therapy. Ir J Occup Ther 46(2):130–140. https://doi.org/10.1108/IJOT-08-2018-0013

Veatch RM, Guidry-Grimes LK (2020) The basics of bioethics, 4th edn. Routledge, New York, London

Utilitarianism: A Nursing Perspective

Michael Igoumenidis

Abstract

Utilitarianism is a moral theory focusing on consequences and defining ethical conduct on the basis of the well-being that these consequences produce. Maximisation of collective well-being is a central mandate for proponents of utilitarianism. Many classical and modern writers have explored this theory and its related concepts from a theoretical standpoint, and practical applications are often visible in the ways society functions. Utilitarian approaches are regularly used in the field of health care, and they have been amplified in the face of the recent COVID-19 pandemic measures. Lockdowns, triage decisions and compulsory vaccination can all be seen as drawing on utilitarian principles, aiming at the greatest collective well-being. The nursing profession's values may seem at odds with utilitarian logic in many instances, but its usefulness cannot be overlooked within the complex health-care systems of modern society.

The aim of this chapter is to explain and discuss the theory of utilitarianism and its relationship to nursing practice, using a case study and the recent pandemic as a background example. It starts by presenting the main theories and concepts related to utilitarianism. I then present some of the most common criticisms that are used against utilitarianism. The discussion then moves to applications of utilitarianism in practice, particularly in the field of health care, before turning its focus on the nursing profession

Keywords

Aggregation · Consequentialism · Impartiality · Utilitarian calculus · Utility · Welfarism

Introduction and Case Study

When the COVID-19 pandemic emerged in 2019, Margaret had been a practicing nurse for 10 years, with the last 5 years in an Intensive Care Unit (ICU) setting. The effect of the pandemic was strongly felt by the nursing profession, and Margaret was no exception. As the pandemic rose in severity, medical staff became ill, health systems were overburdened and shortages of ICU beds and protective equipment became common. Triage decisions were necessary, creating moral distress to those involved. Margaret witnessed cases of COVID-19 patients who received inadequate care and died, for resources were scarce. Eventually she grew exhausted, both physically and emotionally, and utterly disillusioned with her role as a nurse. When vaccines against COVID-19 became available, Margaret was one of the many vaccine-hesitant nurses, expressing distrust in the government and the health-care system that had let her down. Soon, the government imposed a COVID-19 vaccination requirement on all health-care workers, suggesting that unvaccinated staff would be suspended from work. Margaret's attitude moved from hesitancy to refusal. She participated in protests against mandatory vaccination, demanding that the government respect her bodily autonomy and her individual choice. She engaged in social media discourses, in which she claimed that she was "just a cog in the machine" of a social system that was indifferent to individuals, their rights and their personalities. Indeed, she felt that a few overstressed and overworked nurses' opinions were insignificant in front of society's benefit, the supposed "greater good" that this system promotes.

The greater good is a central concept in the moral theory of utilitarianism. This theory is one of the most important consequentialist approaches to ethics, aiming for the betterment of society as a whole. In general, it advocates for the greatest benefit for the greatest number of people. Margaret's concerns represent some of the most common criticisms of utilitarianism: firstly, that it allows for morally problematic decisions and actions (such as the imposition of mandatory vaccination, overriding the right of individuals to refuse vaccination, on public health grounds) so long as the resulting well-being outweighs the harm incurred (in other words, *the ends justify the means*); secondly, that society's greater good cannot be easily defined, and unanimously agreed upon; and, thirdly, that individual rights and individual differences can be sacrificed in the name of utilitarian impartiality (each individual counts as one and only one). In many instances, official responses to the COVID-19 pandemic revealed just how much our society is based on, by and large, uncontested utilitarian principles—with mandatory vaccination being a very negative manifestation of these principles, as implied in Margaret's reaction. But is she right to believe this? Is utilitarianism indeed the driving philosophical force of public policies, and did the pandemic provided the opportunity for its influence to increase?

The aim of this chapter is to explain and discuss the theory of utilitarianism and its relationship to nursing practice, using the case of Margaret and the recent pandemic as a background example. The chapter begins by presenting the main theories and concepts related to utilitarianism, as well as the most common criticisms that are used against it. The discussion then moves to applications of utilitarianism in practice, particularly in the field of health care, before turning its focus on the nursing profession. It examines the antithesis between utilitarian perspectives and nursing ideals, and, finally, it presents society's responses to the pandemic from a utilitarian point of view, with an emphasis on lockdowns, ICU bed rationing and mandatory vaccination. Throughout this discussion, it will be shown that, despite instances where utilitarianism and nursing ideals seem to conflict, this theory is consistent with the main goals of effective nursing care.

Main Concepts and Theories

Utilitarianism has a rich history as many writers have dealt extensively with criticizing utilitarian principles, presenting different approaches and revising its main concepts and theories. It is acknowledged as one of the "big three" traditional moral theories, together with Deontology and Virtue Ethics (Felzmann 2017). While there are many distinct utilitarian approaches to what constitutes a morally right action, they all share the basic idea of *utility maximization*. The concept of utility is quite elusive, tied to different meanings depending on context, but it is generally linked to the notions of good, benefit and well-being. Utility-maximising actions and policies are those that produce the largest amount of well-being. Again, depending on context, utility maximisation can refer to either the greatest well-being for the greatest number of people, maximisation of benefit over burden or minimisation of burden when it is impossible to create benefit. For reasons of simplicity, the principle of utility can be formulated as follows: actions and policies are morally right if they bring about the greatest benefit and the least harm.

This simple formulation leaves much to be desired. Is it possible to define benefit and harm in a consistent way? Does the greatest benefit refer to maximisation of individual or rather collective well-being? Since there are different kinds of benefit, is there a correct way to make trade-offs and comparisons between them? How can utility be measured? Are morally right and wrong actions to be judged on the basis of their *actual* consequences, or on the basis of their *foreseeable* consequences? These considerations shall be further discussed in the next sections. But whatever the answers may be, there are some basic elements inherent in the theories of utilitarianism, namely, consequentialism, welfarism, aggregationism and impartiality, and it is worth considering them in advance.

Utilitarianism is a modern form of teleological theory (in ancient Greek, *telos* means "end" or "goal")—it focuses on bringing about particular kinds of ends or goal—i.e. maximising well-being or benefit for the greatest number. Virtue theory, for example, is an ancient teleological theory that focuses on the perfection of human nature as the desired end or goal.[1] As already noted in the Introduction, utilitarianism is a form of *consequentialism*, so consequences constitute the main focus of interest in all utilitarian approaches. An accurate calculation of consequences would be useful in deciding which actions are morally right, but it is not always possible either to calculate or to foresee consequences. In any case, they should be evaluated based on the well-being they produce for individuals and communities. This is representative of another basic element of utilitarian theories, namely, *welfarism*. This doctrine holds that positive well-being is intrinsically good and should be promoted, and negative well-being is intrinsically bad and should be avoided. There are many different ways to acquire well-being, and some level of subjectivity is always involved in its definition, but the goal of well-being maximization is a clear mandate within the utilitarian way of thinking. It refers to the principle of *aggregation*, another inherent element in utilitarianism, which calls for the summing or averaging of well-being as a guide to ethical behaviour. Aggregationism has been criticized for pursuing a mere sum of individual welfare levels, thus ignoring any distributive considerations and sacrificing the interests of some members of society for the sake of the greatest collective well-being. On the other hand, this view implies that a given quantity of well-being is equally valuable irrespective of the individuals to whom this well-being is attributed. This shows that utilitarian approaches employ a principle of *impartiality*, in the sense that each individual counts as one, and no one's interests are more important than anyone else's.

Throughout the next section on the historical context of utilitarianism, there will be plenty of opportunities to see how these basic elements and the utilitarian principles have been postulated, transformed and refined.

Brief History of Utilitarianism

Classical Utilitarianism
Utilitarianism was originally proposed in the eighteenth century by English philosopher Jeremy Bentham, who drew on ideas going back to hedonism, a Greek school of philosophy founded in the fourth century BC by Socrates' student, Aristippus of Cyrene. Hedonists designated the pursuit of pleasure and the avoidance of pain as universal aims of all people, acknowledging that pleasure can take many forms beyond merely sensual gratification. Bentham examined the concepts of pleasure and pain in a more systematic way (the so-called utilitarian or felicific calculus), proposing that they could be measured according to seven criteria: intensity, duration, certainty, extent, remoteness, richness and purity (Gandjour and Lauterbach 2003). This calculus was the original attempt to measure well-being in its simplest form (pleasure and pain), so as to decide on the right course of action based on this measurement. Achievement of pleasure and avoidance of pain lead to happiness, and, according to Bentham, it is the greatest happiness of the greatest number that

---

[1] Please see Chap. 9 for a discussion of virtue theory and nursing.

is the measure of right and wrong (Bentham 1988). Bentham also formulated the original principle of utility as "that principle which approves or disapproves of every action whatsoever, according to the tendency it appears to have to augment or diminish the happiness of the party whose interest is in question" (Bentham 2007). Subsequent utilitarians refined this principle, but its core meaning remains the same in all utilitarian approaches.

A student of Bentham, John Stuart Mill, proposed a slightly different version of his teacher's theory. In his seminal *Utilitarianism* (1861), he distinguished between *higher pleasures* (for which a certain level of mental capacity is required) and *lower pleasures* (bodily experiences which animals can also have), thus considering both quantity and quality of pleasure and proclaiming that higher pleasures were intrinsically superior (Mill 2007). By proceeding to this distinction between higher and lower pleasures, Mill demonstrated that well-being takes on many different forms and that there should be a consistent way to compare them so as to take sound maximising decisions. In contrast to the hedonistic approach of his teacher, he proposed that intellectual well-being counts more than sensual well-being in the utilitarian calculus.

Other important work on utilitarianism in the nineteenth century was done by Henry Sidgwick, who saw utilitarianism as a form of hedonism which is concerned with everyone's well-being (*universal hedonism*), arguing that the right course of action towards well-being maximization could be defined by an appeal to moral intuitions (*intuitionism*), a common-sense morality in the form of an everyday moral code that most people live by. In other words, he believed that intuitionism and utilitarianism are two compatible and complementary moral approaches, as people tend to base their decisions on self-evident axioms of rational benevolence that promote overall well-being. However, Sidgwick admitted that this intuitively benevolent disposition is not shared by all members of society and that it is hard to convince individuals with an egoistic nature of the advantages of pursuing the greatest benefit for the greatest number of people.

Contemporary Utilitarianism

Since the early twentieth century, utilitarianism has diverged from the theories of Bentham, Mill and Sidgwick and has undergone a variety of refinements which are further discussed in the next sections. Among the many twentieth-century writers whose work employs utilitarian perspectives, it is worth mentioning two indicative texts by John Harris and Peter Singer.

Harris's first widely read paper was entitled *The Survival Lottery* (1975), in which he proposed a purely utilitarian scheme that would minimize suffering by sacrificing randomly chosen individuals and using their organs for transplants, thus saving multiple lives over the ones sacrificed. This thought experiment rests on three assumptions: first, there is no moral difference between killing persons (to retrieve their organs) or letting them die (if they are in need of organs); second, each life has equal value, and therefore, in Harris's utilitarian calculus, saving two or more lives by sacrificing one is always preferable; and, finally, transplant procedures have been perfected to such a degree so as to allow for a complete recovery of the persons receiving organs (Harris 1975). Under these assumptions, Harris describes a scheme where all individuals are assigned a number and drawn out of a lottery when an organ donation is needed and are expected to willingly put aside self-interest for the rest of society if their number is up. The idea is rational, but it is certainly met with fierce criticism on account of the wrongness of taking innocent lives, even for a higher purpose.

In his *Animal Liberation* (1975), Peter Singer famously advanced a utilitarian case against harming animals—such as by using them for food—arguing that, in assessing the consequences of our actions, it is necessary to take the interests of animals seriously, because of their ability to experience suffering. Singer's theory is not about animal rights; ethical behaviour is determined by consequences, and not by any appeal to right. If violating a right in a particular case produces greater well-being than respecting that right, then the ethical course of action is to violate it. His argument is that factory farming is related to painful experiences for billions of animals, whereas humans could eat less meat (and thus obliterate the need for mass meat production) without seriously diminishing their well-being (Singer 1975). If animals had pleasant lives, such as in free-range farms, and relatively painless deaths, then animal slaughtering for food would be much more permissible from Singer's utilitarian perspective. However, it should be noted that, consistently with this perspective, harm against both non-human animals and human beings is permissible, as long as there are good consequences that outweigh this harm. If humans could not eat anything other than meat, the painful lives and deaths of mass production animals would not weigh as much, as eating meat would be required for human survival. And if the use of animals, or even non-consenting humans in medical experiments could produce a large amount of collective well-being, such as the cure for a disease that affects many humans, then it would be morally right to proceed with the experimentation (Singer 1975).

This brief overview does not do justice to the work of Harris, Singer, or other writers who have developed utilitarian theories and principles, but it is a starting point for understanding the impact that utilitarianism has on contemporary ethical thinking, despite its problematic aspects.

Variants of Utilitarianism

Differentiated utilitarian perspectives and ensuing discussions have created distinct types of utilitarianism. The most important ones are briefly presented below.

Act and Rule Utilitarianism

One main distinction is between *act* utilitarianism and *rule* utilitarianism. Act utilitarianism takes individual actions directly into account, judging benefits and harms on a case-by-case basis and allowing anything that maximises well-being. This direct approach is purely consequentialist, as the right course of action is simply defined as the one that yields the best consequences in any given situation. Act utilitarians reject moral rules that classify actions as right or wrong in advance and stress the importance of specific contexts in ethical decision-making. This is the type of utilitarianism which is most frequently associated with the criticism of "anything goes" morality; no single action can be treated as immoral, as long as it results in the greatest amount of well-being for the greatest number of people.

On the other hand, rule utilitarianism constitutes an indirect consequentialist approach. It places emphasis on moral rules, judging actions with respect to their abiding by these rules and not directly by their consequences. Rule utilitarians believe that well-being maximisation rests on carefully formulated rules which should be universally applied. Thus, rule utilitarianism attempts to overcome act utilitarianisms' absoluteness by including deontological (duty-based) elements, in the form of rule-following, into the conversation about the greatest benefit and by shifting the emphasis from the individual level to wider social contexts. At an individual level and in specific contexts, breaking a rule could indeed produce the greatest possible well-being; but from a wider perspective, if everyone broke the rule, it would lose its meaning, and morality would become a matter of individual judgments. Society needs rules that have better long-term consequences, and exceptions can be made for specific groups of situations—not on a case-by-case basis.

Consider Harris's *Survival Lottery* again. In this thought experiment, society could formulate rules that maximise overall well-being by regularly sacrificing individual well-being—that is, taking the lives of randomly chosen persons. In specific contexts, these sacrifices may indeed fail to produce the expected benefit (if, for instance, the transplant recipients are all very elderly), or they may incur much harm (if the person sacrificed happens to have many dependent members in the family, as opposed to the elderly recipients). An act utilitarian would examine each sacrifice separately before proceeding, whereas a rule utilitarian would obey the lottery's commands, trusting that the established system yields the greatest well-being in the long run, by saving many more lives than the ones it takes.

Philosophers such as J.J.C. Smart argue that only act utilitarianism is a true form of utilitarianism, as stringent rules with no exceptions are features of deontological ethics; and if exceptions to rules are allowed, then rule utilitarianism would eventually collapse into act utilitarianism (Smart and Williams 1973), as more and more exceptions would lead to case-by-case appraisals. Therefore, rule utilitarianism must seek rules with a reasonable degree of flexibility built into them, but not so much as to become act utilitarianism in disguise.

Preference Utilitarianism

In contrast to classical theories, in which "good" was defined as whatever produced "the greater happiness" (hedonistic utilitarianism), modern views of utilitarianism assert that utility (well-being) is defined in terms of satisfaction of personal interests or individual preferences. This position can be described as *preference* utilitarianism (or *preferentialism*). It was mainly advanced by British philosopher R.M. Hare (1981), who claimed that well-being cannot be defined objectively and called for recognition of subjective desires, because people's preferences are dependent on their unique personal experiences. To be sure, it is difficult to make assessments at the individual level and decide which preferences count the most. It is also difficult to discern between those preferences associated with actual needs and others associated with mere desires. Another difficulty is that individuals attribute different importance to their preferences—Mill's division between higher and lower pleasures is too arbitrary to reach legitimate conclusions. However, preference utilitarianism seems to be the most widely accepted variant of this theory in modern ethical schools of thought.

In general, preferences seem to count more when they are informed and rational. However, there are cases when this is not possible, as with very young children, mentally incapacitated adults or non-human sentient beings. Consider again Peter Singer's *Animal Liberation*. Singer is a proponent of preferentialism, regardless of whether these preferences are rational or not. He does not attribute rights to animals (he argues that the concept of rights is unnecessary when considering ethics), but he respects their preferences, despite being based on instincts rather than rationality (Singer 1975). Singer's preference utilitarianism asserts that ethical decisions should be made from the point of view of an "impartial spectator" (Singer 1993). Under utilitarian impartiality, a person's interests cannot take precedence over anyone else's interests. In the preference utilitarian calculus, what counts is the satisfaction of the most preferences, weighted in accordance with the strength of the preferences. Therefore, the strong preference of billions of animals not to live in cruel conditions and be slaughtered in a painful way would outweigh the comparatively weak preference of humans to have meat in their diets.

In discussing theories and variants of utilitarianism, some of its strengths and limitations have already been pointed out. In what follows, some main criticisms against utilitarianism are further considered.

Criticisms Against Utilitarianism

In essence, utilitarianism is a simple theory; morally right actions are defined by good overall consequences, which are themselves defined on the basis of the aggregate well-being that they produce. However, many practical issues remain unsolved and set the ground for various criticisms against this theory. It is not possible to provide a full account of all these criticisms here, but some general remarks are in order. There are weaknesses in all four basic elements of utilitarianism, namely, consequentialism, welfarism, aggregationism and impartiality.

First of all, there is the issue of subjectivity in defining good consequences and calculating produced well-being. Different persons may attribute different value to certain outcomes under different circumstances, thus rendering arbitrary any attempt to create and use a utilitarian calculus. In choosing the right course of action, it is difficult to compare different kinds of well-being and reach decisions that maximize it.

A second difficulty lies in the predictive power of such a calculus; the actual consequences of an action may differ from desired or expected consequences, and good intentions cannot compensate for unforeseeable damage that may occur. For instance, if everyone followed Singer's logic and stopped consuming mass-produced meat for the sake of animals' well-being, it is hard to predict how many jobs would be lost and, consequently, how many persons would experience a serious decrease of their own well-being.

A third difficulty lies in the fact that the utilitarian notions of impartiality and aggregation have also been sources of criticism. Utilitarianism transforms society into a mass-person, losing sight of its constituent parts. Philosophers such as Thomas Nagel (1970) and John Rawls (1971) have noted that utilitarian approaches do not take seriously the distinction between persons. The pursuit of collective well-being disregards individuality, in the sense that no one's interests should matter differently from a utilitarian perspective. In a similar vein, Robert Goodin (1988) wonders whether utilitarianism permits individuals to have special obligations towards their closer relationships, as most people intuitively favour and care more for their loved ones than for distant, unknown persons. This attitude seems inherent in human nature, but it is not accepted as the right moral choice from a utilitarian perspective, which calls for a rational prioritization aimed at well-being maximization. Individual interests matter only in relation to their contributions to the general good, and, therefore, individual rights are disregarded for the mass-person's sake. Harris's Survival Lottery is indicative of this problem, as anyone's life could be sacrificed if more lives are to be saved.

Even proponents of utilitarianism admit that this theory is far from perfect, but the alternatives are even less satisfying; deontology rests on rigid assumptions, whereas virtue ethics becomes too vague and subjective in many regards.[2] Therefore, and despite their problematic aspects, utilitarian theories exercise a great influence on society's functioning, as discussed below.

Utilitarianism in Practice

As noted in the Introduction, nurse Margaret from the case study seems to endorse the above-mentioned criticisms of utilitarianism. She feels she is "just a cog in the machine" and that her individual preferences are not respected. Her view shall be further discussed in the next sections, first within a general societal context, and then with an emphasis on health care and nursing.

General Applications

In deciding upon public policy, some version of utilitarianism arguably provides the ethical background for political economy judgments, either explicitly or implicitly. Social costs and social benefits are taken into account, and decisions usually rest on expected outcomes' evaluations. Though not always effective, redistribution of money to the poor who need it more than rich persons do is a utilitarian policy, since

---

[2] For a brief discussion on deontology, please see Chap. 7. For a discussion of virtue ethics, please see Chap. 9.

accumulation of wealth has a decreasing marginal utility. Society's concern for future generations is also based on utilitarian principles; for instance, the threat of global warming requires urgent action and sacrifices of varying importance from present generations for the greater benefit of future persons who will inherit this world. Utilitarian impartiality transcends geographical and chronological boundaries, as well as personal identities.

In a general context, it is difficult to discern just how much of utilitarian rhetoric is translated into specific policies, or how consistent these policies are. The implementation of utilitarianism is better understood when examined in narrower contexts, such as the context of health-care research and practice.

Applications in Health Care

For a start, clinical research is an inherently utilitarian undertaking. Clinical trials are dedicated primarily to promoting the medical good of *future* patients by means of scientific knowledge derived from experimentation with *current* research participants (Miller and Brody 2003). To be sure, the Declaration of Helsinki states that the primary goal of new knowledge can never take precedence over the rights and interests of individual research subjects. Therefore, risk-benefit analysis is a key responsibility of research ethics committees reviewing clinical trials (Muthuswamy 2013). Yet this means that there is a reasonable risk to which individual research participants can be exposed, provided that the expected benefit is deemed sufficient. In his book *For the Common Good: Philosophical Foundations of Research Ethics*, Alex John London puts it as follows:

> A trial can pose an acceptable degree of risk to participants even if those risks are not offset by the prospect of direct medical benefit to participants themselves. Rather, such risks can be justified if they are offset by the prospect that they are necessary to generate sufficiently valuable information. This seems to countenance the permissibility of trading risk of harm to a small group of study participants if it will purchase sufficient social benefit for others.
> (London 2022, p. 185)

The practice of public health promotion is also utilitarian. Successful policies lead to health maintenance and risk avoidance for the greatest number of individuals possible, ideally the entire population. As with utilitarianism, public health seeks to achieve an effect at the greatest possible level; this goal sometimes calls for interventions that negatively affect some individuals but improve the collective health of the population (Nixon and Forman 2008). Utilitarian demands become more evident in crisis situations where public health is under serious threat, as in the COVID-19 pandemic, and this shall be analysed further in the last section of this chapter.

Finally, when it comes to resources allocation, utilitarian principles are widely used in modern health-care systems. Reimbursement decisions are based on cost-effectiveness and cost-benefit analyses, whose basic theoretical framework lies in the assumption that resources should be allocated consistent with maximising well-being, such as deaths averted or quality-adjusted life-years gained (Marseille and Kahn 2019). For instance, a patient with a rare disease may not receive publicly funded care if it is deemed too expensive for the predicted outcomes (as it often happens with rare diseases), because this money can be used for the satisfaction of other health-care needs, for greater numbers of people and in a more cost-effective manner. Utilitarian principles are also used in scarce resources allocation decisions, such as organ transplants or ICU beds, where the main goal is to identify recipients who would maximise total utility; in this way, specific groups of people—such as the elderly—may take on a lower priority for life-extending health interventions.[3]

Utilitarian Perspectives in Nursing

Where do nurses stand on the use of utilitarian principles in health care? With regard to the pandemic response, Margaret's views are shared by many others in the nursing profession, as will be discussed later in this section (see section "Mandatory Vaccination" below). But even without crisis situations, utilitarian approaches can appear to be at odds with some of the core nursing values.

Dilemmas Related to Nursing Ideals

The basic ethos of nursing calls for individualised care and treats each patient's interests as paramount. A purely utilitarian approach does not disregard individual interests, but it is prone to sacrifice them for the sake of greater benefit, as explained above. The mass-person's well-being is far more important, and resources should be used in a maximising way. Given that health-care resources are always limited, allocation decisions are necessary. Policymakers set the amount of resources that health professionals have at their disposal to allocate in the real world, and the latter determine the exact amount of resources that individual patients should receive in terms of interventions, time and skill mix (Igoumenidis et al. 2020). In any case, resources are often exceeded by patients' needs and demands.

In general, nurses should have no problem with this. They know that they could do better with more staff and better equipment, but they also recognise that policymakers protect the interests of the whole population; some patients may not receive optimal care, because there are other, more cost-effective priorities. Still, this recognition has a much greater emotional impact when its effect is seen in practice, and this is something that only nurses and other health-care professionals experience—not policymakers. Heightened levels of moral distress, burnout and compassion fatigue among nursing personnel are frequently associated with disrespect for patients' rights, prioritisation of care, ineffectiveness of services and prolonging patient suffering (Salari et al. 2022). Nurses cannot merely act on the basis of weighing needs and maximisation of potential well-being (i.e. the greatest benefit

---

[3] For a discussion of resource allocation and rationing in nursing, please see Chap. 3.

for the greatest number of patients). They are also expected to show empathy, to react on feelings of right and wrong and to judge for themselves whether they abide by core nursing values.

Good nursing care is founded on individualisation, treating each patient as an individual person, with their own personal characteristics. This is consistent with the moral approach of *care ethics*[4] which goes against utilitarian reasoning and impartiality, focusing instead on small-scale relationships and natural care by inclination. It has been proposed that care ethics makes a valuable contribution to ethics as applied to nursing care (see footnote 4). The shortcomings of such a situational approach are clearly acknowledged; it may be too demanding, too intuitive and emotional, and it disregards the simple ethical principle of benefit maximisation, all for the sake of specific individual patients. However, its proximity to traditional nursing values cannot be overlooked. Modern nursing practice should include care ethics considerations as a micro-level counterbalance to the macro-level utilitarian decision-making processes.

This does not mean that care ethics is the only suitable approach to nursing ethics or that utilitarianism is incompatible with bedside care. When faced with an ethical dilemma, the most beneficial consequences often serve as a moral compass. Accurate calculations of benefit or utility are not feasible at the micro-level of bedside care, but knowledge, experience and intuition can guide nurses to consider what the best outcomes may be. Consider the classical example of withholding the truth from certain patients about their diagnosis or prognosis, as it is argued that this benevolent deception helps patients to keep their optimism, reduce anxiety and continue with family and life events. Health-care professionals uphold the principle of autonomy so they have a *prima facie* (at face value) duty of honesty to the patient; but exceptions are sometimes permitted, based on the principles of beneficence and non-maleficence.[5] The nurse who decides to withhold the truth has considered these principles and concluded that, for this particular patient, the good consequences of deception outweigh this loss of autonomy. Disrespect for the patient's right to be informed is excused on the grounds of greater good. From a utilitarian perspective, it is an acceptable exception to the duty of honesty—though many critics argue that utilitarianism is too permissive about the ethics of deception.

In general, it is possible that utilitarian approaches are useful in the context of everyday nursing practice, provided they are balanced with traditional nursing moral values and individual-based care. When this balance is lost, many health-care professionals may experience similar feelings to those described by Margaret in the case study scenario. And, certainly, a public health crisis such as the COVID-19 pandemic tends to trigger overtly utilitarian responses, as it is discussed below.

---

[4] For a detailed discussion of care ethics in nursing practice, please see Chap. 10.

[5] For a detailed discussion of principles and nursing ethics, please see Chap. 7.

Pandemic Policies from a Utilitarian Point of View

In health crises there are clinicians and policymakers who advocate a complete shift of the focus of care from patient-centred deontology to population-centred utilitarianism (Michalsen et al. 2020). The COVID-19 pandemic created unique conditions in which the need for utilitarian thinking became more obvious. Still, the use of utilitarian principles was met with many criticisms, and it was described as "inhumane" (Browning and Veit 2021).

Lockdowns and Other Restrictions

In the COVID-19 pandemic, as with any infectious disease outbreak, the greatest priority lay in preventing further spread of the disease. Emergency public health measures were rooted in *negative* utilitarian principles, in the sense that minimising harm and suffering took precedence over maximising pleasure. Many countries employed lockdowns and restrictions to public areas, such as mandatory use of facemasks, to avoid the continued spread of COVID-19. The right to personal liberty was compromised for the greater good, whereas infected people were subject to even more limitations, being isolated for varying periods of time and often with no respect for their right to confidentiality. From a utilitarian point of view, liberty and rights are only important insofar as they secure well-being. Some East Asian countries have been highly effective at containing the virus; compared to liberal Western countries, they appeared more ready and willing to sacrifice individual rights, using methods such as tracing contacts and enforcing self-isolation, with severe penalties for failure to comply (Savulescu et al. 2020). Eastern countries were criticised for being overly authoritarian, whereas Western countries were criticised for relying too much on personal responsibility—Sweden in particular stands out for its soft approach, focusing on voluntary rather than mandatory measures (Björkman 2023). But in all instances, utilitarian logic was applied; the difference is to be found in the intensity of its application.

Lockdowns and other restrictions were deemed necessary to prevent the spread of the virus; but whether these produced the maximum utility possible is hard to estimate. The virus had generally more serious effects for subpopulations such as the elderly and the immunocompromised, so public health measures first and foremost were aimed at protecting these more vulnerable members of society. The measures partly succeeded, but they also had profound effects on the daily lives of the majority of people worldwide. Economic consequences were inevitable, international development came to a grinding halt and financial instability became a major concern. Many people lost their jobs or were forced to change their working habits, and evidence showed an increase in mental health problems and in incidents of domestic violence. Thus, continuing pressure to ease lockdowns so as to restart economic growth and mitigate social isolation effects can also be seen as utilitarian-motivated. On a utilitarian basis, decisions would be much more straightforward if there were more data available.

However, there was no comprehensive cost-benefit analysis proving that the negative effects of restrictive measures were outweighed by their positive outcomes and quality-adjusted life-years gained. It is difficult to calculate utility for every situation, especially when decisions must be taken as soon as possible. No one can know whether COVID-19 restrictions actually served the greater good, from a purely utilitarian perspective. They were enforced on the basis of available scientific evidence, though heavily influenced by public sentiment and moral intuitions. Protecting vulnerable members of society is an expression of common-sense morality, in line with Sidgwick's refined theory of utilitarianism. To be sure, there were disagreements, protests and lack of discipline, and many people failed to understand the necessity of preventive measures (or simply did not care); but, in the end, different views were isolated, and society's mass person carried on with this intuitive utilitarian approach.

Triage Decisions

No one can blame Margaret or any other person for feeling coerced by having to follow the restrictive rules of the pandemic and exercise social distance; at the same time, no one can blame governments for trying to protect public health in a crisis situation. On the other hand, governments and health-care systems can be accused of having been inadequate to cope with the increasing numbers of infected people. Health-care professionals were overwhelmed by demand for their services, especially in ICU settings, where life-saving equipment such as ventilators became scarce. All this resulted in harsh triage decisions, which added to health professionals' workload and stress.

In reality, prioritisation of some kind is always necessary in the context of modern health-care provision, as discussed in the previous section, and utilitarian approaches are useful in setting up priorities. The fact that direct life and death dilemmas rarely arise does not mean that there are no difficult allocation decisions in everyday practice. Understaffed nursing units are commonplace in many healthcare systems, and patients do not always receive comprehensive care. Does this mean that they are expendable? It is true that policymakers at the macro-allocation level can always provide more resources, but this cannot take place infinitely. The pandemic necessitated a redistribution of priorities and intensified the use of utilitarian approaches, arguably against patients with low probabilities of survival or small marginal treatment benefit. But the alternative options would be either to use lottery approaches (such as the one John Harris (1975) had proposed), or to provide care on a "first-come, first-served" basis, which is also reminiscent of lottery logic. A third option would be to increase the system's capacity, with more ICU beds, ventilators and properly trained staff, as Margaret implicitly requires. Ultimately, however, resources are not infinite. Critical care needs utilitarian thresholds; otherwise, less urgent health needs would be neglected, either in pandemic situations or otherwise.

Mandatory Vaccination

Expansive responses to COVID-19 worldwide resulted in the rapid manufacturing of safe and effective vaccines. However, a high rate of vaccine hesitancy and refusal among populations internationally was observed, including among health-care professionals such as nurse Margaret. In a global scoping review, which included 51 studies, the overall pooled prevalence of vaccine refusal among 41,098 nurses was 20.7% (23.4% in 2020 and 18.3% in 2021), and the major refusal reasons cited were concerns about vaccine safety and side effects, as well as mistrust in experts, authorities or pharmaceutical companies (Khubchandani et al. 2022). Many governments embraced positive or negative incentives, such as rewards for getting vaccinated or exclusion from social activities for the unvaccinated, and also mandates for specific social groups, including nurses and other health-care workers.

Mandatory vaccination for health-care workers is justified on the basis of the non-maleficence principle; remaining unvaccinated potentially exposes highly vulnerable patients and coworkers to the virus, whereas an infected, unvaccinated health-care worker stays home and unfairly shifts more work burden on to vaccinated coworkers (Myers et al. 2023). Individual autonomy and the right to bodily integrity should be generally respected, but, as the utilitarian argument goes, they can also be sacrificed for the greater benefit. Vaccination is a minor inconvenience and poses negligible risks. Besides, health-care professionals have fiduciary duties to their patients and to the community as a whole, so protecting them from avoidable harm is a well-established moral obligation (Maneze et al. 2023). Margaret feels frustrated with the government and its policymakers; she has lost her trust in the system she is part of and probably does not think clearly of her situation and her duties. These remarks do not justify mandatory vaccination, but they partly explain why educated and responsible individuals may fail to consider the greater good.

Irrespective of mandates, utilitarian arguments can ground an individual moral obligation to be vaccinated. Herd immunity is a collective good, as everyone benefits from it (Giubilini et al. 2018). Any single vaccination does not make a significant difference to vaccination coverage rates, but, from a broader perspective, individual contributions enable the desired collective effect. Derek Parfit is one of the most influential contemporary writers exploring utilitarian ideas, and he provides the following example:

> A large number of wounded men lie out in the desert, suffering from intense thirst. We are an equally large number of altruists, each of whom has a pint of water. We could pour these pints into a water-cart. This would be driven into the desert, and our water would be shared equally between all these many wounded men. By adding his pint, each of us would enable each wounded man to drink slightly more water - perhaps only an extra drop. Even to a very thirsty man, each of these extra drops would be a very small benefit. The effect on each man might even be imperceptible. (Parfit 1984)

In spite of this imperceptibility, it can be argued that all individuals share the same obligation to add their pints of water to the cart, just as they share an obligation to be vaccinated so as to bring about the best outcome: herd immunity. This course of action is by and large based on utilitarian moral intuition, but, in any case, counter-arguments are difficult to maintain. Why would someone go against a moral imperative that maximises benefit at a minor cost, in terms of inconvenience and risk? Individual liberties and decisions should be respected in general, but not when they are associated with harm to third parties. Utilitarian J. S. Mill's harm principle states that "the only purpose for which power can be rightfully exercised over any member of a civilised community, against his will, is to prevent harm to others" (Mill 2002). The state should not have to impose mandates on Margaret or anyone, but it is often necessary for reasons of harm prevention.

Conclusion

In a highly individualistic modern society, utilitarianism has many opponents. Public sentiment often goes against it, as people feel threatened by the indifferent mass-person it represents. In a study investigating moral judgments among older adults during the pandemic, participants were generally not willing to violate the personal rights of others to produce the best overall outcomes (Antoniou et al. 2021). Even when serious threats exist, people tend to uphold fundamental rights at the expense of societal interests. The bad reputation of utilitarianism is unfortunate, since, according to its proponents, it not only holds the key to deciding how to best face the COVID-19 pandemic (or other such pandemics), but also how to respond to non-pandemic diseases (Browning and Veit 2021).

In reality, the basic utilitarian principles are silently accepted by the majority of society. Even without perceiving it, people conform to its simplicity—well-being maximisation. If one were to ask Margaret whether she preferred the end of the pandemic or to remain unvaccinated, she would probably choose the former. Of course, there are some whose selfishness outweighs concern for the greater good, but this should not be the case for nurses and other health-care professionals. Despite its shortcomings and the dilemmas it creates at an individual level, a utilitarian approach is the only effective way of maximising well-being in the world. From a nursing perspective, utilitarianism is a useful and balanced theory, fit for purpose in the complex and changing health-care systems of modern society.

> **Key Learning Points**
> - Utilitarianism is a moral theory which focuses on consequences and advocates for the greatest benefit for the greatest number of people.
> - Utilitarianism is praised for its impartiality but it is also blamed for its disregard of individuality.
> - In health care, utilitarian approaches are used in clinical research, public health policies and allocation of health resources.
> - Pandemic policies such as lockdowns, patient prioritisation and mandatory vaccination are based on utilitarian principles.
> - Utilitarianism seems to conflict with traditional nursing values, but it is a useful approach in the context of modern everyday nursing practice.

References

Antoniou R, Romero-Kornblum H, Young JC et al (2021) Reduced utilitarian willingness to violate personal rights during the COVID-19 pandemic. PLoS One 16(10):e0259110. https://doi.org/10.1371/journal.pone.0259110

Bentham J (1988) Preface. In: Harrison R (ed) Bentham: a fragment on government (Cambridge texts in the history of political thought). Cambridge University Press, Cambridge, pp 3–32

Bentham J (2007) An introduction to the principles of morals and legislation. Dover Publications, New York

Björkman A (2023) The Swedish COVID-19 control measures and the national commission report. Acta Paediatr 112:8–10. https://doi.org/10.1111/apa.16582

Browning H, Veit W (2021) Utilitarian lessons from the COVID-19 pandemic for non-pandemic diseases. Am J Bioeth 21(12):39–42. https://doi.org/10.1080/15265161.2021.1991035

Felzmann H (2017) Utilitarianism as an approach to ethical decision making in health care. In: Scott PA (ed) Key concepts and issues in nursing ethics. Springer, Cham, pp 29–41

Gandjour A, Lauterbach KW (2003) Utilitarian theories reconsidered: common misconceptions, more recent developments, and health policy implications. Health Care Anal 11(3):229–244. https://doi.org/10.1023/B:HCAN.0000005495.81342.30

Giubilini A, Douglas T, Savulescu J (2018) The moral obligation to be vaccinated: utilitarianism, contractualism, and collective easy rescue. Med Health Care Philos 21(4):547–560. https://doi.org/10.1007/s11019-018-9829-y

Goodin RE (1988) What is so special about our fellow countrymen? Ethics 98(4):663–686

Hare RM (1981) Moral thinking. Its levels, method and point. Oxford University Press, Oxford

Harris J (1975) The survival lottery. Philosophy 50(191):81–87. https://doi.org/10.1017/S0031819100059118

Igoumenidis M, Kiekkas P, Papastavrou E (2020) The gap between macroeconomic and microeconomic health resources allocation decisions: the case of nurses. Nurs Philos 21(1):e12283. https://doi.org/10.1111/nup.12283

Khubchandani J, Bustos E, Chowdhury S et al (2022) COVID-19 Vaccine refusal among nurses worldwide: review of trends and predictors. Vaccines (Basel) 10(2):230. https://doi.org/10.3390/vaccines10020230

London AJ (2022) For the common good: philosophical foundations of research ethics. Oxford University Press, New York

Maneze D, Salamonson Y, Grollman M et al (2023) Mandatory COVID-19 vaccination for healthcare workers: a discussion paper. Int J Nurs Stud 138:104389. https://doi.org/10.1016/j.ijnurstu.2022.104389

Marseille E, Kahn JG (2019) Utilitarianism and the ethical foundations of cost-effectiveness analysis in resource allocation for global health. Philos Ethics Humanit Med 14(1):5. https://doi.org/10.1186/s13010-019-0074-7

Michalsen A, Vergano M, Quintel M et al (2020) Epilogue: critical care during a pandemic—a shift from deontology to utilitarianism? In: Michalsen A, Sadovnikoff N (eds) Compelling ethical challenges in critical care and emergency medicine. Springer, Cham, pp 157–166

Mill JS (2002) On liberty. Dover Publications, New York

Mill JS (2007) Utilitarianism. Dover Publications, New York

Miller FG, Brody H (2003) A critique of clinical equipoise. Therapeutic misconception in the ethics of clinical trials. Hastings Cent Rep 33:19–28

Muthuswamy V (2013) Ethical issues in clinical research. Perspect Clin Res 4(1):9–13. https://doi.org/10.4103/2229-3485.106369

Myers M, Dunikoski L, Brantner R et al (2023) An ethical anaylsis of the arguments both for and against COVID-19 vaccine mandates for healthcare workers. J Emerg Med 64(2):246–250. https://doi.org/10.1016/j.jemermed.2022.11.005

Nagel T (1970) The possibility of altruism. Clarendon Press, Oxford

Nixon S, Forman L (2008) Exploring synergies between human rights and public health ethics: a whole greater than the sum of its parts. BMC Int Health Hum Rights 8(2). https://doi.org/10.1186/1472-698X-8-2

Parfit D (1984) Reasons and persons. Oxford University Press, Oxford

Rawls J (1971) A theory of justice. The Belknap Press of Harvard University Press, Cambridge, Massachusetts

Salari N, Shohaimi S, Khaledi-Paveh B et al (2022) The severity of moral distress in nurses: a systematic review and meta-analysis. Philos Ethics Humanit Med 17(1):13. https://doi.org/10.1186/s13010-022-00126-0

Savulescu J, Persson I, Wilkinson D (2020) Utilitarianism and the pandemic. Bioethics 34(6):620–632. https://doi.org/10.1111/bioe.12771

Singer P (1975) Animal liberation: a new ethics for our treatment of animals. Random House, New York

Singer P (1993) Practical ethics, 2nd edn. Cambridge University Press, Cambridge

Smart JJC, Williams B (1973) Utilitarianism: for and against. Cambridge University Press, Cambridge

Virtue Ethics and Nursing Practice

9

Derek Sellman

Abstract

Virtue ethics is an approach that focuses on character with the assumption that a person of good character will tend to behave in ways consistent with their character. A virtue ethics for nursing is therefore concerned with the character of individual nurses and seeks ways to enable nurses to develop character traits appropriate for actions that enhance wellbeing. This chapter offers some insights into the nature of virtue ethics from an Aristotelian perspective and includes an outline of the virtue of *phronesis* (practical wisdom) which provides guidance in situations where it is not obvious what action would be the virtuous action. Virtue ethics is contrasted with modern ethical theory (deontology and utilitarianism). Some ways in which virtue ethics can enhance professional nursing practice are considered.

Keywords

Virtue · Aristotle · Kindness · Compassion · Phronesis (practical wisdom) · Nursing

Introduction

This chapter is about the idea of virtue ethics. In recent times virtue ethics has come to be considered as one of the big three ethical approaches alongside deontology and utilitarianism. However, as Lachman (2006) indicates, virtue ethics has made fewer inroads into applied and professional ethics precisely because it does not profess to offer the type of formulaic approaches to (often complex) moral issues

D. Sellman (✉)
Edmonton, AB, Canada
e-mail: anne.scott@universityofgalway.ie

that modern moral theory tends to adopt. If this is true, then it might be reasonable to ask what it is that virtue ethics can offer nurses as they go about their everyday practice. The short answer is that, at a minimum, virtue ethics can help redirect focus away from mere rule following towards consideration of what counts as good for human beings. It does so by encouraging the cultivation of those character traits that promote actions that are fair, honest, kind, compassionate, and so on: actions that contribute to human wellbeing. Thus, virtue ethics might be described as an approach that is concerned primarily with character and with human goods.

At the outset it should be recognised that virtue ethics is not one thing but rather can be understood as an umbrella term for sets of ideas that share a common foundation. In this respect virtue ethics does not differ from other ethical approaches including but not limited to deontology and utilitarianism; there are factions in both of those theories that diverge in regard to particular points and interpretations. Nevertheless, as is commonly understood, there are some fundamental premises that underpin different versions of both deontology and utilitarianism, and the same can be said for virtue ethics. If the deontologist is characterised as claiming that an act is good if it is in accordance with duty and the utilitarian is characterised as claiming that an act is good if it brings about the best consequences, then the virtue ethicist might be characterised as claiming that an act is good if it is a virtuous act. These characterisations are, of course, oversimplifications, and while it is not the purpose of this chapter to discuss deontology or utilitarianism,[1] both theories will be mentioned in order to help explain some of the nuances of virtue ethics and how it differs from those two theoretical approaches. The essential point here is that just as there are different versions of deontology and utilitarianism, so there are different versions of virtue ethics.

The one thing that underpins virtue ethics is the emphasis on character; and this focus on the character of the agent is what distinguishes virtue ethics from most other approaches to ethics.[2] Some versions of virtue ethics characterise this difference as a difference of the primary question: so that whereas most ethical theories seeks to answer the question 'what should I do?', virtue ethics asks instead 'how should I be?' This distinction suggests either that what a person does is less important than how a person is, or that virtue ethics does not provide action guidance. Neither suggestion is as straightforward as critics claim, and, as will be outlined in this chapter, both not only oversimplify many of the ideas about virtue ethics but also overstate the purported advantages of modern moral theory. Danielle's experience, described in the case study below, is illustrative and will be referred to throughout the chapter in order to explore some key elements of virtue ethics.

---

[1] Chapter 8 is dedicated to a perspective on utilitarianism.
[2] One exception is 'the ethics of care' or 'care-based ethics' which forms the focus of Chap. 10.

Case Study

Danielle is a student nurse half-way through her final clinical placement on Azalea ward, a busy surgical unit. Like all student nurses, she has had a mentor in each of her previous placements, but she has never before met anyone quite like Belanna, her mentor on Azalea ward. It is a very busy ward, yet unlike most of the other qualified nurses Danielle has worked with, Belanna seems always to know what to do whatever the situation. She always has a kind word to say to everyone from the most difficult and demanding patient to the most arrogant and obnoxious of doctors; from the ward cleaner to the hospital chief executive, and even in the most challenging of situations, she always seems to be able to find a way to ensure that everyone's dignity is upheld, that no one gets left unattended, and that no one feels neglected or humiliated. Belanna is kind, compassionate, and caring but does not flinch from confronting situations that might otherwise undermine those ideals of practice. Yet she has no pretensions and does not think that what she does is anything special, in fact she thinks that she does not do anything different from that which anyone in her position would do. She seeks and welcomes feedback from students, patients, families, and co-workers and goes out of her way to ensure that everyone who arrives on Azalea ward has a positive experience. At first Danielle thought that this was too good to be true, or that it was all an act that would collapse at the first sign of frustration, but after 6 weeks on the placement, Danielle recognises that there is something about Belanna that marks her out as a particularly good nurse. Danielle decides that Belanna represents the type of nurse that she (Danielle) wants to become.

What Is Virtue Ethics?

So what is virtue ethics? Virtue ethics is the term given to an approach that has a focus on character. More specifically, it focuses on the character of the actor or agent. Hence virtue ethics is sometimes referred to as agent-based ethics. This is to be contrasted with act-based ethics in which the primary focus is on the act. As indicated earlier, act-based ethics asks the question: 'what should I do?' while agent-based ethics tends towards asking: 'how should I be?'—although it should be noted that not all versions of virtue ethics make this distinction. Armstrong (2007), for example, claims an action-oriented account of virtue ethics for nursing, while Crisp (2007) and Hursthouse (1997) both hint that the latter question is subsumed within the former and so engage seamlessly with action guidance in their accounts. A more nuanced distinction might be had by noting that act-based theories tend towards accounts in which action is in accordance with an external principle or from a rule derived from a general principle, while agent-based approaches tend to emphasise the role of character in formulating decisions for actions. So the deontologist may ask, 'which duty takes precedence in this situation?'; the utilitarian may ask 'what action will lead to the best consequence?', and the principlist may ask 'which principle applies here?'[3] In contrast, guidance for action in agent-based ethics requires the agent to seek to become a certain sort of person, a person with the virtues to lead them to act in ways that the virtuous person would act. So, following Hursthouse (1997), the virtue ethicist might ask 'if I act in such and such a way, would I be acting in a way that was virtuous?' The assumption here is that by becoming, for example, a just, courageous, and honest person, the individual will tend towards acting in just, courageous, and honest ways out of habit or, perhaps more importantly, from inclination. This is to say that the just, courageous, and honest person will act in ways that reflect their character. And this is exactly what Danielle is witnessing when she sees her mentor (Belanna) in action. The reason Belanna seems to know what to do whatever the situation is that she is a kind, compassionate, honest, just, and courageous person and this is exemplified in her actions. Belanna acts in ways that reflect her character.

It is often said that people act characteristically. That is, we expect people to act in ways consistent with the type of person we take them to be. We tend to identify friends, colleagues, and peers in terms of their characteristics. We all know people who we can describe as kind or honest or courageous, and the more they continue to act in ways that are kind and honest and courageous, the more we appreciate and admire their integrity and their character. Similarly, most of us can identify individuals who might be described in more negative terms; we might thus identify some people as tending towards one or more of dishonesty, ruthlessness, unhelpfulness, unreliability, and so on. Many of Danielle's earlier mentors, while not particularly dishonest or unkind, did not seem to possess the same confidence in being the type of nurse who acts, as Belanna does, by inclination in kind or honest ways. Most of Danielle's earlier mentors did aim to do the right thing but sometimes doing the right thing seemed to require them to follow rules or general guidance. Of course, general rules are helpful, but at times merely following the rules seemed to result in nursing actions that might be perceived as, if not exactly unkind, then at least less than kind or less than compassionate. Danielle has a vivid recollection of the distress experienced by a young patient when informed of the death of her husband in the car accident in which they had both been involved. Danielle has often wondered if being told the truth in the matter-of-fact manner in which the news was delivered was a kind thing to do, but she had been told that being honest was a requirement of both her nurses codes and of the principle of respect for autonomy (justified on the grounds that a patient has a right to know the truth if they are to make autonomous choices).[4] Having now seen the way in which Belanna is honest in her dealings with patients, relatives, and others while at the same time being compassionate and kind is leading Danielle to question whether what she has been told previously about ethical practice is altogether accurate or satisfactory. Danielle is now beginning to recognise that being honest is only one part of ethics. The need to act in ways that are not callous or unkind means that honesty cannot be seen in isolation from other aspects of ethical nursing practice. And the more she observes Belanna in practice,

---

[3] See Chap. 7 for further discussion of principlism and nursing ethics.

[4] See Chap. 6 for an in-depth discussion of patient autonomy in nursing and healthcare contexts.

the more Danielle wants to become like her; and the more she recognises that Belanna acts characteristically in kind, honest, compassionate, fair, and courageous ways; that is, in ways that reflect the type of person, the type of nurse, that Belanna is.

That we can make such judgements indicates that we acknowledge the idea of character, which lends weight to the idea of virtue ethics, because in virtue ethics character guides conduct. In other words, virtue ethicists will want to say that right action follows right character. And it is this primacy of character that distinguishes virtue ethics from other approaches to ethics. In our case study, Belanna seems to represent a nurse with the virtues insofar as her actions appear to stem from her character traits. She acts in kind ways because she is a kind person; she acts in honest ways because she is an honest person, and so on.

From this basic tenet of virtue ethics—that individuals generally act in ways consistent with their character traits—it follows that those who wish to act in virtuous ways should seek to become virtuous persons. In so doing the question 'what should I do?' becomes one that is asked less often because in many situations, just as Belanna exemplifies, what a person should do is what they characteristically will do. But perhaps the language of virtues is off-putting or old-fashioned. Perhaps a change of language might be useful. So instead of a phrase such as 'virtue ethics requires those who wish to act in virtuous ways to become virtuous persons', we might say instead 'virtue ethics requires that those who wish to act for the good need to develop good traits of character'. The virtues of kindness, honesty, courage, and justice are perhaps better understood in modern vocabulary as character traits. And most people identify these as positive traits: traits that are admired and identified as good things in and of themselves and traits that are encouraged in society in general and in nursing (and other healthcare occupations) in particular [see for example, the NMC (2015/2018) (NMC (Nursing and Midwifery Council) 2015) code for nurses].

Some Background Regarding the Idea of Virtue and the Idea of Virtue Ethics

The background information in this section is designed to help the reader gain an appreciation of the origins of the language of virtue.

Aristotle (1953 edn) held that being or doing good required cultivation of *aretê*. Aretê is translated most commonly as 'virtue' but sometimes as 'excellence' or 'moral virtue'. The Ancient Greeks understood aretê in a way that we might now describe as holistic: in other words, a person of aretê (a person of virtue or a person of excellence) would be a person with all the virtues or excellences necessary for a good life. Note that this idea of virtue is a composite—to be a person of virtue is to be a person with the appropriate set of virtues—possession of some but not other virtues would disqualify a person from aretê. Of course, the question then becomes what are the appropriate virtues—a question that has exercised successively, and among many others, Aristotle, Aquinas, and Austen as well as the disciplines of philosophy and psychology ever since. The idea of virtue ethics fell out of favour with the rise of Enlightenment thinking and the Industrial Revolution, following which the Victorians appropriated the word 'virtue' for ideas related to chastity, domesticity, and religiosity. The rise of what we might now describe as modern ethical theory (i.e. ethical theory that has evolved from the deontology associated with Kant and from the utilitarianism of Bentham and Mill) further relegated the idea of virtue ethics until the publication of 'Modern Moral Philosophy' (Anscombe 1958) which is credited as beginning a resurgence of interest in the idea of virtue ethics.

Most versions of virtue ethics draw from the Ancient Greek philosophy of Aristotle—and in this chapter I continue the tradition. (The reader should note that there are other, non-Aristotelian versions of virtue ethics.) One of the difficulties of working with ancient ideas lies in translation. It is not just that the ideas get lost in translation, it is more that many Ancient Greek terms often have no one direct equivalent in English. As noted above, aretê can be translated as 'virtue', 'excellence' or 'moral virtue'. These different translations can represent significant changes in meaning, as can be seen above, where translating the idea of a person of aretê as 'a person of virtue' can be interpreted quite differently from the translation of 'a person of excellence'. Hence the use of one rather than another translation can have significance for interpretation and understanding. There are two more ancient Greek terms that are important in Aristotelian and neo-Aristotelian virtue ethics: *eudaimonia* and *phronesis*. Eudaimonia is most often translated as 'good life', 'happiness', 'human flourishing', or just 'flourishing', phronesis as 'practical rationality' or 'practical wisdom'. My preference is flourishing for eudaimonia and practical wisdom for phronesis.

Eudaimonia

Aristotle considered that all things (including persons) have a purpose and to pursue that purpose is to pursue the good appropriate for the thing that it is—this is the pursuit of eudaimonia. For Aristotle a good chair is a chair that performs as a chair should, so a chair that is unstable, or tends to unexpectedly eject its occupant, would not be a good chair. Similarly, a good horse is a horse that is able to excel in those things that make a horse a horse and not, for example, a snake—thus a good life for a horse qua horse without legs would be unlikely. The good for a human then lies in pursuit of that which is good for humans as humans. For Aristotle it is the virtues that provide the platform for a good life for a person, and it is in striving to cultivate the virtues that humans can excel. Note it is not the pursuit of an individual or a particular virtue but the pursuit of those virtues necessary for human flourishing.

Phronesis

The Ancient Greeks did not separate individual from societal good, at least not in the way that we do in the twenty-first century. Thus Aristotle's list of virtues reflects an Ancient Greek sociology—just as ours, as MacIntrye (2007) argues, should reflect our own sociology. In other words a modern list of virtues should reflect the sociological norms of our time as well as those timeless virtues of honesty, courage, and justice. And for nursing, as I have argued elsewhere, at least some of these virtues can be identified in nursing codes (Sellman 1997, 2011).

Among Aristotle's list of virtues, phronesis (practical wisdom) is the uber-virtue, the one virtue to guide action in the form of knowing when to do the right thing. As Hursthouse (1997) notes, there is much in virtue to guide action. The just person is inclined to act in just ways, the honest person in honest ways, and the courageous person in courageous ways. Yet while this tendency to act in ways consistent with cultivated virtues provides a starting point for good action and for pursuit of the good, there is a need for cultivation of the wisdom to know when and how to act in any one particular situation. This is the role of phronesis (practical wisdom) for without practical wisdom, acting solely according to any one other virtue is likely to leave the actor at the mercy of their emotions. And while emotions are important in virtue ethics, they nevertheless require tempering with practical wisdom if acting for the good is the aim.

Virtue Ethics and Nursing

So what is it that virtue ethics can offer nursing? One common criticism of deontology and utilitarianism (and also of principlism) is the tendency, at best, towards rule or principle following and, at worst, towards cold calculation. We saw the results of rule following without regard to fellow human feeling witnessed by Danielle early on in her preregistration nursing programme. While supporters of modern moral theory recognise the desirability for actions that respond to the human condition in some way, neither deontology nor utilitarianism relies on that as a factor for the measure of the good. At a minimum, virtue ethics can provide that aspect of humanity seemingly absent from extreme forms of deontology and utilitarianism; and better still, and following Hursthouse (1997), virtue ethics can enhance the terms of ethical debate.

Hursthouse notes that ethical debates tend to be couched in terms that emerge from thinking influenced primarily by modern moral theory. For example, ideas of rights, duties, obligations, and so on represent the common language of the abortion debate. Such language, she notes, serves to allow for, sometimes to justify, behaviour that in other circumstances might well be perceived as unkind, hurtful, or even pernicious. She argues that while our relationships can and do flourish in an environment where parties respect human rights, to insist that rights, or any one right, should or must supercede all other considerations, in any given moral discussion, is to undermine something fundamental about what it is to be a moral agent. She also argues that any ethical theory that encourages or permits insensitivity towards others fails in some significant way. For Hursthouse virtue ethics can intercede by inviting agents to acknowledge the general virtuousness or viciousness of their intended action and thereby ensure human goods remain a central focus in our efforts to be moral beings.

What Hursthouse seems to be alluding to here is the use of Aristotle's virtue of phronesis. The practical wisdom involved in deliberating about which actions are virtuous—which actions, that is, promote and contribute to human flourishing—is one of the things that distinguishes virtue ethics from modern moral theory. Actions that approximate fairness, honesty, kindness, compassion, sensitivity, and so on are clearly more consistent with ideas of human flourishing than ways of being that are, for example, dishonest, unfair, and unkind.

We can see how character traits that support the idea of human flourishing can be overturned, if we return to Danielle's experience of seeing truth-telling being argued for as some sort of pre-eminent principle for guiding action. Telling the truth (being honest) is generally a good thing, and not only does it appear in some form in nursing codes; it is a principle supported by most ethical theories. For a deontologist, truth-telling would seem to be a prima facie (on first impression) obligation regardless of the consequences—so from a deontological perspective, despite the distress caused to the patient, telling the truth looks like it was the right thing to do. For the utilitarian wanting to act in terms of a good outcome, telling the truth might have been considered the right thing to do, if the belief was that an outcome in which the patient did not hold the false belief that her husband was alive, was the best outcome—but lying might also be considered as the right thing to do, if the best outcome is considered to be that the wife does not become distressed. The virtue ethicist would not hold onto either the deontological or the utilitarian approach but would want to deliberate about right action based on which action would be the virtuous action. Consequences and obligations—particularly role obligations—would, of course, enter into that deliberation but so too would the exercise of practical wisdom. Recognising that being brutal with the truth will likely cause unnecessary distress and might be regarded as callous or unkind, the virtue ethicist might devote more time to allowing the patient to come to understand what has happened to her husband: recognising also that being honest does not require being brutal with the truth but does require support and understanding. Danielle wonders how Belanna would have dealt with the situation. In asking this question, Danielle is asking the very question that virtue ethics considers appropriate in situations where what right action requires is not obvious, or in situations where, as here, actions supportive of the virtue of honesty might clash with actions supportive of the virtue of kindness.

Danielle admires Belanna and wants to try to become the type of nurse that Belanna is. This desire to be a particular type of nurse—a good nurse defined by pursuit of the virtues—is perhaps the first step in becoming that type of nurse and adopting a virtue ethics approach to practice. Danielle wants to develop her character so as to become a kind, honest, fair, courageous, and compassionate person. She may not find this easy at first, but if Aristotle is right in saying that by practicing being virtuous we can become virtuous, then Danielle will need to practice being, for example, kind, honest, fair, compassionate, and courageous. This will likely require vigilance in observing herself in action, honesty in reflecting on her actions, and humility in seeking feedback on her actions, until such time as her actions become characteristically kind, honest, fair, compassionate, and courageous—and she may not always get it right. Nobody is perfect and our fictitious Belanna may well be an unattainable ideal. Yet in striving to become virtuous, having an idealised picture of the virtuous nurse may help to guide actions in those situations when seemingly different virtue actions might clash or when it is not clear what should be done in a particular set of circumstances. In asking 'how would Belanna act?' Danielle would be learning to develop the practical wisdom that is the hallmark of the virtuous agent; and one day, perhaps, others may come to admire Danielle and seek first to imitate her ethical practice and then to become virtuous practitioners themselves.

The Situationist Argument Against Character

One of the central ideas of virtue ethics is that human beings have, and can develop, a persistent character that guides, or even determines, action. Situationists question this assumption and point to empirical research to support their contention that character has less effect on behaviour than does context. They claim that we are prone to misattribute human behaviours as expressions of character. They posit that this continuing triumph of belief over evidence leaves us vulnerable to misunderstanding the nature of moral behaviour, which in turn sustains a general belief that wrong doing is solely a matter of individual responsibility. The situationists point to, for example, Darley and Batson's (1973) Good Samaritan study (where a reduction in the amount of 'hurriness' rather than anything else was seen as the main factor predicting helping behaviour) and Zimbardo's (1971) Stanford prison experiment (where 'guards' and 'inmates' quickly fell into role specific and disturbingly harmful behaviours unrepresentative of their supposedly true and regular characters). Both studies powerfully illustrate the human tendency towards attribution failure, as both provide strong indications that behaviour is determined as least as much, if not more, by situation than by character alone. These experiments, and many like them, show not bad people doing bad things but regular, every day, flawed human beings doings things that are less or more helpful or less or more harmful—determined, at least in part, by the situation in which they find themselves.

Of course, nurses are ordinary everyday people too, and are capable of doing harmful things as the reports into the events of Mid-Staffordshire illustrate (Francis 2010, 2013). Here we have reports of nurses acting in callous, unhelpful, inconsiderate, and seemingly indifferent ways towards patients. While most commenters are quick to apportion blame to individual nurses, Paley (2014) argues for a recognition of the effect situation can have on people's behaviour before rushing in to lay responsibility solely at the feet of individual nurses. If Paley and the situationists are right, then the implication is that character may be less able to withstand circumstance than is generally imagined. If this is true, then the implications for nursing and for the idea of a virtue ethics are profound.

Using the Situationist Critique to Enhance the Development of Character

However, even if the situationists are right, this does not spell the end of character, or the end of a virtue ethics for nursing. On the contrary, an understanding of the corrosive effects of situation on character can be used to provide a platform from which a virtue ethics for nursing can be developed and from which individual nurses can cultivate appropriate virtue.

Situationists might argue that if we want people to act well (i.e. in fair, honest, courageous, caring, and compassionate ways), then all that is needed is to provide situations that encourage good action and discourage harmful action. So if an increase in Darley and Batson's hurriness equates with a reduction in helping behaviour, then the remedy should be obvious; an increase in helping behaviour can be facilitated by a reduction of hurriness. In other words, if there is sufficient nursing staff to ensure that nurses are not constantly hurrying from one task to the next in the context of a seemingly never-ending and always-expanding set of things to get done before the end of shift, then they will be less hurried and more likely to stop to check that, for example, Mrs. Patel has fresh water to drink or that Mr. Rwani has the help he needs to get to the bathroom. In this scheme, it matters not if the individual healthcare workers are fair, honest, courageous, caring, or compassionate individuals—all that matters is that when those workers are less distracted, less busy, less hassled, they are more likely to take notice of, and help, fellow human beings in distress. Some might argue that the utility value in arranging situations such that it is easier for people to act in fair, honest, courageous, caring, and compassionate ways is greater than that to be gained from attempts to inculcate those types of actions as dispositions in people, while leaving them at the mercy of situations in which acting in ways consistent with those dispositions is the difficult option.

But there is a caveat needed here. If we arrange situations to encourage right action, then we are not encouraging virtuous action so much as automated action. There is nothing wrong with this if it is action for the good except that, outside of the carefully controlled situation, those who only know how to act within the controlled situation will struggle to know what are good rather than harmful actions. They will be acting in a purely behavioural response-to-stimuli manner which does nothing to cultivate virtue. So situation alone will not assist in developing the type of practical wisdom envisaged in a virtue ethics of an Aristotelian kind. More will be needed, including a personal desire, to become a better person—a better nurse—one who has developed the character traits that tend towards, for example, kind and compassionate actions as matter of inclination.

Conclusion

In this chapter I have offered a glimpse of what it might mean to be a good nurse in the sense understood in terms of virtue ethics. I have hinted at what a virtue ethics for nursing might look like, and I have indicated how an individual nurse might begin to go about developing an appropriate set of virtues for nursing. Virtue ethics may not provide all the answers to nursing's pressing ethical problems, but as I have suggested in this chapter, neither do any of the other ethical approaches. I suppose from this it can be seen that I have pragmatic tendencies. At the very least, I believe that a case can be made for introducing virtue ethics into nursing, as a way of offsetting the worst excesses of the mere rule following tendencies of modern ethical theory and its principle-based offspring.

Among the criticisms of virtue ethics is its purported failure to provide action guidance. I hope that I have answered some part of that criticism by showing that a nurse who wishes to be kind, compassionate, caring, fair, honest, and so on, in their work as a nurse, can do so from the perspective of virtue ethics. One advantage I see in so doing is that the nurse with the virtues will tend to act in ways consistent with their character from inclination, rather than against inclination. That is, the need to pretend to be kind, for example, will diminish over time as being kind becomes part of the person, part of the nurse. And this, it seems to me, provides a genuineness that may become absent when following rules and principles without due regard for the potential negative effects on patients' and others' flourishing.

I have noted too that situationists argue that we are sometimes—perhaps even often—misled into thinking that people act from their character rather than from the forces of the situations in which they find themselves. In my view this does not detract from the value of a virtue ethics for nursing. Rather, it indicates that the next step in virtue ethics is to arrange situations so that both right action is the easiest thing to do *and* the development of virtue in practitioners is encouraged. So often our best intentions are constrained, sometimes corrupted, by situational factors outside of our control. If this is true, then it seems that what nurses need to focus on is to help create environments that are supportive rather than discouraging of the expression of the virtues in practice. But until this time individual nurses can use a virtue ethics of nursing to enhance ethical nursing practice in ways that are appropriate to their own particular spheres of influence. And to avoid the burden of thinking that each nurse must become the ideal virtuous nurse, remember that Belanna is a fiction used to illustrate an ideal, an ideal to which we might aspire rather than attain. After all, no one is perfect.

Key Learning Points
- The focus on character distinguishes virtue ethics from most other approaches to ethics.
- Acting in virtuous ways from inclination is consistent with calls for authenticity in nursing practice.
- Virtue ethics cannot answer all nursing's pressing ethical problems (but neither can any one other approach to ethics).
- Virtue ethics is implied in much of the language used by nursing's regulatory and professional bodies.
- Virtue ethics requires individuals to develop their character for the good.

References

Anscombe E (1958) Modern moral philosophy. Philosophy 33(124):1–19
Aristotle (1953) The Nicomachean ethics. Penguin, Harmondsworth
Armstrong AE (2007) Nursing ethics: a virtue-based approach. Palgrave, Basingstoke
Crisp R (2007) Roger Crisp. In: Peterson TS, Ryberg J (eds) Normative ethics: 5 questions. Automatic Press/VIP, pp 13–24
Darley JM, Batson CD (1973) "From Jerusalem to Jericho": a study of situational and dispositional variables in helping behaviour. J Pers Soc Psychol 27(1):100–108
Francis R (2010) Independent inquiry into care provided by Mid Staffordshire NHS Foundation Trust January 2005—March 2009. The Stationery Office, London
Francis R (2013) Report of the mid Staffordshire NHS foundation trust public inquiry. Executive summary. The Stationery Office, London
Hursthouse R (1997) Virtue theory and abortion. In: Statman D (ed) Virtue ethics: a critical reader. Edinburgh University Press, Edinburgh, pp 227–244
Lachman VD (2006) Applied ethics in nursing. Springer, New York
MacIntrye A (2007) After virtue: a study in moral theory, 3rd edn. University of Notre Dame Press, Notre Dame
NMC (Nursing and Midwifery Council) (2015/2018) The code. Standards of conduct, performance and ethics for nurses and midwives. Nursing and Midwifery Council, London. https://www.nmc.org.uk/standards/code/read-the-code-online/
Paley J (2014) Cognition and the compassion deficit: the social psychology of helping behaviour in nursing. Nurs Philos 14(4):274–287
Sellman D (1997) The virtues in the moral education of nurses: Florence Nightingale revisited. Nurs Ethics 4:3–11
Sellman D (2011) What makes a good nurse: why the virtues are important for nurses. Jessica Kingsley, London
Zimbardo PG (1971) Stanford prison experiment: a simulation study of the psychology of imprisonment conducted at Stanford University. https://www.prisonexp.org/. Accessed 21 May 2023

Care Ethics and Nursing Practice

Ann Gallagher

Abstract

Care ethics, also known as ethics of care, is one lens with which to view ethics as applied to nursing and care more generally. The beginning of this particular approach to ethics as applied to care is attributed to the work of Carol Gilligan and Nel Noddings in the early 1980s. Care ethics has evolved primarily in North America and Europe with different strands and input from philosophers and social scientists. This chapter traces the development of care ethics, summarises key elements, and focuses on the work of two theorists—Joan Tronto and Chris Gastmans—and the implications for nursing ethics. A short case study from an ethics education research project suggests the value of applying insights from care ethics to everyday practice situations. The strengths and limitations of care ethics are discussed, and it will be concluded that, whilst care ethics makes a valuable contribution to ethics as applied to care, other perspectives enhance this approach.

Keywords

Care ethics · Relationality · Vulnerability · Dependency · Dignity · Responsibility

Introduction

There has been scholarship on ethics as applied to care since the 1800s. Fowler (2016) points out that, from 1890 to the 1960s, approximately 50 texts were published on nursing ethics. Many of these were written by nurses, but some were authored by social workers, priests, or physicians. The topics within these texts are

A. Gallagher (✉)
Department of Health Sciences, Brunel University London, London, UK
e-mail: Ann.Gallagher@brunel.ac.uk

still relevant today, with discussions of confidentiality, truth-telling, the atmosphere of the hospital (what we would now refer to as ethical climate), and duties towards patients, the family, and the doctor and towards the nurse herself, her friends, her hospital and school, and other nurses. Fowler argues that early nursing ethics:

> ...effectively removes nursing's ethics from the realm of a "bedside ethics" alone to one that reaches into both the problems of society and the structure of society. These early requirements are the precursors to contemporary nurses' concern for health disparities. However, an examination of these historical requirements in social-ethical and social justice content, as well as the nursing ethics historical literature, indicates that nursing's perspectives on social justice do not align very well with the bioethical discourse on distributive justice and are far closer in spirit to the contemporary work by, Baier, Held, Kittay and colleagues [...] Tronto and others who look closely at structural inequalities far more broadly than concerns for the costs and access to healthcare. (Fowler 2016 p. 11)

Baier, Held, Kittay, and Tronto are but some of the leading theorists who have contributed to a particular approach to ethics as applied to care. This has become known as both 'care ethics' and 'ethics of care'. This one approach albeit with different varieties by different authors—primarily in Europe and the United States—emphasises the primacy of relationships of care. It is presented as remedying some of the deficits of bioethical approaches that focus on justice, principles, and professional detachment. It is, however, but one lens that illuminates ethical aspects of nursing and care practices more broadly.

In this chapter, I will provide an overview of the evolution of care ethics and an explanation of the 'core' elements of care ethics. I will discuss the implications of the work of two care ethics theorists—Joan Tronto and Chris Gastmans—for nursing practice and consider the potential of care ethics to throw light on ethical aspects of a care situation. I will conclude by summarising some of the strengths and limitations of care ethics.

The Evolution of Care Ethics

The beginning of care ethics is generally attributed to the publication of Carol Gilligan's book *In a Different Voice: Psychological Theory and Women's Development* in 1982. Whilst early writings from nurse scholars and from feminist and other philosophers (e.g. Mayeroff 1971) had features of care ethics, it was Gilligan's work that is credited with initiating the particular approach which has become known as both 'care ethics' and 'ethics of care'. Around the same time, Nel Noddings published *Caring: A Feminine Approach to Ethics* (1984) which had much in common with the themes identified by Gilligan and later care ethicists. Michael Slote (2007, p. 10) has argued that it was Noddings, rather than Gilligan, who 'was the first person to attempt to spell out an ethics of care'. Nevertheless, it is Gilligan who is most often referred to as the originator, and her research is most illuminating as background to the approach.

Gilligan's research challenged some of the findings of earlier work by American psychologist Lawrence Kohlberg and his perspective on stages of moral development. She reports findings from the presentation of a dilemma, devised by Kohlberg, to two 11-year-old children, Jake and Amy. They were asked to respond to a series of dilemmas including one where a man (Heinz) is considering whether to steal a drug to save the life of his wife and which he cannot pay for. Amy and Jake are asked to share their perspectives and arguments as to whether Heinz should steal the drug (Gilligan 1982, p. 25–26). Their responses provide insights regarding the structure of their moral thinking.

Gilligan explains how Jake proceeds to respond logically as he sees the problem as 'sort of like a math problem with humans' (p. 26). He constructs the problem as one of a conflict between 'the values of property and life' and concludes that Heinz should steal the drug. Jake was of a view that a judge 'should give Heinz the lightest possible sentence'. Amy, on the other hand, responded to the dilemma differently and appeared uncertain. She didn't think Heinz should steal the drug and wanted to explore other options, for example, borrowing the money for the drug or taking out a loan. Amy was mindful of the effect of a theft considering the consequences of stealing the drug: the life of Heinz's wife might be saved; however, he might then be imprisoned and unavailable to care for his wife. She thought they should have a conversation and try and find other ways to fund the drug (p. 28).

Gilligan points out that, unlike Jake, Amy does not see the dilemma as a maths problem but rather as 'a network of connection, a web of relationships that is sustained by a process of communication' (p. 32). Gilligan's analysis of the response highlights well the distinction between ethics as underpinned by logic and law and a 'different voice' of care. Amy's response suggests 'a world comprised of relationships rather than of people standing alone, a world that coheres through human connection rather than through systems of rules, she finds the puzzle in the dilemma to lie in the failure of the druggist to respond to the wife' (p. 29). Her approach is to consider resolving the situation through negotiation with the pharmacist or by appealing to other people who may be able to help.

Many examples discussed in Gilligan's text illustrate different ways of thinking about ethics. She suggests that men and women may assume a different approach to the moral life which creates 'misunderstanding which impede communication' (p. 173). Gilligan's work signals a shift from a focus on justice to one of networks of care and relationships.

We arrive at two distinct ethical perspectives set out in the conclusion to Gilligan's (1982) text (p. 174): an 'ethic of justice' is underpinned by equality, requiring that all be treated the same, whereas, an ethic of care is based on nonviolence, focusing on not hurting others. Gilligan writes that:

> .. *both perspectives converge in the realization that just as inequality adversely affects both partners in an unequal relationship, so too violence is destructive for everyone involved* (p. 174).

This dialogue between fairness and care not only provides a better understanding of relations amongst genders but also gives rise to a more comprehensive portrayal of adult work and family relationships.

Gilligan's early research and conclusions regarding two different approaches to ethics and moral development continue to be very influential. However, limitations of her research have also been highlighted. Tronto (1993), for example, points out that Gilligan's work does not challenge the boundary between private and public life and between justice and caring. An undesirable consequence is that relegating caring to private life it is considered to be outside the political realm and not considered as part of public life. Tronto argues that the work of Gilligan—and also that of Kohlberg—'maintain the position of the relatively privileged' (p. 96), whereas valuing care should be considered as both a moral *and* a political process.

Theories strengthening the idea that the ethics of care is a defensible alternative to an ethics of justice—or should be combined—have been developed by philosophers and feminists such as Tronto and Fisher (1991); Tronto (1993, 2013), Held (1993, 2006), Kittay (1999, 2002), and Ruddick (1989). In 2014, a series of lectures were convened at the Oxford Institute of Population Ageing and the Oxford Martin School, by Jaco Hoffman, Andries Baart, and Frans Vosman. The lectures marked 35 years of the care ethical theory development. The conveners recently reflected on progress and provided an update on the evolution of this approach in *The Ethics of Care: the State of the Art* (Vosman et al. 2020). The book includes contributions from international scholars on themes such as the role of emotions and politics of care, vulnerability and trust, realism in ethics, the social contract, empirically grounded ethics of care, and application to practices of care including social work and palliative care. The book contributes to 'the internationalisation of care ethics' (p. 3), which addresses critiques such as anthropocentrism of care ethics and the centrality of politics to care ethics: 'Care ethics uncovers the fact that caring and being cared for are practices that are crucially political in nature'.

In relation to nursing care specifically, ethicists such as Chris Gastmans, Per Norvedt, and Helen Kohlen continue to develop this approach.

It is not possible to do justice to the work of all of these care ethicists and philosophers, so I focus on two. Before discussing the contribution of Joan Tronto and Chris Gastmans—with reference to an aspect of Kittay's work—elements of care ethics will be discussed.

The Core of Care Ethics

There is much diversity in care ethics and many rich perspectives continue to be developed. It is difficult to determine exactly what is agreed as constituting the approach. Political theorist, Collins (2015), helpfully sets out a care 'slogan' and four claims. The slogan is 'dependency relationships generate responsibilities'. The four claims which, Collins argues, 'capture what is distinctive about care ethics' are detailed below with some suggestions as to how they relate to care practices and to other approaches to applied ethics:

Claim 1

'Ethical theory should positively endorse deliberation involving sympathy and direct attendance to concrete particulars'—this claim suggests a requirement fulfilled by most ethical perspectives with potential application to care practices. It seems unimaginable that an ethical theory could be worthy of consideration that accommodated unsympathetic and inattentiveness to concrete particulars. Ethical approaches that accommodate human sympathy and an emotional component of the moral life, such as virtue ethics, will also satisfy this claim.

Claim 2

'To the extent that they have value to the individuals involved, relationships ought to be (a) treated as moral paradigms,[1] (b) valued, preserved or promoted (as appropriate to the circumstance at hand) and (c) acknowledged as giving rise to weighty duties'.[2] The relational focus of care ethics is different to most other ethical approaches. It is not, for example, a focus of the four principles approach[3] or utilitarianism.[4] However, it is a key feature of 'relational ethics' (Pollard 2015; Austin 2006).

Claim 3

'Care ethics sometimes call for agents to have caring attitudes, that is, attitudes that: (1) have as their object something that has interests, or something that might affect something that has interests; and that (2) are a positive response (e.g. promoting, respecting, revering) to those interests; and that (3) lead the agent's affects, desires, decisions, attention, and so on to be influenced by how the agent believes things are going with the interest-bearer'. Care ethics in the context of care practices always calls for agents to have caring attitudes that focus on a positive response to the interests of others. This is an element that is, arguably, shared with virtue ethics[5] whereby the virtue of care is a moral disposition that contributes to the flourishing of the care recipient and the caregiver (Banks and Gallagher 2009).

---

[1] By 'moral paradigm' Collins (2015) means that caring relationships should be extended beyond relatives, that is, we should adopt the same kind of attitude to non-relatives (see page 35).

[2] For a discussion of the nurse–patient relationship as a lens to view the moral/ethical domain of nursing practice, please see Chap. 1.

[3] For a discussion of the four principles approach to ethical judgement and decision-making, please see Chap. 7.

[4] For a discussion on utilitarian approaches to ethical judgement and decision-making, please see Chap. 8.

[5] Please see Chap. 9 for an introduction to virtue ethics.

Claim 4

'Care ethics calls for agents to perform actions (1) that are performed under the (perhaps tacit) intention of fulfilling (or going some way to fulfilling) interest/s that the agent perceives some moral person (the recipient) to have; (2) where the strength of the demand is a complex function of the value of the intention, the likelihood that the actions will fulfil the interest, and the extent to which the interest is appropriately described as 'a need.' Responses to the needs of others, particularly those who are considered most vulnerable and dependent, is a central feature of care ethics and has to be, arguably, the focus of any ethical perspective applied to care. Approaches to ethics that can be described as teleological, with a *telos* or end in mind, have some similarities although the nature of the end aspired to will differ. In care ethics, Collins refers to interests and need. In utilitarianism, the end aspired to is happiness or the good of the majority.[6] In virtue ethics, the end aspired to is human flourishing (Banks and Gallagher 2009).

Collins goes on to argue that, whilst the four claims capture the distinctiveness of care ethics, they require an overall unifying principle. This is described as 'the Dependency Principle' which has four components: 'there is an important interest that is unfulfilled; an agent is sufficiently capable of fulfilling that interest; the agent's most efficacious measure is not too costly; and [...] the agent's fulfilling the interest would be the least costly of any agent's doing so' (p. 97).

The four claims as outlined by Collins present the core features of, and ethical justification for, care ethics. They can also be more fully fleshed out when considered in relation to the Dependency Principle (see Collins 2015 Chap. 8). However, they are somewhat elusive as normative prescriptions for everyday care practice and are not so clearly distinct from other approaches to ethics as applied to care. There are clearly similarities with virtue ethics and relational ethics, for example, and differences with autonomy-focused approaches to ethics. What is particularly valuable about care ethics is the recognition that care is crucially important and that any analysis of care requires both ethical and political insights. One of the most important care ethicists, Joan Tronto, brings her moral and political expertise to bear on care sharing insights and implications for individuals, organisations, and global communities.

Perspectives on Care Ethics: Joan Tronto

The year 2023 marked the 30th anniversary of Joan Tronto's (1993) text *Moral Boundaries*. Many of the features of Tronto's version of care ethics have direct and obvious implications for nursing and other care practices and have been discussed elsewhere, for example, in a text marking the 20th anniversary of *Moral Boundaries* (Gallagher 2014). Three features of Tronto's work are discussed here: her description of the phases of care and the ethical attitudes that accompany them, her

---

[6] For an introduction to Utilitarianism, please see Chap. 8.

discussion of the role of care and caregivers, and an explanation for unethical practice. First, let us look at the definition of 'care' proposed by Tronto and Fisher (1991, p. 40):

> *On the most general level, we suggest that caring be viewed as a species activity that includes everything that we do to maintain, continue and repair our "world" so that we can live in it as well as possible. That world includes our bodies, ourselves, and our environment, all of which we seek to interweave in a complex, life-sustaining web.*

Tronto (1993) points out that their definition intentionally highlights that caring includes caring for objects that are not human, that it is not restricted to individuals or 'dyads' but rather should be thought of as part of wider social networks, that it is 'defined culturally', and that it is ongoing. Tronto (1993, Chap. 4) outlines the initial four phases of care and the ethical attitude that accompanies each (Table 10.1).

Two additional phases of care were added by Tronto in other works. In her 2015 essay *Who Cares? How To Reshape a Democratic Politics,* Tronto writes (p. 14):

> *The first four phases of care imagined a citizen as someone who is attentive, responsible, competent and responsive: "caring with" imagines the entire polity of citizens engaged in a lifetime of commitment to and benefitting from these principles. "Caring with" is our new democratic ideal.*

This fifth phase of care involves trust and a feeling of solidarity with other citizens. Tronto goes further and redefines democracy:

> *Democracy is the allocation of caring responsibilities and assuring that everyone can participate in those allocations of care as completely as possible.* (Tronto, 2015 p. 15)

Banks (2021, p. 89–90) discusses a sixth phase, attributed to Tronto. which is 'the integrity of care', arguing that 'good care' requires the bringing together of the previous five phases. Judgements require the needs assessment in social, political, and personal contexts.

Table 10.1 Tronto's dimensions or phases of care

Dimensions/phases of care	Ethical attitude
Caring about—This involves the 'recognition that care is necessary' and includes concern, worry about someone or something. This could include making a donation to a charity where a need has been recognised	**Attentiveness**—Noticing need for care
Taking care of—This next step of the caring process involves taking responsibility for tasks relating to the provision of care and looking after someone. This could include arranging care for a child or elderly relative	**Responsibility**—To improve the situation of someone
Caregiving—The 'direct meeting of care needs' involves delivering care to someone and includes the activities of nurses and other caregivers	**Competence**—Having the knowledge, skills and values necessary to meet the goals of care
Care-receiving—This final phase of care focuses on the care recipient, on the difference care makes and on their response to care and their feedback	**Responsiveness**—Saying 'thank you', responding positively to care delivery

People 'care about' many issues, individuals, and artefacts; however, they may go no further than notice a need for care. 'Taking care of' requires more of an investment. It requires taking responsibility to improve the situation of another. This could involve making a donation to a charity or, more personally, making arrangements for a loved one to receive care from a domiciliary, residential, or day care facility. The third phase—'caregiving'—requires a direct engagement with care. It requires competence to deliver care adequately. The fourth phase of 'care-receiving' involves the responsiveness of those receiving care where, that is, they are able to provide a response. Those who are unconscious, who are psychotic, too young, or who have severe dementia may be unable to appreciate the experience of receiving care or to recognise the difference care makes.

Regarding the role of care and caregivers, Tronto (1993, p. 117) clearly articulates the importance and devaluation of care in society. Her view clearly also has a political dimension:

Care is difficult work, but it is the work that sustains life [...] The fact that care-givers can see an essential truth about the value of care, though, does not negate the fact that care is reduced to a lesser importance in society as a whole. When we look at the distribution of such rewards as money and prestige, it is clear that we value much else before care. (p. 179)

Tronto goes on to state that recognition of the value of care is a societal, moral and political priority and change needs to come about to realise this truth (p. 179).

Despite a recognition of the importance of care, it is sometimes the case that there are care deficits where care recipients are neglected, humiliated, and abused (Francis 2013; Bubb 2014). Some of these violations may arise, according to Tronto, when there are inadequate resources or when the caregivers' own needs are unmet. They may come to resent the care recipients they are charged with delivering care to. Tronto writes (Tronto 1993, p. 143):

[...] *care-givers are often enraged about their own unmet needs. If they are unable to recognise this rage, care-givers are likely to vent their anger on those for whom they care. Perhaps some rage is appropriate, but when it subverts the process of care itself, then it poses a serious moral problem.*

The theme of care deficits and mistreatment is also examined by Eva Feder Kittay (Kittay 2002), most particularly in relation to institutional care for those with learning disabilities. She argues that where caregivers are exploited, they may become 'victimisers' as well as victims. 'In such a society', she writes, 'care will be minimal, and callous caretakers will be inevitable' (p. 269). She goes on to say:

[...] *abusive behaviour by those who are charged with providing care is facilitated not only by the social devaluation of persons with mental disabilities, but also by the devaluation of the caregivers themselves. If we want to remove the prejudice and lack of understanding that blights the lives of people with mental retardation we can begin by treating their caregivers as if their work mattered (because it does) and as if they mattered (because they do).* (p. 270)

Kitay goes on to argue that caregivers need better work conditions, compensation, and encouragement to provide good care to care recipients.

Caring for the caregivers is an understandable and important priority. So too is understanding the reasons for unethical behaviour in care practices. This is particularly pressing in the light of recent high-profile care scandals. What is most helpful from the perspectives of Tronto and Kittay is the extension of explanations beyond individual blame to societal and political explanations. Tronto's (2013) recent work has developed what Barnes et al. (2015 p. 4) refer to as 'the political character of feminist virtue ethics'. The next section discusses the perspective of a European philosopher and theologian who is well-known for his work in nursing ethics.

Perspectives on Care Ethics: Chris Gastmans

Chris Gastmans has been actively involved in researching philosophical and empirical aspects of ethics as applied to care for over two decades. His research and scholarship have been influential in interpreting elements of care ethics for everyday nursing practice (see, e.g. Gastmans et al. 1998; Gastmans 1999, 2013; Vanlaere and Gastmans 2011). Three of his papers will be the focus of this section: collaborative work with de Casterlé and Schotsmans on nursing as a moral practice and the concepts of 'good care' (Gastmans et al. 1998), writing on 'dignity-enhancing care' (Gastmans 2013; Gomez-Virseda and Gastmant 2022).

In the 1998 article, Gastmans, de Casterlé, and Schotsmans develop a model for 'nursing considered as a moral practice' with three main components: the caring relationship (a condition of nursing practice), caring behaviour ('integration of virtue and expert activity), and 'good care' described as 'the final goal of nursing practice'. Regarding the caring relationship, Gastmans et al. (1998) discuss the perspectives of the nurse as caregiver and the care recipient. They write:

> *Caring generally can be considered as a specific way of relating oneself to the other in a relational context, with attention given to the maintenance and the development of the other (patient) and oneself (nurse).* (p. 49)

Gastmans and his co-authors emphasise the *otherness* of the patient and the importance of recognising the uniqueness and value of the patient with a view to helping him/her to grow and to maximise 'his or her own life development' (p. 49). An important feature of this discussion is the focus on self-care. It is argued that nurses need to care for themselves if they are to care well for patients. Building on the work of Tronto (1993) and Noddings (1984), they argue that care receivers play an important part in the way care is interpreted and judged in relation to their care needs. Caring behaviour, according to Gastmans et al. (1998), involves the integration of virtue (altruistic virtue of care with cognitive and affective-motivational features) and expert activity (including technical competencies).

Nursing is defined as:

[…] *a relation-based practice that is directed to providing good care to (usually sick) human beings.* (p. 52)

For Gastmans and his co-authors, 'good care' is the 'goal and foundation of nursing practice'. To better understand and illuminate what is meant by 'good care', they draw on European philosophical perspectives on 'being human' (p. 59). Their approach elaborates on six dimensions of the patient: the physical, the relational, the social, the psychological, the moral, and the spiritual. Understanding the concept of 'good care' is also described as requiring engagement with insights from psychology, philosophy, sociology, nursing, and medicine. Overall, then, nursing is described as a practice with three components: the caring relationship, the integration of virtue and expert activity, and 'good care as the goal of nursing practice'. Good care involves engagement with six dimensions. Gastmans and colleagues argue that:

> *Care is more than simply the sum of the various aspects that can be differentiated in the concept. A comprehensive description of good care involves a number of dimensions and is not simply the juxtaposition of detached properties and domains of thought. Constructing an ethical concept such as good care is impossible without drawing on data from the diverse human sciences such as philosophy, psychology, sociology, nursing science and medicine. But from an ethical point of view, the various components cannot be considered separately from each other—they influence and invoke each other.* (Gastmans et al. 1998, p. 66)

Another version of care ethics, proposed by Chris Gastmans, is described as 'dignity-enhancing care' (Gastmans 2013). Recent scholarship by Gómez-Vírseda and Gastmans (2022) has applied this approach to 'euthanasia in persons with advanced dementia'. The three core ideas or concepts of dignity-enhancing care are proposed as central: dignity, care, and vulnerability. Gastmans writes that much scholarship in medical ethics has focused on the four principles approach—respect for autonomy, beneficence, non-maleficence, and justice. However, this approach (principlism[7]) is concerned with questions such as 'what is to be done?' or 'what act or decision is to be taken? […] Gastmans argues that care does not involve isolated decisions but rather that those 'caring for patients go through a whole process of care'. He argues that we need to engage with three components: lived experience (vulnerability), interpretative dialogue (care process), and normative standard (dignity). These three components are aspects of an 'ethical framework to inspire our reflection on the ethical essence of nursing' (p. 146). Further interrogation is required in relation to each of these concepts, and some of this will be developed in the next section.

---

[7] For an introduction to principlism in nursing ethics, please see Chap. 7.

A Practice Situation: Case Study

The following is an example from focus group data relating to a care situation from a research project which evaluated three different approaches to ethics education for residential caregivers (Gallagher et al. 2017; Gallagher and Cox 2015). The residential caregivers assumed the role of care recipients, and care was delivered by student nurses. The context was a meal time where a care recipient attempted to eat a slice of cheesecake with the use of one hand:

> *I just kept picking up that whole entire thing where it was quite sticky and really gooey and it's cheesecake, I just want to plough in. And I just couldn't get anything. And before I'd realised it, her hand had just come across the table, she hadn't even looked at me, and she was just like that, and she just carried on talking. And just from that simple movement I was able to feed myself my cheesecake. And that was brilliant because there was not 'Oh do you want any help with that?' it was just a gentle little ... yeah, to make it blatant to everyone ... it was just a little slide of a hand, place the fingers on it and just carried on talking ... nobody ... I didn't actually even notice that she'd done it until I'd actually finished.* [RIPE project Focus group 5]

The student nurse caregiver shared her view of the same situation:

> *I didn't want to take away her ability to eat the cheesecake, cos I could have gone 'Give me the cheesecake, I'll help you' or you know 'Let me spoon it ...' I wanted to enable [care recipient] to eat her cheesecake herself, you know she had the ability to do it with her good hand. And I thought it would empower her more to eat the cheesecake herself and just have this ever so slight intervention.* [Focus group 5]

These two extracts provide an example of a caregiver assessing what the care recipient needed and acting in a way that she thought empowering. The caregiver acted spontaneously and non-verbally in response to a perceived need. From a care ethics point of view, it could be argued that the student caregiver was sensitive to the vulnerability of the care recipient and to the potential for indignity. As the care recipient suggested, her deficit was not made public, and attention was not drawn to it which could lead to a loss of dignity. In terms of the relevance of other care ethics concepts and dimensions, we might draw on Tronto's four phases of care, focusing on caregiving and care receiving and the associated 'attitudes' of competence and responsiveness.

In terms of the six dimensions of good care outlined by Gastmans et al. (1998), the physical, relational, and moral appear most pertinent. They point out that the provision of care to maintain and improve the patient's physical condition is an essential part of good care. They discuss the serving of meals explicitly:

> *Having a meal is more than the functional consumption of food for purely physical ends. The serving of meals in a health care institution is, in our opinion, a very important case in point that must be elevated above its merely nutritional function in order to maintain its human character [...]. By approaching the patient's body in a prudent and respectful way, nurses can bear witness to their own striving toward care and human dignity.* (p. 60)

The example also relates to the relational dimension where space needs to be made for the development of a caring relationship. As meals are taken, as in this case in a social context, there needs to be sensitivity as to how the intervention will be perceived by other care recipients. A subtle, non-verbal intervention appears attuned to the needs of the care recipient. As this example comes from a simulated care ethics education intervention, there may be a question of authenticity of the experience. However, both care recipient and caregiver were able to articulate the impact of the example as 'good care'. Concepts, then, such as vulnerability, dignity, care, competence, relationality, and responsiveness, appear to be applicable to this simulated practice example and resonate strongly with the care ethics literature. If this were to be considered through another ethical lens, different concepts may be considered, for example, the four principles' approach (Beauchamp and Childress 2013). The focus would then perhaps have been on respect for autonomy, weighing benefits with potential harms and justice. If we were to draw on a virtue ethics approach, virtues in addition to care could be considered such as prudence, respectfulness, and kindness.

Care Ethics and Nursing Ethics: Strengths and Limitations

The strengths of care ethics in relation to care practices seem obvious as it addresses fundamental ethical aspects of care. It is difficult to imagine how ethical discourse relating to care could proceed without reference to vulnerability, dignity, receptivity, and the concept and value of care itself. However, challenging aspects of the approach have also been discussed. Sander-Staudt (undated), for example, suggests six potential criticisms of care ethics: that it is a 'slave morality', that it is empirically flawed, that it is 'theoretically indistinct', that it is parochial, that it is essentialist, and that it is ambiguous.

- *Care ethics as a 'slave morality'*—Sander-Staudt advises that the term 'slave morality' is attributed to the philosopher Nietzsche who argued that people who are oppressed tend to 'develop moral theories that reaffirm subservient traits as virtues'. The view that care ethics supports the oppression of women is deserving of further attention. As Sander-Staudt states: 'This objection further implies that the voice of care may not be an authentic or empowering expression, but a product of false consciousness that equates moral maturity with self-sacrifice and self-effacement.'
- *Care ethics as empirically flawed*—This critique focuses on the robustness of Gilligan's research. It is alleged that her sample is too narrow and homogenous.
- *Care ethics as theoretically indistinct*—It has been argued that care ethics is not clearly distinct from other ethical approaches and shares many of the same values, for example, equality, autonomy, and justice. It has particular similarities with virtue ethics particularly when care is construed as a virtue.
- *Care ethics as parochial*—This criticism stems particularly from claims by Nel Noddings that care obligations were primarily to those who are close rather than

to distant people. There is a concern that 'without a broader sense of justice, care ethics may allow for cronyism and favouritism toward one's family and friends.'
- *Care ethics as essentialist*—There is criticism of a tendency within care ethics to focus on a 'dyadic model of a (caregiving) mother and a (care-receiving) child, on the grounds that it overly romanticises motherhood and does not adequately represent the vast experiences of individuals'. Differences within gender groups tend to be overlooked and the complexity of sexual identity and sexual orientation downplayed. Black and lesbian women, for example, are likely to be different to white heterosexual women. Recent discussions of the relationship between care ethics and 'intersectionality' (Ward 2015) engage constructively with this criticism.
- *Care ethics as ambiguous*—The accusation of ambiguity stems from the view that care ethics does not provide concrete guidance on what to do. In response to this criticism, Sander-Staudt points to a range of principles that are central to care ethics relating to, for example, the origin and fundamental need for care, the nature of care relations, and the 'scope of care distribution'.

Conclusion

Care ethics or ethics of care is an approach to ethics in care that continues to evolve with contributions from philosophers and social scientists. Although some theorists have chosen to focus on the gendered aspect of care ethics, most do not. Increasingly there is also a recognition that embracing care does not exclude a commitment to justice and that care needs to be considered in the public as well as in the private and professional domains, hence an emphasis on both the moral *and* political underpinnings of care. The six phases of care and accompanying attitudes identified by Joan Tronto and her discussion of the role of caregivers and explanations for unethical practice [along with Kittay (2002) provide helpful insights]. Chris Gastmans' discussion of 'good care' and 'dignity-enhancing care' can also be applied to everyday care situations. The six criticisms of care ethics discussed by Sander-Staudt (undated) need to be kept under review as the approach evolves.

As care ethics is currently an umbrella for a disparate range of theoretical accounts, it seems unlikely that it will replace well-established approaches such as the four principles' approach, deontology, utilitarianism, rights-based ethics, or virtue ethics. However, it is hoped that this chapter illustrates the richness of the concepts and elements that contribute to an understanding of 'good care'.

Key Learning Points
- There has been scholarship relating to ethics and care, most particularly nursing, since the mid-1800s.
- The beginning of 'care ethics'—also known as 'ethics of care'—is attributed to the work of Carol Gilligan and Nel Noddings in the early 1980s.
- The scholarship of Joan Tronto and Chris Gastmans has been highlighted as providing helpful insights that illuminate ethical aspects of everyday care.
- Six criticisms of care ethics, as presented by Sander-Staudt (undated), should be reflected on and discussed by all who consider the potential of care ethics as an effective applied ethics for everyday care.
- At this point, care ethics should not be considered as an alternative to other approaches to applied ethics in care but rather be seen as a rich approach that challenges more individualistic, gendered, and apolitical approaches.
- Care ethics continues to evolve and is likely to continue to contribute to our understanding of ethical and political dimensions of good care over the longer term.

References

Austin W (2006) Engagement in contemporary practice: a relational ethics perspective. Testo Contexto Enferm Florianopolis 15:135–141

Banks S (2021) Ethics and values in social work, 5th edn. Bloomsbury, London

Banks S, Gallagher A (2009) Ethics in professional life: virtues for health and social care. Palgrave Macmillan, Basingstoke

Barnes B, Brannelly T, Ward L, Ward N (eds) (2015) Ethics of care: critical advances in international perspective. Policy Press, Bristol

Beauchamp TL, Childress JF (2013) Principles of biomedical ethics, 7th edn. Oxford University Press, New York

Bubb S (2014) Winterbourne view—time for change: transforming the commissioning of services for people with learning disabilities and/or autism. https://www.england.nhs.uk/wp-content/uploads/2014/11/transforming-commissioning-services.pdf. Accessed 1 Oct 2016

Collins S (2015) The core of care ethics. Palgrave Macmillan, Basingstoke

Fowler M (2016) Heritage ethics: towards a thicker account of nursing ethics. Nurs Ethics 23(1):4–6

Francis R (2013) The mid-Staffordshire NHS Foundation Trust public inquiry: final report. http://webarchive.nationalarchives.gov.uk/20150407084003/http://www.midstaffspublicinquiry.com/report. Accessed 1 Oct 2016

Gallagher A (2014) Moral boundaries and nursing ethics. In: Olthuis G, Kohlen H, Heier J (eds) Moral boundaries redrawn: the significance of Joan Tronto's argument for political theory, professional ethics, and care as practice. Peeters, Leuven, pp 133–152

Gallagher A, Cox A (2015) The RIPE project protocol: researching interventions that promote ethics in social care working papers in the health sciences spring. http://www.southampton.ac.uk/assets/centresresearch/documents/wphs/AGRIPE.pdf

Gallagher A, Peacock M, Zasada M, Coucke T, Cox A, Janssens N (2017) Care-givers' reflections on an ethics education immersive simulation care experience: a series of epiphanous events. Nurs Inq 24(3):12174. https://doi.org/10.1111/nin.12174

Gastmans C (1999) Care as a moral attitude in nursing. Nurs Ethics 6(3):214–223
Gastmans C (2013) Dignity-enhancing nursing care: a foundational ethical framework. Nurs Ethics 20(2):142–149
Gastmans C, Dierckx de Casterlé B, Schotsmans P (1998) Nursing considered as moral practice: a philosophical–ethical interpretation of nursing. Kennedy Inst Ethics J 8(1):42–69
Gilligan C (1982) In a different voice: psychological theory and women's development. Harvard University Press, Cambridge
Gómez-Vírseda C, Gastmans C (2022) Euthanasia in persons with advanced dementia: a dignity-enhancing care approach. J Med Ethics 48(11):907–914. https://doi.org/10.1136/medethics-2021-107308
Held V (1993) Feminist morality: transforming culture, society and politics. University of Chicago Press, Chicago
Held V (2006) The ethics of care: personal, political and global. Oxford University Press, Oxford
Kittay EF (1999) Love's labour: essays on women, equality and dependency. Routledge, New York
Kittay EF (2002) When caring is just and justice is caring: justice and mental retardation. In: Kittay EF, Feder EK (eds) The subject of care: feminist perspectives on dependency. Rowman & Littlefield Publishers Inc., Lanham, pp 257–276
Mayeroff M (1971) On caring. Harper Perennial, New York
Noddings N (1984) Caring: a feminine approach to ethics and moral education. University of California Press, Berkeley
Pollard CI (2015) What is the right thing to do: use of a relational ethic framework to guide clinical decision-making. Int J Caring Sci 8(2):362–368. http://www.internationaljournalofcaringsciences.org/docs/13_pollard.pdf
Ruddick S (1989) Maternal thinking: toward a politics of peace. Bellentine Books, New York
Sander-Staudt M (undated) Care ethic internet encyclopedia of philosophy. http://www.iep.utm.edu/care-eth/
Slote M (2007) The ethics of care and empathy. Routledge, Oxon
Tronto JC (1993) Moral boundaries: a political argument for an ethic of care. Routledge, London
Tronto JC (2013) Caring democracy: markets, equality and justice. New York University Press, New York
Tronto J (2015) Who cares? How to reshape a democratic politics. Cornell University Press, Ithaca and London
Tronto JC, Fisher B (1991) Toward a feminist theory of care. In: Able E, Nelson M (eds) Circles of care: work and identity in women's lives'. State University of New York Press, Albany, p 40
Vanlaere L, Gastmans C (2011) To be is to care: a philosophical–ethical analysis of care with a view from nursing. In: Leget C, Gastmans C, Verkerk M (eds) Care, compassion and recognition: an ethical discussion. Peeters, Leuven, pp 15–31
Vosman F, Baart A, Hoffman J (eds) (2020) The ethics of care: the state of the art. Peeters, Leuven
Ward N (2015) Care ethics, intersectionality and post structuralism. In: Barnes B, Brannelly T, Ward L, Ward N (eds) Ethics of care: critical advances in international perspective. Policy Press, Bristol, pp 57–68

Part III

Ethical Issues in Caring for Specific Groups, and in Specific Contexts

Ethical Issues at the Beginning of Life

11

Janet Holt

Abstract

This chapter explores the ethical and legal issues faced when caring for pregnant women. A case study involving four women who have used or are contemplating using reproductive technologies forms the basis of the chapter to illustrate and discuss the issues raised. The issue at the heart of the debate is the question of when life begins and what sort of status we should afford to the entity that develops from a fertilised ovum through various stages to be a fully formed baby. Beginning with an exploration of this concept of when life begins and begins to matter, assisted conception, surrogacy, and prenatal diagnosis are discussed. This is followed by a consideration of the notion of choosing children including the creation of saviour siblings. The final section of the chapter considers the complex ethical issue of abortion particularly on the grounds of foetal abnormality. Differing views on the moral status of the embryo are explored along with common reasons for justifying abortion. The chapter concludes with a glimpse into the future, with an examination of new and emerging technologies.

Keywords

Assisted conception · Abortion · Prenatal diagnosis · Saviour siblings

Introduction (Including Case Study)

Over the last 50 years, technological advances and new treatments have been developed in the care of pregnant women. There have also been changes in the law to allow abortion under some circumstances and sophisticated treatments for

J. Holt (✉)
School of Healthcare, University of Leeds, Leeds, UK
e-mail: hcsjh@leeds.ac.uk

© The Author(s), under exclusive license to Springer Nature Switzerland AG 2024
P. A. Scott, S. M. Scott (eds.), *Key Concepts and Issues in Nursing Ethics*,
https://doi.org/10.1007/978-3-031-54108-7_11

infertility, all of which give rise to ethical questions focusing on the very essence of human life. Beginning with a discussion of when life begins, this chapter will explore some of the ethical issues in contemporary healthcare including assisted conception, surrogacy, prenatal diagnosis, the creation of saviour siblings, and the controversial subject of abortion. A case study involving four women in different stages of their reproductive lives will be used to illustrate and inform the debate. The chapter concludes with a consideration of new and potentially controversial techniques emerging in reproductive medicine.

Clare, Saadia, Ruth, and Liz are friends who were at secondary school together over 10 years ago. They now live in different parts of the country but meet up for a reunion every year. At their most recent meeting, two of the friends are pregnant, Clare with her first child and Saadia with her second. Saadia knows that the baby is a boy who they are going to name Amir. Saadia's first child, Yusuf, now 4 years old, was born with beta thalassaemia, an inherited condition which means that he has to have regular blood transfusions. Saadia explains that she had undergone IVF (in vitro fertilisation) in this pregnancy to ensure that her baby would be a tissue match for Yusuf. Immediately after birth some blood will be taken from the umbilical cord and the cells in it used to treat Yusuf and hopefully cure his condition.

Clare is in the early stages of her pregnancy and tells her friends that she is worried about the tests she has recently had to exclude foetal abnormality. Clare has a brother with Down's syndrome and knows how difficult her parents found caring for a disabled child. But she is very uncomfortable with the idea of termination and says she doesn't know what she would do if she was told there was something wrong with her baby. Liz, who has had four children in 6 years, is adamant that she wouldn't want another child and says that she just couldn't cope. While she understands Clare's views, she says she wouldn't be concerned at all about having a termination and thinks that it is her right as a woman to have this choice.

Ruth tells her friends that she hadn't planned to have any more children, feeling that her family is complete with the two she has. But recently her sister has undergone treatment for breast cancer and has been advised to freeze some of her eggs as the treatment is likely to affect her fertility. Ruth asks her friends what they think about surrogacy and wonders if she should offer to have a child for her sister.

The women in this scenario face a number of challenges concerning the way in which they view the moral status of the foetus, the use of assisted conception and prenatal diagnosis, the creation of saviour siblings, and the ethical dilemma of abortion. Central to all of these and other ethical problems in reproductive technology is the fundamental question of when life begins; this is where we will begin this exploration.

When Does Life Begin?

There are several different claims about when human life comes into existence. These claims are important as they are relevant to the question of what status should be afforded to the human embryo and ultimately what can be done to it. For some people, life begins at conception, that is, when the sperm fuses with a mature ovum to form the early embryo. In many respect this is the most obvious point to identify as the beginning of life, as the fertilisation of the ovum by the sperm, each containing 23 chromosomes, causes the creation of a new life. For some people this means that the embryo, from the moment of conception, should have the same degree of protection as any other human being.

But fertilisation does not always produce an embryo, and on rare occasions (approximately 1 in 700–800 pregnancies per year), the fertilised ovum does not develop normally, and while there is a mass of rapidly growing cells called a hydatidiform mole, no embryo develops. As a molar pregnancy is likely to develop into a choriocarcinoma,[1] it is usually removed as soon as a diagnosis has been made. To suggest that the mole should not be removed would be a difficult argument to sustain, firstly because there is no embryo and, secondly, because of the potential dangers of not removing it. We cannot even describe a fertilised ovum as being the beginning of a unique new life, as there is still a possibility of twins being formed from the single fertilised ovum as late as 2 weeks following conception. Nevertheless people holding what are described as pro-life views, such as members of the Society for the Protection of Unborn Children (SPUC), unequivocally state that life begins at conception because at that point "Human life begins at fertilisation.... Once fertilisation has taken place, the new cell conceived by mother and father, is a new human being with a complete genome" (Society for the Protection of Unborn Children 2023).

Before the advent of ultrasound, much significance was placed on the first time a woman felt the foetus move, usually around 16–20 weeks. Reference to foetal movements can be found in the Gospel of Luke in the Bible. Luke describes a meeting between Mary, pregnant with Jesus, and Elizabeth who was pregnant with John the Baptist. On hearing Mary's voice, Elizabeth says that "the babe leaped within her womb" (Luke 1:41 Holy Bible 2023). It is not surprising that this was associated with the beginning of life as a moving foetus clearly indicated a "live" foetus. In traditional Roman Catholic theology, the first foetal movements had even more significance, in that they indicated the moment when the soul is created in the embryo. Aristotle believed that a male body was formed at 40 days but that of a female took 90 days to be formed. Thomas Aquinas, a thirteenth-century theologian developed Aristotle's theory further by proposing that God creates the soul within the embryo at 40 days for males and 90 days for females (Gillon 2001). From this we can conclude that for Aquinas, male foetuses were valuable at an earlier stage than female ones. While a moving foetus is undeniably a "live" foetus, modern ultrasound techniques show foetal movements are present much earlier in pregnancy than when the woman begins to feel them, or than suggested in historical accounts.

In 1984 an influential committee chaired by Dame Mary Warnock debated the ethical and social implications of infertility treatment and embryo research following the birth of the first "test tube baby" (Department of Health and Social Security (DHSS) 1984). An important point to emerge was the significance of the primitive

---

[1] A fast-growing cancer in the uterus originating in tissue that would normally form the placenta.

streak, that is, the beginning of the individual biological development of the embryo and the last point at which twinning can occur. The primitive streak represents early development of cells that will develop into neural tissue, the very first stages of the nervous system, and hence the root of consciousness. As the primitive streak develops on day 15, one of the Committee's recommendations was that embryo research should only be allowed up to 14 days after fertilisation. However, the International Society for Stem Cell Research (ISSCR) has recently discussed setting aside the 14-day rule and extend culture of human embryos beyond this time period. But setting new guidelines has proven to be problematic as scientists and ethicists in ISSCR to date have been unable to reach a consensus on the format (Adashi and Cohen 2022). While ensuring experimentation would only be carried out on embryos before the appearance of any neural tissue, this could be interpreted as meaning that embryos up to this point are seen to be less valuable than those over 14 days.

Even if it is not possible to argue that life definitely begins at conception and that a new individual is created at that point, it does still seem plausible to recognise the importance of conception. Following this line of argument, we might say that while there is a continuum of human development, the embryo even in the earliest stages has the genetic material of a human and, given the right conditions, will develop into a human being. Therefore, the embryo should be afforded the same rights and protection as any human being. This is called the potentiality argument.

Harris (1985) points to two problems with this argument. Firstly, the fact that something will become X is not a good reason for treating it now as if it were X. For example, an acorn, given the correct conditions has the potential to grow into an oak tree but does this mean that we should treat an acorn the same as an oak tree? Or to put it another way, do you think that squashing an acorn is the same as cutting down an oak tree that is a 100 years old? Even using acorns and oak trees as the example still has a moral nuance. We may have more reservations about cutting down an ancient tree without due cause than standing on the acorn accidentally or otherwise. The second problem relates to the ova and sperm individually, as clearly they too have the potential to become human beings. Generally speaking we do not take much care over the fate of "unwanted" ova or sperm. However, following the potentiality argument methods of contraception that destroy ova and/or sperm could be deemed morally wrong, and Roman Catholics, for example, have teaching forbidding the use of contraception based upon this argument.

When Does Life Begin to Matter?

The development of the fertilised ovum into an embryo, foetus, and ultimately a baby, can be thought of as a continuum with stages that merge into each other. Therefore, rather than trying to answer the question "when does life begin", a different approach is to ask "when does life begin to matter". We have already seen that the emergence of the primitive streak is a biological event which marks the development of neurological tissues, and the emergence of the sentient being[2] is linked to this concept. Singer (2012) argues that if a sentient being, human or non-human, can feel pain or distress, then its interests should be given the same consideration as any other human being. So if hurting or destroying sentient beings is considered to be wrong, then sentient beings should not be harmed. However, non-sentient beings cannot be harmed by their destruction as they do not have the capacity to feel pleasure or pain and thus cannot be harmed. Based on sentience, abortion and embryo research are legitimate as long as the embryo cannot feel any pain; as the argument from sentience only prohibits hurting the sentient entity but does not offer absolute protection.

Leaving biological definitions and sentience to one side, a far more complex issue, and one of the most influential philosophical arguments about when life begins to matter, is that of the recognition of self or personhood. The precise meaning is hard to define, but personhood is essentially the things that make us human, or the combination of beliefs, desires, and aspects of personality that make us who we are. From as early as the seventieth century, this has been described as a combination of rationality and self-consciousness (Locke 1997). More recently and directly related to abortion and infanticide, Michael Tooley defined the criterion for personhood as an organism that "possesses the concept of a self as a continuing subject of experiences and other mental states, and believes that it is itself such a continuing entity" (Tooley 1972, p. 29). So for Tooley, in order to have a claim to a right to life, the person must be able to recognise themselves as the same being over time. Therefore, killing a person is wrong as it removes from the individual something they are able to value; but using this distinction, individuals who cannot value their own existence cannot be wronged by killing as they are not deprived of something they are capable of valuing. While this may be a persuasive argument, a key problem with defining personhood as a combination of rationality and self-consciousness is that foetuses, babies, some adults with learning disabilities, those in a permanent vegetative state, and even some with other cognitive disorders such as dementia may not be classified as persons.

Having explored some of the differing views on when life begins and begins to matter, we will now turn to some of the contemporary uses of reproductive technologies and the ethical questions that face Clare, Saadia, Ruth, and Liz. To ensure a tissue match for her son with beta thalassaemia, Saadia has become pregnant using in vitro fertilisation (IVF), while Ruth is considering being a surrogate for her sister's baby.

Assisted Conception

Since the birth of Louise Brown, the first "test tube" baby, in 1978, increasingly sophisticated techniques to assist conception have been developed. Some forms of treatment, such as those that solely use medication, are not usually considered

---

[2] A sentient being is one that can feel pleasure or pain.

controversial. However, other techniques, such as the use of donor sperm and/or ova, IVF, and surrogacy, do raise ethical problems. Opinions on the morality of assisted conception rest on an individual's view of the moral status of the embryo. The idea of creating a life in vitro is considered to be unnatural, and, unsurprisingly, those who hold pro-life views are generally opposed to IVF. What lies at the heart of this debate is whether infertility is considered a disease to be treated the same as any other condition. At the very least, infertility is a malfunction of part of the body much in the way that diabetes is. Treatment of diabetes with insulin, like many other medications, may also be considered unnatural; yet we would not consider this to be a sufficient reason to deny someone having insulin. But while infertility might be thought of as a malfunction of the body, unlike diabetes, the treatment is not life-saving. However, infertility is a cause of suffering and misery to those unable to have much wanted children. There is also the added problem that the treatment is concerned with creating embryos, not all of which will be used. Those that are not may be discarded or used in research. Despite some moral objections to the assisted conception process, it is widely utilised. The Human Fertilisation and Embryology Authority began collecting data in 2019 and since then 1.3 million IVF cycles, and over 26,000 donor insemination cycles have been performed resulting in the birth of 390,000 babies (HFEA 2023).

In the scenario, Ruth's sister is facing infertility because of her cancer treatment, and Ruth wonders if she should offer to have a baby for her. In the UK surrogacy is lawful if, by using IVF, an embryo is created using the ova and sperm of the intended parents. As Ruth's sister will have some of her ova frozen, this is the process they will most likely use. Therefore, Ruth will have the embryo created from her sister and partner's sperm implanted into Ruth's uterus. Surrogacy can also occur when a donated ovum is fertilised with the intended father's sperm, using an embryo created using a donor ovum and sperm, or when the surrogate's ovum is fertilised with the intended father's sperm, usually using the more straightforward process of artificial insemination. In the UK surrogacy is regulated by the Surrogacy Arrangements Act 1985, and while a surrogate can be paid reasonable expenses, engaging in a commercial surrogacy arrangement, where the surrogate is paid for the service, is a criminal act (Hoppe and Miola 2014).

While Ruth can be a surrogate for her sister, she would need to consider that not all of the process is legally enforceable. So while Ruth as the person who carries the child will be the birth mother, if she is married, her husband will be assumed to be the father. Furthermore, Ruth is entitled to change her mind once the baby is born and not give the child to her sister. Similarly, her sister may decide that she does not want the child after all and Ruth will then have to keep it. At some stage Ruth and her sister will have to decide what the child is going to be told about the manner of his or her conception and all members of the family will need to understand and agree to this. Ruth may develop a strong attachment to the child and still feel it in some way belongs to her, all of which could upset family dynamics. Conversely the bonds that have developed between Ruth, her sister, and the child might strengthen their relationships. So while Ruth and her sister will enter into a form of contract, much of it is based on trust. Keeping the arrangement in the family might help to establish that trust, but the act is one of altruism and not without complications.

Ruth will also have to decide, possibly in conjunction with her sister, if she will undergo screening tests for foetal abnormality and what they will do should the tests show something wrong with the baby. Clare has already undergone a series of tests and is now anxiously waiting for the results. In the next section, we consider the ethical problems that women like Clare and Ruth face in undergoing prenatal diagnosis.

Prenatal Diagnosis

All women in Ireland and the UK are offered screening tests in pregnancy, to detect foetal abnormality. These usually take the form of blood tests and ultrasound scans. Thus women are given a choice about the tests they want to have and can, if they wish, refuse to have any tests altogether. Until very recently the blood tests taken to detect foetal abnormalities such as Down's syndrome were not very accurate and only gave women a ratio of the likelihood of the foetus being affected. Any woman thought to be at risk was then offered an amniocentesis. This is an invasive procedure where fluid is extracted from the amniotic sac surrounding the foetus and the cells contained within it examined. But now a noninvasive prenatal blood test (NIPT) is available to test for genetic conditions as early as 10 weeks into the pregnancy. These tests are much more accurate and substantially reduce the number of women who need to proceed to amniocentesis with its accompanying risk of miscarriage. In January 2016, the UK National Screening Committee recommended that the test be made available to women in the UK. Research into the benefits and costs published in April 2016 (Chitty et al. 2016) claimed the test to be cost-effective and offering improved quality of care and choice for women. From September 2021 NIPT is available through the NHS to test for Down's, Edward's, and Patau's syndromes but only following a higher chance result for Down's syndrome or a joint higher chance result for Edward's and Patau's syndromes from an NHS combined test. It can also be offered if there is a higher chance result for Down's syndrome from an NHS quadruple test.

However, offering easier and noninvasive tests does raise ethical issues. Prenatal testing for some women inevitably leads to difficult decisions about what to do if an abnormality is detected. There is usually no treatment for the foetus in utero, and the woman is faced with the choice of continuing with the pregnancy or having an abortion. This is the dilemma facing Clare in the scenario. If Clare is told her baby has an abnormality such as Down's syndrome, she would be given a choice to continue or to terminate the pregnancy. Giving women the choice respects autonomy and, assuming Clare has capacity, to do otherwise would be legally and morally indefensible. However, this is a very difficult decision to make, and both choices have associated problems. Clare can decide to have an abortion, but evidence shows that while termination of unwanted or unplanned pregnancies are rarely accompanied by psychological and social problems, terminations carried out on the grounds of foetal abnormality are different. These are often planned and wanted pregnancies, and typically termination is carried out later in pregnancy; when the termination is more difficult to cope with and obvious to family and friends (Gonzalez-Ramos et al. 2021). If Clare decides to continue with the pregnancy, she faces an uncertain future having personal experience of how difficult caring for a child with disabilities can be.

It is plausible that women may agree to tests, particularly those that are noninvasive such as NIPT and ultrasound scans, without fully considering the potential outcomes. A recent literature review, exploring-decision making factors in prenatal testing, identified that attitudes towards abortion play a significant role in deciding whether to have prenatal testing (Di Mattei et al. 2021). In this review of 46 papers, women who were more likely to have an abortion were also more likely to undergo prenatal testing. However, the authors also note that some women do undergo prenatal testing in order to prepare for a child born with a genetic abnormality. So while making a decision to continue with a pregnancy or not is described as a "choice", it maybe one that women like Clare would prefer not to make at all. Perhaps the notion of choice regarding termination is misplaced and would be better considered before any testing takes place. In this way, women could freely enter into the testing process being clear that they not only have a choice about having the tests but also, depending on the results, what this may lead to. Currently, this seems even more important with more widespread use of NIPTs in antenatal care.

For many women the idea of not giving birth to a child with disabilities is a benefit, but others express concerns about prenatal screening programmes being 'seek and destroy' missions and a form of eugenics. Because of its history, eugenics, the practice of genetically improving humans, is generally considered to be a bad thing. Selgelid (2014), however, argues that while prenatal diagnosis in some respects does fit the criteria of eugenics, for those not opposed to abortion on moral grounds, eugenics per se is not necessarily a bad thing. Advocating an approach far removed from the state-controlled policies of the past, Selgelid describes an era of new genetics where individuals freely choose to have prenatal diagnosis and act on the information obtained from the tests, a position that he considers to be entirely different to past coercive practices, such as state-sponsored sterilisation of people with undesirable genetic traits. Nevertheless, despite legislation to ensure equality in our society, there are still concerns that wider use and availability of prenatal genetic testing could make life difficult for people with disabilities. Abortion following prenatal diagnosis has been described as expressing discriminatory attitudes not just about the condition but also about those who have it (Dufner 2021). Therefore, abortion on the grounds of foetal abnormality could result in fewer people with disabilities being born. Also, those whose birth could have been prevented, by the use of prenatal diagnosis and selective abortion, could be considered less valuable and more vulnerable to prejudice and discrimination.

Saviour Siblings

Where there is a known genetic or inherited condition, an alternative to prenatal testing and termination is to offer the woman IVF with preimplantation genetic testing (PGT), so that only healthy embryos are implanted into the uterus. Saadia has undergone this procedure to ensure that her second child will not only be free of the inherited disease but will also be a tissue match for Yusuf. This is known as the creation of a saviour sibling. In the UK, the Human Fertilisation and Embryology Act 2008 allows saviour sibling selection as long as the recipient has a serious medical condition which can be treated by cord blood, bone marrow or other tissues (Human Fertilisation and Embryology Authority 2021).

The advantage for Saadia is that no harm will be done to her baby and the cord blood containing stem cells may be the only hope of a cure for Yusuf. A further advantage is that the embryo selection takes place prior to implantation. The cells for testing are removed 2–3 days after conception, so the embryo is in a very early stage of development. As discussed above, for some people, the embryo at this stage has less value, and therefore this process is morally more preferable than an abortion at a later stage in the pregnancy. Of course this is not the case for those who believe that life begins at conception, and such individuals would raise objections to this process seeing it as morally no different to an abortion.

Saadia has been fortunate in that an embryo has been successfully created that is a tissue match for Yusuf. But this does not always happen, and there have been cases where despite repeated attempts, a tissue match has not been achieved. There is also the problem of what to tell Amir about the manner and reason for his birth. Opponents of saviour siblings argue that the process reduces children to a commodity and thus not considered as ends in themselves.[3] Amir may feel that his parents did not want him for his own sake, but given the lengths his parents went to, this could suggest they are committed parents. Therefore there seems no reason to suspect that Amir will not be loved as much as Yusuf. Indeed it could be argued that, as he has been so instrumental in the treatment of his brother, he may feel particularly valuable and loved. But there is the possibility that the treatment does not work and that Amir is unable to save Yusuf. Or that he feels pressurised into further and more complex donations such as bone marrow at a later date which could cause psychological harm. To date there are no published findings of the psychological impact of being a saviour sibling so we can only speculate; but it should be noted that to object to saviour siblings on the grounds of potential psychological harm is a different argument from the pro-life objection to the artificial creation and section of embryos.

---

[3] The requirement to consider persons as "ends in themselves", as fundamental to the principle of respect for persons, is an important element of Kantian ethics.

Choosing Children

One of the problems in allowing preimplantation genetic testing (PGT) is the concern that it will not stay restricted to avoiding disease but lead to allowing individuals to choose other characteristics of their child such as the gender, IQ, or hair colour. With the mapping of the human genome, in the future it may be possible to test an embryo for a number of traits and characteristics that we could select to enhance our potential children. Savulescu (2001), for example, draws no distinction between treatment for disease and enhancement and argues that if one is morally permissible, then so the other should be. Savulescu develops his argument further to say that in the future if such a thing was possible, genetics tests should be used to only select children expected to have the best life possible, which may include a high IQ, an aptitude to play a musical instrument, or achieve sporting prowess. However, giving people the freedom to choose their children in this way could lead to further ethical problems. For example, what if a couple decides they wanted to deliberately create a child with a disability as happened in the USA in 1996. In this case a deaf lesbian couple wanted to have deaf child, so selected a congenitally deaf man as a sperm donor to maximise their chances of this occurring (Wilkinson 2010). Here, the couple took matters into their own hands and achieved the pregnancy without using health services. But suppose a couple asked health providers to do this using IVF and PGT. In order to respect their freedom of choice, would health professionals have to comply with their wishes? Of course it would be possible to enact legislation to prevent unrestrained choices, but even within the constraints of the current techniques, individuals do not have absolute freedom. For example, it is possible to test for sex, but individuals using IVF and PGT are not allowed to select an embryo just on sex alone.

There are a number of objections to the practice of choosing children, not least of which are the inequalities that would potentially occur in society. Children could be created who would have an unfair advantage over others. Also, in a publicly funded healthcare system, it is unlikely that all individuals would be able to access what would undoubtedly be expensive procedures. Therefore, only people with the ability to pay may be able to choose their children, creating an elite and potentially entirely different species; with the children of the poor unable to compete with the enhanced children of the rich (Bostrom 2012). While we can only speculate what the consequences of improvements in scientific techniques might be, we can be sure that that this will give rise to many ethical problems in the future.

The process of IVF and PGT that Saadia has undergone has resulted in a positive outcome, creating a foetus with a tissue match for Yusuf. But for Clare and Ruth, the situation could be very different. Should the tests indicate some form of foetal abnormality, they will be faced with the difficult choice of either continuing with the pregnancy, and possibly giving birth to a baby with disabilities, or ending the pregnancy with an induced abortion.

Abortion

One of the most profound and divisive ethical dilemmas is that of abortion. Historically, abortion has been governed by different legislation across the four countries of the UK. Since 1967 in England, Scotland, and Wales, abortion is a criminal act unless carried out under the grounds of the Abortion Act 1967 (amended by the Human Fertilisation and Embryology Act 1990) (Hoppe and Miola 2014). It is important to consider abortion in this way as abortion is not available to women on demand. Termination of a pregnancy is lawful when there is substantial risk of a child being born with physical or mental abnormality, and while for the other clauses there is a time limit of 24 weeks gestation, in cases of foetal abnormity there is no time limit (Hoppe and Miola 2014). Up until 2019, abortion was unlawful in Northern Ireland (with very few exceptions), but changes in legislation decriminalised the procedure, and The Abortion (Northern Ireland) Regulations came into force in March 2020 in line with the rest of the UK. The Republic of Ireland had one of the most restrictive bans on abortion in the European Union, but in 2018 this was overturned in a public referendum allowing abortion up to 12 weeks of pregnancy and after 12 weeks in some exceptional circumstances including foetal abnormality.

Notwithstanding the law, moral opinion on abortion is sharply divided with opposing views described as pro-life and pro-choice. In a nationally representative sample of members of the general public, there are likely to be few people who believe that abortion should never be carried out in any circumstance, or that it should be freely available on demand at any stage of pregnancy. But there are likely many with more nuanced views. For example, an individual may consider themselves to be largely pro-life but agree that abortion should be allowed in cases of rape, or if there is foetal abnormality. Others may lean more towards a pro-choice stance but feel it important that there should be an upper time limit in pregnancy, after which it should not be allowed. Essentially the foundation for the opinions lies in the debate on the moral status of the embryo and foetus, discussed at the beginning of the chapter; those who believe that life begins at conception generally oppose abortion at any point in the pregnancy. Holding a more nuanced view of abortion can however be very complicated. If, for example, an individual believes that life begins at conception, they would need to be able to argue why the manner of conception, i.e. rape, is relevant and can be used to justify killing the foetus. With modern visualisation techniques, the appearance and movement of embryos and foetuses can be easily shown, and there can be no doubt that abortion does mean killing the entity. However, the crucial issue for those who agree with abortion is being able to justify on moral grounds that it is the more preferable course of action.

Some arguments for and against abortion are rights-based with the woman's right to choose in opposition to the foetus's claim to a right to life. The arguments here focus on moral rights, as in law a foetus is not afforded any rights while still in utero. In the scenario Liz shows no reservations about abortion and says she believes it is her right as a woman to have the choice. Liz may believe that the foetus isn't an independent entity and simply part of the woman's body and therefore she has the right to make any decisions about what happens to it. This is the line taken in a famous paper *In Defense of Abortion*, published in 1971 by Judith Jarvis Thomson. Through a series of thought experiments, Thomson asks the reader to imagine waking up to find that a famous violinist has been plugged into your kidneys for 9 months of life support (Thomson 1971). Thomson concludes that the foetus's right to life does not override a pregnant woman's right to control her own body and, thus, abortion is permissible.

Clare on the other hand is apprehensive about the thought of abortion, and even though she recognises that the foetus does not have legal rights, she feels that it is a gradually developing entity and can't distinguish between one stage of its development and the next. Clare thinks of the foetus she is carrying already in terms of being a baby, with the same moral status and right to protection as herself. Although her situation is complicated by the results of the prenatal diagnostic tests, the heart of the matter is still the same. If Clare firmly believes that a foetus has a right to life irrespective of any disabilities, she is unlikely to change her mind about this should the tests prove to be positive. This is the root of the complex problem of abortion, where individuals disagree on whether abortion is a matter of personal choice for a woman, or, that a foetus, as a potential person, has the right to life and should not be killed in any (or at least in very few, carefully defined) circumstances. Despite a vast philosophical, theological, and clinical literature on the subject, it seems impossible that a definitive solution will ever be found to satisfy both the supporters and opponents of abortion.

The Future

This is a fast-moving area with scientists and clinicians working on new and improved techniques such as NIPTs and gene editing on early embryos. This technique, approved by the HFEA in February 2016 for research purposes, has the aim of preventing miscarriage and increasing IVF success, though greater understanding of early embryo development. CRISPR (clustered regularly interspaced short palindromic repeats) technology, for example, used in gene editing has the potential to be used in treating diseases, gene therapy to eliminate inherited conditions, and the production of vaccines. The Nuffield Council (Nuffield Council on Bioethics 2016) identifies a number of ethical issues in its use and aims to develop advice, conclusions, and recommendations. For example, recent work with animals in laboratory conditions has resulted in cloning 581 mice from a single cell, and using the technique of parthenogenesis, mice have been successfully created from unfertilised mouse eggs without using sperm (Loike and Kadish 2022).

Cases of postmenopausal women becoming pregnant through IVF, while rare, are reported in women as old as 72 (Marszal 2016), while the HFEA reports an increasing trend in women freezing their ova to delay parenthood for nonmedical reasons (HFEA 2023). In 2016, the Newcastle Fertility Centre was licensed to perform so-called three-person IVF for women with mitochondrial disease. The technique allows healthy mitochondria from a woman donor to be combined with the DNA of the parents. The subsequent new genetic material will be passed on through future generations. In April 2023, it was reported that the first babies had been born following this technique, although no further details have been released to protect confidentiality (Sample 2023). There are also instances of controversial legal decisions regarding assisted conception. One example is the case decided in July 2016 involving a 60-year-old woman being given permission to use IVF in an attempt to become pregnant, using the ova her daughter had frozen before her death from bowel cancer (BBC 2016). Around 100 womb transplant have been carried out around the world, and approximately 50 babies born subsequently. In August 2023, the first successful womb transplant in the UK was reported, giving rise to the possibility of women having successful pregnancies through IVF post-hysterectomy and even in the future for transgender women (Kirby 2023). Ethical and legal controversy surrounds each of these examples. However, similar to the issues discussed above, some will argue that research resulting in new methods, particularly with the possibility of treatment, is positive and morally justifiable. But for others, interference with what may be considered the essence of life itself will remain morally wrong.

Conclusion

Overall, the use of reproductive technologies has laudable aims—either to help those unable to do so to have children, to create children free from disease, disability, or, with a tissue match, to treat their sick siblings or to offer women the choice to continue with or terminate a pregnancy. However, as has been shown in the discussion, there are a myriad of ethical problems that arise from such technologies, accompanied by a diverse range of opinions on the morality of their use. What is at the heart of this debate is the fundamental question of when life begins, and what sort of status we should afford to the entity that develops from a fertilised ovum, through the embryonic and foetal stages, to a fully formed baby. Modern visualisation techniques that show this development, particularly at the very earliest stages, bring detailed images where there can be no doubt about the entity as a living being with human characteristics. All of which adds to the dilemma and complexity of the ethical problems faced by women, such as those in the scenario above. There are no easy answers to these problems. National bodies, such as the HFEA, and the law can be used to enact legislation to govern the use of procedures or address cases bought before the courts; but this will only result in legal responses and practical solutions, leaving the central ethical issues unanswered.

Key Learning Points
- There are differing claims about when life begins and when life begins to matter.
- An argument based on sentience permits early abortions and embryo research as the embryo is not hurt.
- Defining personhood as a combination of rationality and self-consciousness has negative implications for individuals who lack capacity.
- Surrogacy is lawful in the UK when the ova and sperm of the intended parents are used and when the sperm or ova of a donor is used.
- Parents are not allowed by the HFEA to choose the characteristics of their children, but saviour siblings can be created where there is an inherited disease in the family.
- Arguments for and against abortion demonstrate conflict between a woman's right to choose what happens to her body and the foetus's right to protection from harm.

References

Adashi EY, Cohen IG (2022) Who will oversee the ethical limits of human embryo research? Nat Biotechnol 40(4):463–463

BBC (2016) Woman wins appeal to use dead daughter's eggs. http://www.bbc.co.uk/news/health-36675521. Accessed 5 Dec 2023

Bostrom N (2012) Human genetic enhancements: a transhumanist perspective. In: Holland S (ed) Arguing about bioethics. Routledge, Abingdon

Chitty LS, Wright D, Hill M, Verhoef TI, Daley R, Lewis C, Mason S, McKay F, Jenkins L, Howarth A, Cameron L, McEwan A, Fisher J, Kroese M, Morris S (2016) Uptake, outcomes, and costs of implementing non-invasive prenatal testing for Down's syndrome into NHS maternity care: prospective cohort study in eight diverse maternity units. Br Med J 345:i3426. https://doi.org/10.1136/bmj.i3426

Department of Health and Social Security (DHSS) (1984) The Warnock report. HMSO, London

Di Mattei V, Ferrari F, Perego G, Tobia V, Mauro F, Candiani M (2021) Decision-making factors in prenatal testing: a systematic review. Health Psychol Open 8(1):2055102920987455

Dufner A (2021) Non-invasive prenatal testing (NIPT): does the practice discriminate against persons with disabilities? J Perinat Med 49(8):945–948

Gillon R (2001) Is there a new ethics of abortion? J Med Ethics 27(suppl. 2):ii5–ii9

Gonzalez-Ramos Z, Zuriguel-Pérez E, Albacar-Riobóo N (2021) The emotional response of women when terminating a pregnancy for medical reasons: a scoping review. Midwifery 103:103095. https://doi.org/10.1016/j.midw.2021.103095

Harris J (1985) The value of life. Routledge, London

HFEA (2023) Fertility treatment 2021: preliminary trends and figures. HFEA, London

Hoppe N, Miola J (2014) Medical law and medical ethics. Cambridge University Press, Cambridge

Human Fertilisation and Embryology Authority (2021) ND pre-implantation genetic testing for monogenetic disorders (PGT-M) and pre-implantation genetic testing for chromosomal structural rearrangements (PGT-SR). HFEA. Accessed 20 Aug 2023

Kirby J (2023) Womb transplants for trans women 'many years off'—UK surgeon. Independent. https://www.independent.co.uk/news/uk/richard-smith-imperial-college-london-university-of-alabama-sweden-mailonline-b2397710.html. Accessed 6 Dec 2023

Locke J (1997) An essay an essay concerning human understanding. Penguin, London

Loike JD, Kadish A (2022) The reproductive technology advances no one asked for. The Scientist. https://www.the-scientist.com/news-opinion/opinion-the-reproductive-technology-advances-no-one-asked-for-70160. Accessed 6 Dec 2023

Luke 1:41 Holy Bible (2023) King James Version. https://www.kingjamesbibleonline.org/Luke-1-41/. Accessed 19 Aug 2016

Marszal A (2016) Indian woman gives birth at 70 with help of IVF. The telegraph. http://www.telegraph.co.uk/news/2016/05/10/indian-woman-gives-birth-at-70-with-help-of-ivf/. Accessed 5 Dec 2023

Nuffield Council on Bioethics (2016) Genome editing. Nuffield Council, London

Sample I (2023) First baby with DNA from three people born after new procedure. The Guardian. https://www.theguardian.com/science/2023/May/09/first-uk-baby-with-dna-from-three-people-born-after-new-ivf-procedure. Accessed 6 Dec 2023

Savulescu J (2001) Procreative beneficence: why we should select the best children. Bioethics 15:413–426

Selgelid M (2014) Moderate eugenics and human enhancement. Med Health Care Philos 17(3):2–12

Singer P (2012) The metaphysical status of the embryo: some arguments revisited. In: Holland S (ed) Arguing about bioethics. Routledge, Abingdon

Society for the Protection of Unborn Children (2023). https://www.spuc.org.uk/50questions. Accessed 8 Aug 2023

Thomson JJ (1971) A defense of abortion. Philos Public Aff 1(1):47–66

Tooley M (1972) Abortion and infanticide. Philos Public Aff 2(1):37–65

Wilkinson S (2010) Choosing tomorrow's children. Oxford University Press, Oxford

Ethical Issues in Mental Health Nursing

12

Grahame Smith

Abstract

This chapter explores mental health nursing practice within an ethics context. It teases out the ethical challenges that mental health nurses can face on a daily basis. A short case study highlights potential solutions to those challenges.

For mental health nurses, having the power to control and being expected to control people diagnosed with a mental disorder can be morally distressing, especially where situations do not always have clear outcomes. The case study part of the chapter will consider how in these difficult circumstances mental health nurses can control and potentially restrict service user freedoms in a way that reduces moral distress and is beneficent and sensitive. A challenge for the contemporary mental health nurse is to know how to wield this power in a way that acknowledges their societal responsibilities while at the same time respecting the rights of the individuals they are required to control. It is important to recognise that restricting freedoms through the use of sanctioned coercion can be a good thing; however, this is dependent on coercion being used by the mental health nurse in a way that is sensitive to the needs of the mental health service user and is recovery-focused.

Keywords

Mental health nursing · Coercion · Ethical reasoning · Values-based practice · Expert practice · Emotional intelligence

---

G. Smith (✉)
School of Nursing and Allied Health, Liverpool John Moores University, Liverpool, UK
e-mail: G.M.Smith@ljmu.ac.uk

© The Author(s), under exclusive license to Springer Nature Switzerland AG 2024
P. A. Scott, S. M. Scott (eds.), *Key Concepts and Issues in Nursing Ethics*,
https://doi.org/10.1007/978-3-031-54108-7_12

Introduction

This chapter will explore mental health nursing within an ethics context. It will tease out the ethics of mental health nursing practice, presenting common ethical challenges mental health nurses face on a daily basis, providing a case study example which will highlight potential solutions to those challenges.

On a daily basis, mental health nurses make clinical decisions. These decisions have an ethical dimension; however, this ethical dimension is not always acknowledged (Smith 2016). It does not necessarily follow that this lack of acknowledgement means mental health nurses are not ethical practitioners; clearly their practice will be framed by ethical rules and frameworks (Nursing and Midwifery Council (NMC) 2018). It is more the case that ethical reasoning and clinical decision-making have become so entwined it is hard to distinguish the difference, if indeed there is a difference. The competent mental health nurse will be adept at top-down ethical reasoning, using rules and frameworks; however, to be expert they will need also to be bottom-up ethical reasoners (Smith 2016; Cohen 2004). In addition, mental health nursing practice has a unique aspect compared to other nursing fields of practice. In this field of practice it is the case that:

> .... a *fully conscious adult patient of normal intelligence may be treated without consent, not for the protection of others (though this is also possible) but in their own interests.* (Fulford 2009, p. 62)

Being able to control people who have been diagnosed with a mental health condition is nothing new. Indeed there is an historical context for such intervention which this chapter will explore. Restricting services users'[1] freedoms can be morally distressing, even where it is justified and especially where situations do not always have clear outcomes (De Veer et al. 2013). In the case study part of the chapter, we will consider how in these difficult circumstances mental health nurses can restrict service user freedoms beneficently and sensitively.

The Context of Mental Health Nursing

Over 30 years ago, the main ward door on an acute mental health ward in the English health system was not routinely locked. Fast forward to the twenty-first century and these doors are now routinely locked. The practice of locking the main ward door is not in itself unusual. What is unusual is that they are kept locked all the time, which in some ways can be seen as a return to the restrictive practices of the past (Ashmore 2008). Keeping the door unlocked was a key component in the process of creating a therapeutic environment (Ashmore 2008). Bowers et al. (2010) describe a journey of 'door locking where in the 1960s and 1970s it was unusual to permanently lock

---

[1] While recognising the debate in the literature around nomenclature patient/client/service user, see, for example, Chap. 6 of this book, the term service user is the term used in this chapter, as that in most common usage in mental health care contexts in both Ireland and the UK.

the main ward door. By 2010 42% of ward doors were permanently locked. In 2015 the Care Quality Commission (CQC) reported that '86% of wards (1109) had locked doors' (p. 34) (Care Quality Commission (CQC) (2015).

Locking doors certainly creates a potential ethical tension between keeping mental health service users' safe, protecting the vulnerable, and eroding freedoms and being paternalistic (Bowers et al. 2010). At this juncture it would be useful to consider within an historical context why society has this imperative. Morse (1977) makes the following observation:

> *For hundreds of years, the Anglo-American legal system has been developing special rules for dealing with problems caused by the inherently perplexing phenomenon of mentally disordered behavior.* (Morse 1977, p. 529)

In *Madness: A Brief History* (2002), Roy Porter describes madness as being potentially as old as mankind. Porter (2002) supports this view by citing the ancient art of trepanning, where holes were drilled into a person's skulls to allow 'devils' to escape. At this time madness was viewed as a punishment, where the gods would smite people with madness for committing a perceived wrong (Porter 2002). In early Christian times, madness could be good or bad. It was good in the case of saintly visions. Inevitably it was only bad, satanic possession that needed to be dealt with and exorcised (Porter 2002). Around the Enlightenment (1620s–1780s), madness was starting to be viewed by some as a nervous system defect. This was the start of viewing madness as a medical condition. During this period locking up people who were viewed as mad would only happen if their family or the local community could not take care of them and sometimes if they were viewed as being dangerous (Porter 2002). According to Porter (2002) in England only 5000 people out of a population of ten million were held in asylums in 1800. At this time the medical discipline of psychiatry started to form, with the requirement that asylums were licensed and that they had a medical presence.

The standards of care in these facilities varied greatly irrespective of whether they were funded privately or by charitable donations. Physical punishment was not uncommon; however, some asylums offered rest and recuperation (Porter 2002). The legal system started to create special rules for people who were not necessarily committing crime but whose behaviour was pejoratively viewed as not being the norm (Morse 1977). Demonstrating 'abnormal' behaviour in itself was not an issue; it only became an issue to control when the person was also viewed as not being socially responsible (Morse 1977). Creating special rules to manage what we would now view as mental distress was the start of society perceiving mental health conditions as a risk (Morse 1977). Society wanting to control behaviour that is perceived as a risk is nothing new. Throughout history political philosophers have explored this issue; however, they have always paid scant attention to risky behaviour arising from a person's mental distress (Wolff 2006).

Over time, as societal norms and rules developed, people on a day-by-day basis were expected to abide and sign up to these rules—even if this was a tacit process. The aim of these rules was to prevent people engaging in destructive behaviours including self-destructive behaviours (Wolff 2006). By abiding by these rules, a person was given certain freedoms. If they broke these rules, such as committing a crime, these freedoms could be taken away as a form of punishment (Wolff 2006). This position does not consider rule-breaking behaviour where a person may break the rules due to a mental disorder. Where it is briefly considered, the general view is that people with a mental disorder who break the rules should not be punished; they should be protected, even if this process restricts freedoms and in effect looks like a form of punishment (Wolff 2006).

In the early days of the asylums, nursing as a profession did not exist, neither did psychiatry as a medical discipline. It is only since the 1930s that mental health nursing started to become recognised as a future field of nursing practice (Nolan 1993). Mental health nursing within a UK context has always been closely aligned with the medical discipline of psychiatry; as this discipline started to form in the 1800s mental health nursing practice also stated to take shape (Porter 2002; Nolan 1993). It is important to recognise mental health nurses have not always been called mental health nurses, throughout the ages they have had different titles such as keeper and attendant (Nolan 1993).

The role of the keeper started to emerge during the 1800s with the emergence of the asylums. The job of the keeper was to look after the institution, control the 'inmates', and, where required, be a servant to the doctor who was in charge of the asylum (Nolan 1993). As the asylums became more numerous and at the same time started to focus on the treatment of mental distress, the keeper role started to transform into the role of attendant (Nolan 1993). At this time there was the belief that mental health conditions should and could be treated and possibly 'cured' (Porter 2002). The role of the attendant was to assist in the delivery of these cures, which included anything from good basic care, exercise, and good nutrition, to activities such as fettering (tying people down) and blood-letting (Porter 2002; Nolan 1993). Similar to be the keeper role attendants tended to be un-trained; however, this changed in 1889 when attendants were required to attend a national training course. From 1923 female attendants started to be called nurses, and male attendants began to gain this title from 1926 (Nolan 1993).

With the change of title from attendant to nurse, there was a greater emphasis on the delivery of good basic care. More technical elements of care were in their infancy (Nolan 1993). Over time the notion of healing and curing within mental health care started to incorporate psychiatric medication and talking therapies as important elements. Observation and control of people incarcerated in asylums were also important; however, they became less explicit and more implicit as treatments such as fettering started to disappear (Nolan 1993; Roberts 2005). Treating mental distress in this way was continuing to be influenced by the medicalisation of madness, involving describing different forms of mental distress and developing different forms of treatments (Porter 2002). With the promise of treatment came the promise that irrationality could be controlled. At the forefront of controlling irrationality was the mental health nurse (Roberts 2005). Fast forward to the present day, the challenge, for the contemporary mental health nurse, is to know how to wield this power to control in a way that acknowledges their societal responsibilities, while at the same time respecting the rights of the individuals they are required to control.

The Moral Domain of Practice

Having the power to control and being expected to control people with mental health conditions have been shaped by the historical development of mental health nursing practice; it has also been shaped by the media and by public perceptions (Smith 2016). Over recent years the media have covered high-profile incidents of people with mental health conditions in a way that portrays people with mental health conditions as being more risky than so-called normal people (Wood et al. 2014; Johnson 2013). In addition, mental health services are usually portrayed as failing. This tends to be based on the view that they did not control the individual and in turn prevent the incident from happening (Wood et al. 2014; Johnson 2013). Driven by this societal expectation that people with mental health conditions should be controlled, mental health legislation has also been applied in a more controlling manner, such as the increase in compulsory admissions to mental health services (Roberts 2005; Johnson 2013).

Of course contemporary mental health nursing has moved away from the brutalities of the past in the way that people with mental health conditions were confined, conformed, and treated (Nolan 1993; Roberts 2005). The emphasis of contemporary mental health nursing practice is to be evidence-based and to be ethical, which includes abiding by the nursing profession's ethical rules (Smith 2016; Nursing and Midwifery Council (NMC) 2018). That does not mean that interventions which confine and conform do not take place, or that some treatments are not controversial—such as electroconvulsive treatment (ECT). However, if these practices are used in an unethical way, mental health nurses are held to account (Nursing and Midwifery Council (NMC) 2018). It is important to recognise that these practices have an explicit and an implicit dimension. Explicit interventions include the use of mental health law, physical restraint, environmental control such as seclusion and locking wards, and the use of medication (Roberts 2005). Implicit interventions are more subtle; they are day-to-day interventions which the nurse may not recognise as having a controlling element. These include such interventions as observing and monitoring the service user, making clinical judgements and recording them, assessing (including the assessment of risk), psychosocial interventions, and reviewing a service user's care (Roberts 2005). The impact of both explicit and implicit interventions is that the service user knows they are being monitored. They know that if they do not conform and exhibit 'normal behaviours', their freedoms could be restricted. They also know they have to demonstrate conformity; in other words they have to control themselves (Roberts 2005).

Explicit interventions can be viewed as directly coercive, overtly restricting a service user's freedoms, whereas implicit interventions allow an element of choice. However, the service user is being pressured to behave in ways that the mental health nurse and society expect them to behave (Smith 2016; Roberts 2005). Having this sanctioned power to coerce and apply pressure emanates from a service user being labelled as having a mental health condition. Irrespective of the heated debates surrounding, the use of these labels the outcome is the same. The mental health nurse has the power to control the individual with a diagnosed mental health condition (Roberts 2005). A check and balance to the use of this power is that the mental health nurse will follow the rules, including legislation, polices, and professional codes (Smith 2016). The challenge with a rules-based approach is that it is more suited to making clinical decisions when a situation is not complex, when there is plenty of time to make the decision and the outcome is relatively certain (Smith 2016). The reality of everyday clinical practice is that this is not usually the case. Certainty of outcome, for example, can be a luxury rather than a given. Irrespective of this uncertainty, the mental health nurse will still have to make decisions which have to be justified; this may include providing evidence of the right motives and/or the right outcomes (Nursing and Midwifery Council (NMC) 2018).

Ethical decision-making within a mental health nursing context is not just a rational process; it is also an emotional process, one that requires a high degree of self-awareness (Roberts 2004). This is coupled with the need to maintain a therapeutic relationship, which is the medium for treatment (Smith 2016). In the process of navigating an ethical way through this complexity, the mental health nurse will rely on their professional knowledge and their ability to reason (Smith 2016). Reasoning and professional knowledge are not separate activities. They complement each other. They do not happen in a vacuum. Ethical reasoning which builds on good professional knowledge (bottom-up reasoning) will have external points of reference (top-down reasoning) (Cohen 2004). External points of reference include professional frameworks and codes, legal frameworks, policies, clinical guidelines, and ethical theories (Smith 2016). These rules are there to guide the mental health nurse. However, the rules and frameworks do not always provide specific answers, even if the nurse would like this to be the case; there is always a level of interpretation required (Smith 2016). In addition, these rules and frameworks can provide conflicting advice, and on this basis the nurse not only has to interpret; they also have to know which rules to apply, when to apply them, and how they should be applied (Smith 2016).

Being ethical is a balancing act regardless of the expertise of the mental health nurse. There is a constant need to respect autonomy[2] while recognising that mental health care can be inherently paternalistic and controlling (Smith 2016). Making sense of autonomy within mental health care is a challenge, especially as most ethical theories were developed with the rational person in mind. However, principlism[3] does take a position on the person who has a mental health condition. Beauchamp and Childress (2013) highlight that being paternalistic is justified as the person's

---

[2] Please see Chap. 6 for an in-depth discussion of patient/client autonomy within the nursing and health care context.

[3] Principlism describes an approach to ethical decision-making using ethical principles; such as the four-principle approach of Beauchamp and Childress (2013) cited above. For an in-depth discussion of principlism within the nursing context, please see Chap. 7.

condition prevents rational deliberation, free choice, and action, and therefore the person is nonautonomous. Paternalism is justified on the grounds of beneficence or nonmaleficence. This position appears quite straightforward. The weakness of this approach, however, is that judgement of whether a person is nonautonomous is based on the mental health nurse using what appears to be facts, such as 'mental illness' and 'lack of capacity'. These concepts are 'values turned into facts' or value-laden judgements (Fulford 2009). The effect being that restricting a service user's freedom is dependent on the viewpoint of a moral agent and the one who holds the power, the mental health nurse (Fulford 2009).

Establishing whether a mental health service user is nonautonomous is an ethically complicated matter. Some authors such as Roberts (2004) offer a pragmatic solution to the ethical challenges inherent within mental health care by combining a principle-based approach with other ethical approaches. Taking this pragmatic approach gives the nurse the scope to look first at the uniqueness of their practice, as a bottom-up reasoner, and then decide which ethical theories enable them to reach an agreed solution, as a bottom-up to top-down reasoner (Cohen 2004; Roberts 2004). An example of such an approach may be where a mental health service user demonstrates risky behaviour and the mental health nurse wants to keep them safe, a good outcome which links to a number of ethical theories. The mental health nurse has the sanctioned power to restrict their freedoms; however, as a bottom-up to top-down reasoned, they will recognise the importance of achieving a good outcome for all parties. The outcome will need to keep the service user safe while at the same time maintaining the therapeutic relationship, essentially being person-centred. To achieve this the nurse will use practice-orientated skills, such as the use of the therapeutic self, to explore and deliver a solution which is least restrictive.

Ethical Challenges

It is important to recognise that coercion can be a good thing. The Department of Mental Health and Learning Disability (2006) Report, now known as City 128 Report, was an extensive piece of research focusing on understanding and identifying the mental health nursing interventions that produce both a controlled and therapeutic environment. The report infers that coercive strategies when used to benefit the service user can be a good thing (Department of Mental Health and Learning Disability 2006). This is, however, dependent upon these strategies being used in a way that is sensitive to the needs of the mental health service user.

The City 128 Report does not specifically look at implicit interventions; neither does it consider mental health nursing in the community. However, it does highlight that 'sensitive' coercion which reduces the emotional intensity of mental distress is a good thing, thereby placing this notion within an ethical context. A good starting place to consider what sensitive coercion may look like or how it should be applied would be to explore the notion of coercion in more depth. There are a number of political philosophers who have written about the issue of coercion. Likewise there are a number of articles within the field of mental health nursing that touch upon the issue of coercion. The obvious difference between these perspectives is that political philosophers focus on coercion within a 'rational person in society' context, whereas mental health nurses are trying to understand coercion within an 'irrational person in society' context. This does not mean lessons cannot be learnt from both perspectives; however, there is a need to reconcile and interpret one perspective with the other. The work of the political philosopher Ripstein (2004) provides a solid base in which to start this process.

Coercion can be seen as a way of getting individuals to do or not do something. It also diminishes the individual's freedoms, and on this basis it is a violation of an individual's rights (Anderson 2011). This also includes the threat of being coerced. Carr (1988) highlights that the threat of coercion ultimately restricts an individual's freedom; in effect their freedoms are dependent on meeting certain conditions. Generally coercion, including the threat of coercion, is justified and authorised where it prevents societal harms (Ripstein 2004). According to Ripstein (2004) 'both the use of official force and the claim of states to tell people what to do are justified because, in their absence, arbitrary individual force prevails, even if people act in good faith' (p. 3).

The authorisation of coercion is transferrable to mental health nursing practice. If it is used in accordance with mental health law, it can be seen as justified. If it is not sanctioned, it is not justified (Ripstein 2004). However, while coercing someone who is 'rational' usually relates to preventing societal harms, it can also be a form of punishment. Someone who is deemed to have a mental health condition can be coerced not only to prevent societal harms, but also to prevent them from harming themselves, on the basis of the best interests argument (Morse 1977; Roberts 2005). Acting on behalf of someone, in their best interests, can make understanding the coercive nature of mental health nursing practice more difficult: 'I'm not really using coercion I am acting in their best interests' (Roberts 2005). This is usually justified by, 'the person is irrational and no longer free and therefore I have to act and restrict what a rational person would call freedoms, and if they were rational they would agree with my actions' (Smith 2016; O'Brien and Golding 2003).

The work of O'Brien and Golding (2003) tries to move this debate forward by first defining coercion within a mental health nursing context; 'any use of authority by the mental health nurse to override the choices of the service user' (p. 68).

O'Brien and Golding (2003) then assert that coercion in all its forms is only justified where:

- The service user lacks capacity.
- The harms prevented or benefits provided outweigh the harms caused by the coercive act.
- The least coercive (described in policy as least restrictive) intervention that will promote good or prevent harm is used.

O'Brien and Golding (2003) are contending that 'best interests' should not be a catch-all phrase which justifies the uses of coercion (p. 172). O'Brien and Golding (2003) make a valuable contribution to the debate; however, measuring capacity, weighing outcomes, and deciding on the least restrictive strategy are values and ones that are dependent on the viewpoint of the nurse (Fulford 2009). As an example a service user wants to leave the ward, but they are openly expressing ideas of harm to self and others, and they lack capacity. To keep the service user on the ward would increase the chances of preventing harm. It would also increase the chances of treating the underlying mental disorder and therefore potentially reducing the risk of harm, an act that would benefit the service user (Roberts 2004). If persuading the service user does not stop them leaving the ward, you move on to locking the door and so on, it sounds pretty straightforward (O'Brien and Golding 2003). And yet there is an emotional dimension to these interventions. Stopping the service user leaving can be distressing for both the service user and the nurse. It can also impact negatively upon the therapeutic relationship, which is the medium for treatment (Smith 2016). The nurse has to be rational and reasoned. They also have to be emotionally intelligent, with the ability to facilitate an open dialogue with the service user that shows an understanding of the power differences inherent within the relationship (Roberts 2005).

The work of O'Brien and Golding (2003), you could argue, provides a minimum standard of how coercion should be justified, a way of preventing the abuse of the nurse's power. In addition it has to be recognised that when delivering care in complex situations, what works in one situation may not work in another. Coercion is no different. A set of actions in one situation could be described as being beneficial, whereas in another but similar situation, the same set of actions could be described as being harmful. The mental health nurse, when using coercion, has to be sensitive to the individual nature of a situation, to ensure that the coercion is indeed beneficial. Being sensitive is based on responding in the right way. To do this the nurse will have to have the right character traits such as kindness, patience, tolerance, and compassion to name a few (Armstrong 2006; Nursing and Midwifery Council (NMC) 2018). In addition to these character traits, the nurse will need to possess practical wisdom, the ability to make the right choice at the right time (Armstrong 2006; Smith 2016).[4] By using coercion in a reasoned and emotionally sensitive way, the outcomes of its use should benefit all parties.

A Case Study

This section will highlight, through the use of a case study, how the mental health nurse can emotionally and rationally reason through a number of ethical challenges.

Sam is 25 years old and lives at home with his mother. He has recently completed a further education course in business management, and he is looking for a full-time job. He still works part-time at the local supermarket; however, his goal is to manage his own supermarket. Since completing his business management course, a number of people including his mother have mentioned that he has become a 'bit

---

[4] For an in-depth discussion of character traits, practical wisdom, and nursing practice, please see Chap. 9.

excitable'. Sam does not know what this means, he just feels incredibly happy. He is aware that the 'voices' are talking to him more often and he has a secret; he has stopped taking his medication. He made the decision to stop taking his medication because he felt he would concentrate better and he was fed up with putting on weight. He also decided not to tell anyone especially his mother as she would be upset with him.

A couple of weeks ago, Sam did not arrive at work. His manager phoned Sam's mother wondering where Sam was. This phone call was out of concern as he had noted that Sam was looking increasingly distracted and he was also not attending to his hygiene, which was out of character for Sam. His mother, in a panic, immediately phoned the police, just as Sam walked through the door. Sam became angry, accusing his mother of plotting behind his back and trying to stop him reaching his potential as a chosen one. Sam's mother was frightened and as she was still on the phone to the police she asked for their help. Within minutes the police arrived, and Sam, out of frustration and fear, struggled with the police. Sam was assessed in the police cells first by a police surgeon and then by a member of the mental health liaison team. It was agreed that Sam should be admitted to hospital. Sam was reluctant; however, he felt quite fearful being in a police cell, so he agreed to be admitted for a period of 'assessment'. Sam arrived on the ward, and he was offered medication which he refused and then went to bed. The next morning Sam was seen by a doctor and a nurse. He told them he wanted to go home. He was told that they would consider his request; however, he needed to tell them about the events leading up to his admission. Sam told them about being special and that he hears voices. He is not sure whether they are angels or just entities called the 'helpers'. Sam also mentioned that since he had stopped taking his medication, he has started to realise that agents called the 'shadows' were stopping him from achieving his goals. He was asked about his goals. Sam said his main goal was not clear until he was in the police cell, and then he realised his goal was to 'purge the shadows'.

After being assessed Sam asked again about going home. He was told that he would need to stay on the ward for the time being and he really needed to start taking his medication again. Sam became angry and stormed out of the office towards the ward door. He tried to push through the door. It was locked, and this frustrated Sam, and he started to kick the door. People were suddenly telling him to calm down and offering him medication. He lashed out. Suddenly he was on the floor; he knew he had been injected with medication. After being moved to a single room, he started to cry. He briefly heard a nurse mention he was on a section of the Mental Health Act. He did not care. He wanted to be left alone.

John is a third year mental health student, and it is his first day on the ward today. Sam is mentioned in the morning handover and a brief overview is given. Sam is a 25-year-old male with a diagnosis of schizophrenia. He is on a section 3 of the Mental Health Act (compulsory admission to mental health services for treatment); he hears voices and has delusions about being a 'messiah-like figure'. He stopped taking his medication around 4 months ago. This is his second psychotic episode. The first episode happened around 5 years ago and he did not need hospitalisation.

After the handover John says hello to Sam and goes to shake his hand, suggesting they have a chat. Sam tells John he is like the others and he does not want to talk. At the lunch time medication round, Sam initially refuses his medication but takes it when he is reminded that he is on a section of the Mental Health Act. Once he has taken his medication, he opens his mouth to show he has taken it without prompting, and then leaves the trolley area muttering 'you are not sticking another needle in me'. On his next shift John decides that he will have a good chat with Sam. John approaches Sam and starts a conversation; Sam immediately mentions that he will talk if he has to, 'because you're the boss; otherwise leave me alone, and phone my Mum—I want some clean clothes, but I do not want to talk with her as she put me in here'.

John recognises that Sam has been through a tough time. He also recognises that Sam is controlling his own behaviour, possibly out of the fear of being coerced again (Roberts 2005). John talks to his mentor about Sam to explore the best way forward. His mentor explains to John that Sam has been coerced; however, it will have always been for his benefit. In Sam's notes it mentions that he has been debriefed after the 'restraint' incident (National Institute for Health and Clinical Excellence (NICE) 2015). John wonders if this is the case why Sam still appears to be upset and possibly resentful. John's mentor starts to explore with John the idea that even if a reasoned approach is used, this does not mean it will instantly remove conflict. John starts to embrace this idea of ambiguity: that not all things fit nicely into systems and models (Cohen 2004; Smith 2016). He is aware that the nursing team recognise that coercion is an ethical issue; the facts were explored before it was applied, it was adherent to professional, ethical, and legal rules and theories, and the team explored all alternative options including reflecting on the outcome (Smith 2016). John asked his mentor if he thought the use of coercion was right. His mentor said, 'yes, in certain circumstances, however even though it could be right, at an emotional level it may feel wrong'. His mentor went on to explain that coercion was more than just restraining and using medication; it could be about observing and monitoring, which has the effect of the service user controlling their behaviour to fit in (Roberts 2005).

Taking this advice into account, John started to think about the emotional impact of coercion and how he could work with Sam's perspective. John decided he would use a values-based approach when working with Sam, to first understand Sam's perspective and then to resolve any ethical conflict through working with Sam's story and values in a person-centred way (Fulford 2009). John meets with Sam again and takes the opportunity to encourage Sam to talk about his experiences. Through this process of listening to Sam's story, John starts to gain an emotional insight into Sam's experiences and how it feels to be coerced (Roberts 2005). John also recognises that Sam's distress is not all about the act of coercion; it is also about feeling powerless. John realises there are lessons to be learnt, ones that give him the opportunity to understand what therapeutic approaches to use when working with Sam (Roberts 2005; Smith 2016).

Reflecting on their conversation John recognises the importance of working with both facts and values: 'the two feet principle' (Fulford 2009). Using this approach *can help to resolve ethical conflict especially when using coercion, it is also recovery-focused* and promotes independence (Sustere and Tarpey 2019). *In the long term by engaging with Sam in this way, John acknowledges that he will:*

- *Promote Sam's well-being through being compassionate.*
- *Maximise opportunity for Sam and reduce feelings of social isolation.*
- *Empower Sam to start to take control and be independent.*
- *Facilitate and support Sam to find meaning and purpose outside of the hospital setting.*

Conclusion

The clinical decisions that mental health nurses make have an ethical dimension which is sometimes not acknowledged. This does not mean that mental health nurses are not ethical practitioners. It is more the case that ethical reasoning and clinical decision-making have become so entwined it is hard to distinguish the differences between the two. To be expert the mental health nurse has to be adept at both top-down and bottom-up ethical reasoning. Being able to do this means the nurse takes a more holistic approach which is person-centred and pays careful attention to the service user's needs, while at the same time acknowledging the regulatory and ethical frameworks that must influence and regulate mental health nursing practice.

Historically there has also been a propensity for society to expect the mental health nurse to have a controlling element to their practice. Controlling can be explicit, but, it can also be implicit. To make ethical sense of this controlling element, a number of authors offer a pragmatic ethical approach which could potentially give the mental health nurse the opportunity to look first at the uniqueness of their practice, as a bottom-up reasoner, and the latitude to decide which ethical theories enable them to reach a reasonable and workable solution.

There is also an emotional dimension to mental health nursing, especially where the therapeutic relationship is the medium of treatment. Being emotionally sensitive is based on responding in the right way, using the right character traits, and possessing practical wisdom. Even when using coercion the mental health nurse should be emotionally sensitive and by doing so the outcomes should benefit all parties.

> **Key Learning Points**
> - The ethical dimension of clinical decision-making within mental health nursing practice can sometimes be hidden.
> - Expert mental health nurses engage in ethical reasoning which is simultaneously top-down and bottom-up reasoning.
> - Mental health nurses have the explicit and implicit power to control mental health service users; however, to achieve good outcomes for all parties the mental health nurse has to use this power sensitively.

References

Anderson S (2011) Coercion. http://plato.stanford.edu/entries/coercion/. Accessed 5 Dec 2023

Armstrong AE (2006) Towards a strong virtue ethics for nursing practice. Nurs Philos 7:110–124

Ashmore R (2008) Nurses' accounts of locked ward doors: ghosts of the asylum or acute care in the 21st century? J Psychiatr Ment Health Nurs 15(3):175–185

Beauchamp TL, Childress JF (2013) Principles of biomedical ethics, 7th edn. Oxford University Press, New York

Bowers L, Haglund K, Mir-Cochrane E, Nijman H, Simpson A, Van der Merwe M (2010) Locked doors: a survey of patients, staff and visitors. J Psychiatr Ment Health Nurs 17(10):873–880

Care Quality Commission (CQC) (2015) Monitoring the mental health act in 2014/2015. Care Quality Commission, Newcastle upon Tyne

Carr CL (1988) Coercion and freedom. Am Philos Q 25(1):59–67

Cohen S (2004) The nature of moral reasoning: framework and activities of ethical deliberation, argument and decision-making. Oxford University Press, Melbourne

De Veer AJ, Francke AL, Struijs A, Willems DL (2013) Determinants of moral distress in daily nursing practice: a cross sectional correlational questionnaire survey. Int J Nurs Stud 50(1):100–108

Department of Mental Health and Learning Disability (2006) The City 128 study of observation and outcomes on acute psychiatric wards: report to the NHS SDO programme. City University London, London

Fulford KWM (2009) Values, science and psychiatry. In: Bloch S, Green SA (eds) Psychiatric ethics, 4th edn. Oxford University Press, Oxford, pp 61–84

Johnson S (2013) Can we reverse the rising tide of compulsory admissions? Lancet 381(9878):1603–1604

Morse SJ (1977) Crazy behavior, morals, and science: an analysis of mental health law. S Calif Law Rev 51:527–654

National Institute for Health and Clinical Excellence (NICE) (2015) Violence and aggression: short-term management in mental health, health and community settings—clinical guideline 39. NICE, London

Nolan P (1993) A history of mental health nursing. Stanley Thornes, Cheltenham

Nursing and Midwifery Council (NMC) (2018) The code: professional standards of practice and behaviour for nurses, midwives and nursing associates. NMC, London

O'Brien AJ, Golding CG (2003) Coercion in mental healthcare: the principle of least coercive care. J Psychiatr Ment Health Nurs 10:167–173

Porter R (2002) Madness: a brief history. Oxford University Press, Oxford

Ripstein A (2004) Authority and coercion. Philos Public Aff 33(1):2–35

Roberts M (2004) Psychiatric ethics: a critical introduction for mental health nurses. J Psychiatr Ment Health Nurs 11:583–588

Roberts M (2005) The production of the psychiatric subject: power, knowledge and Michel Foucault. Nurs Philos 6:33–42

Smith G (2016) A practical introduction to mental health ethics. Routledge, Oxon

Sustere E, Tarpey E (2019) Least restrictive practice: its role in patient independence and recovery. J Forensic Psychiatry Psychol 30(4):614–629

Wolff J (2006) An introduction to political philosophy, 2nd edn. Oxford University Press, Oxford

Wood L, Birte M, Alsawy S, Pyle M, Morrison A (2014) Public perceptions of stigma towards people with schizophrenia, depression, and anxiety. Psychiatry Res 220(1):604–608

Ethical Issues in Caring for Older People

13

Riitta Suhonen and Minna Stolt

Abstract

Ethics is a fundamental part of nursing care in all care settings. Ethical issues are prevalent in the provision of nursing care to older people, as growing old may bring several health issues, vulnerability, dependence, and frailty. Such issues bring special requirements of nurses and other healthcare professionals, including sensitivity to ethical issues, reflection on one's knowledge and actions, and the ability to carefully manage ethically challenging situations in the provision of nursing care. The type of ethical issues professionals face while caring for older individuals include how to maintain the autonomy, self-determination, and dignity of the older person. Older individuals also face ethical issues while seeking care or being cared for, including how to maintain their own autonomy and dignity, how to enable shared decision-making, and how to ensure one's wishes are heard and respected. Individuals of all ages have the right to be cared for in a dignified manner, but it is especially important when growing old and having lived a long life across different decades and circumstances. The ethical issues in the care of older people are multifaceted. Fundamental patient rights must be respected and cherished in all nursing care circumstances, and knowledge of these can be increased. This chapter raises current and future ethical issues and challenges in the nursing care of older people, with particular focus on the context of home care and long-term care settings.

R. Suhonen (✉)
Department of Nursing Science, University of Turku, Turku and Turku University Hospital, Wellbeing Services County of Southwest Finland, Turku, Finland
e-mail: riisuh@utu.fi

M. Stolt
Department of Nursing Science, University of Turku, Turku and Wellbeing Services County of Satakunta, Pori, Finland
e-mail: minna.stolt@utu.fi

© The Author(s), under exclusive license to Springer Nature Switzerland AG 2024
P. A. Scott, S. M. Scott (eds.), *Key Concepts and Issues in Nursing Ethics*,
https://doi.org/10.1007/978-3-031-54108-7_13

Keywords

Older individuals · Nursing ethics · Ethical issues · Care context · Care environment · Rights · Responsibilities

Case Study

Nursing care always includes an ethical aspect, and nursing care in different contexts may raise a variety of ethical issues due to the circumstances of individual patients, their health conditions, or environment. The case study encapsulates some of the ethical issues that may arise in caring for an older person in a home care context.

> *Anneli is a retired nurse aged 85 years. She lives at home with her sister who has become Anneli's main carer. Anneli's health is deteriorating. She struggles to eat and is beginning to lose weight. Anneli is also showing some signs of cognitive impairment, and last year she fell and broke her hip. She has had mobility problems since then—but refuses physiotherapy. Her ability to move is deteriorating. Anneli's younger sister Kirsten, herself 75 years old, is becoming increasingly worried for Anneli's health. Kirsten is also worried that if Anneli's health continues to deteriorate she may not be able to care for her in their home. Kirsten is aware that Anneli does not wish to move to a nursing home or any other form of institutional setting. Kirsten aims to act according to Anneli's wishes, supporting Anneli's autonomy, but knows that the vulnerability, inability to move, and cognitive impairment is likely to progress, ultimately making it impossible for Anneli to stay at home.*
>
> *Kirsten starts to discuss possible options with Anneli, including whether professional home care may ease in their situation, or whether they should look for a suitable nursing home near their house. Anneli refuses to talk about any transfer to a nursing home but after discussing with Kirsten the types of support and care available Anneli may see a nursing home as an option.*
>
> *As Anneli trusts that Kirsten aims for what is best for her, she allows Kirsten to ask for a needs assessment from the home care agency. A home nurse visits them and discusses the different options available, based on Anneli's needs and situation. Following much discussion and consideration of the likely trajectory of her health, and the options available, Anneli indicates her preferences and her wish to select the nursing home she is to live in. The nurse aims to lessen Anneli's vulnerability in the difficult transition to residential care, with a respectful dialogue supporting relational autonomy and maintaining Anneli's dignity.*

Introduction

Several ethical issues are fundamental when investigating the nursing care of older individuals, including autonomy, self-determination, respect, dignity, and questions related to decision-making in clinical care (Suhonen et al. 2010). In this chapter these ethical issues will be discussed in connection with clinical care situations.

In caring for older people, nurses face specific ethical issues for which they are more, or less, well prepared, based on their educational background, values, attitudes, and ethical competence (Pennestrì et al. 2023). In the organisations where they work, nurses have various opportunities to observe and have support systems to identify, specify, confront, and address ethical issues (Bartlett and Finder 2018). However, intervening in violations of older individuals' rights, including violations of self-determination and dignity or lack of respectful attitude, requires moral courage from nurses. When living in a nursing home or institutional care context, older individuals or their family members have very few opportunities to influence their situation. The same may apply to nurses if the organisational culture is not conducive to identification and discussion of humane values and ethically appropriate care. Healthcare systems and organisations have some structures for detecting, evaluating, and supervising service and care delivery (Mabel et al. 2023). However, if nursing professionals, care organisations, leaders, and supervisory bodies are not eager to offer channels to highlight different needs or the ethical issues encountered (Pennestrì et al. 2023), they miss the opportunity to learn and make development needs visible. Quality improvement is the ongoing activity in all care and service settings promised in strategies and required based on professionals' ethical codes. The care context of the older person is usually long-term and embraces the whole life-space of the older individual. This calls for vigilance in the care settings for older people.

Growing old and having different health problems is a current topic in many countries, as are global strategies regarding how to live a healthy life (United Nations 2020) and how to live well with long-term health conditions (OECD 2023). Not all individuals will experience healthy ageing; instead, they will be vulnerable (European Commission 2021), for example, due to different health needs, long-term conditions, poverty, powerlessness, social isolation, loneliness, and lack of or unequal access to healthcare (United Nations 2020), and some may have unmet care needs (OECD 2023) and/or an inability to obtain appropriate treatment or nursing care (Rush et al. 2017). Older individuals' vulnerable situations are often the result of multiple intersecting states or conditions including age, gender, and socio-economic circumstances, which potentially expose individuals to risk of harm and even neglect. Given these varied situations, the service system may miss opportunities to support those in difficult situations early enough. This applies particularly to home care (Spasova et al. 2018). The shift from institutional care to home care has been instituted in many European countries, but strategies to support independence, preventive, and rehabilitation services to keep older individuals physically, socially, and mentally active are limited, missing, or underdeveloped (Spasova et al. 2018).

Staying in your own home as you get older is called "ageing in place", and it is mentioned in many national and international policy documents (National Institute on Ageing 2017). For example, care and service plans are negotiated with those older individuals who live at home, identifying the most important needs for services and care. Needs assessment is sometimes difficult for nurses as it requires time and getting to know the older individuals. Recent studies have pointed out several topics related to missed care in the community or home care context (Sworn and Booth 2020) or in institutional care of older people (Kalánková et al. 2021; Kangasniemi et al. 2022), or even neglect (Kangasniemi et al. 2022) of older individuals. This warrants some consideration. Living alone at home with various health problems and without access to assistance can lead to exclusion and neglect, which are issues of ethical concern.

Many older individuals living in long-term care institutions, residential facilities, or at home have some level of cognitive impairment and dementia. In considering caring for this group of people, Denier and Gastmans (2022) introduced the idea of dignified dementia care, including respect for autonomy. One may assume that autonomous individuals have the capacity to process information, are competent, and have the ability to make informed decisions (Husted et al. 2015, pp. 55–58). When cognitive deficits are present, it does not mean that people are not autonomous.[1] However, we need to recognise that autonomy is a fundamental value and can easily be violated. Therefore, it needs to be noted that best practice is a "dialogue concerning what is the right thing to do in actual care practice" (Denier and Gastmans 2022, p. 968). Denier and Gastmans (2022, p. 968) state that "as such, respect for autonomy enters the stage as a positively sensitising and dialogue-enhancing concept, relationally seen from the various different perspectives of the relevant stakeholders". In the case study above, the nurse discusses, with both Anneli and Kirsten, Anneli's health situation and needs, trying to get the full understanding of the situation. She shows respect for Anneli and her preferences and wishes but also takes into consideration Kirsten's views and perceptions regarding Anneli's health, nutritional status, and mobility. Kirsten's ability to continue looking after Anneli in their home is also a matter for consideration.

Nurses frequently face ethical challenges in their work with older people in various healthcare settings (Suhonen et al. 2010). Older individuals also face ethical issues, for example, violation of patient's rights (Podgorica et al. 2021) or fundamental human rights, including equity in healthy ageing (European Network of National Human Rights Institutions 2017; United Nations 2020). The basic notion of rights is as important for someone living in a residential care setting, regardless of their cognitive or physical frailty, as it is for any other member of society (Kelly and Innes 2013, p. 61). Violation of rights may appear as abuse or neglect of older people, examples of which have been found in the older person's own home context (Yon et al. 2017) as well as in different care settings (Yon et al. 2019; Hirt et al. 2022; World Health Organization 2022).

Nursing care is delivered in the prevailing socio-political context. One of the general characteristics present in many contemporary societies is ageism, manifesting as pervasive ageism, which may impact on care delivery (Nemiroff 2022). Nurses' lack of awareness, for example, of the unique clinical manifestations of diseases affecting older adults can lead to indirect ageism due to missed diagnoses or delayed treatments based on age (Hammouri et al. 2022; Suhonen et al. 2018). Our beliefs about older people deeply condition our expectations and what we are prepared to accept as older people and as those who care for them. Therefore, it is an ethical issue whether nursing professionals are influenced by ageism bias or

---

[1] For an in-depth discussion of patient autonomy in the context of healthcare, including the impact of assisted decision-making legislation, please see Chap. 6.

whether they attend to individual patients who need nursing care, from a basis of respect, regardless of the patient's age or situation.

Healthcare professionals including nurses are committed to providing ethically sound and high-quality nursing care—as stated in many ethical and professional codes (World Health Organization 2016; International Council of Nurses, ICN 2021). This chapter raises ethical issues and challenges in the nursing care of older people, focusing particularly on the context of home care and long-term care settings.

Autonomy and Dignity as Fundamental Ethical Issues

Autonomy is one of the fundamental values in nursing ethics and in the care of older people (Bollig et al. 2016). From the point of view of older people, perceived autonomy refers to the opportunities for making their own decisions and choices about their daily lives. In the case study, Anneli's autonomy was respected by enabling Anneli to work through her situation; to consider her deteriorating health, the likely increasing burden this will place on her sister Kirsten, Anneli's main caregiver; and ultimately to choose the nursing home she would live in. This is important to Anneli as she has some criteria which a nursing home should meet to enable her to enjoy living there.

Anneli's wish to stay at home with Kirsten was not possible to support anymore, but still a mutual understanding was achieved in discussion, and Anneli's autonomy was supported. Perceived autonomy has been found to enhance both the quality of life and the health of older individuals living in residential care settings (Moilanen et al. 2021). Autonomy is linked to older people's individual capacities, including their level of independence, physical and mental competence, personal characteristics, and whether family members share and support their perceived autonomy. Older individuals also report that nurses can facilitate or hinder their autonomy in several ways, including providing opportunities for choice, enabling the older person's input into how daily care needs are supported, how activities can be organised, and how they are involved in decision-making regarding their daily activities. The relationship with the nursing staff is of the utmost importance and is perceived as both rewarding and problematic (Bollig et al. 2016).

From a nursing point of view, a recent literature review (Moilanen et al. 2022) reveals several ways to support autonomy. These include protecting older individuals' right to make their own decisions, respecting, and taking into account their hopes and wishes in care and fostering independence. At the same time, we need to acknowledge interdependence as many older individuals are frail and are dependent on others. Nurses acting as advocates, giving information to, and communicating with residents and relatives, have been found to enable autonomy. However, in many situations examined, communication is found to be a one-sided (Paananen and Lindholm 2023), missed, or neglected element of nursing care (Kalánková et al. 2021), thus undermining the ability of the older people concerned to exercise their autonomy. A relational understanding of autonomy, which sees the individual in a network of co-dependent relationships, interacting with others (professionals and/or family members), helps highlight the importance of shared decision-making (Gómez-Vírseda et al. 2019) in enhancing the perceived autonomy of older individuals.

Nursing care may raise awareness of how best to identify the preferences, wishes, and desires of older persons regarding their care, how to connect with family members, and how to use their professional competence to cherish the fundamental value of respect for autonomy. This calls for recognising one type of vulnerability that is present in older persons as the basic vulnerability of a human being: mortality and certainty of death, being subject to progressive deterioration and, thereby, dependency (Denier and Gastmans 2022). Another type of vulnerability is that different care situations may make older individuals vulnerable due to medication or illness-related deficits including challenging behaviour, wandering, or depression. These make "older adults more exposed than others to threats or injustices" (p. 968). We need to recognise that older individuals, like many other groups of people or individuals, are vulnerable because of such circumstances (Denier and Gastmans 2022). To provide ethically sensitive and respectful nursing care, it is important to recognise the issues and circumstances which make individuals vulnerable. Several studies, for example, have shown intentional or unintentional violations of patient rights (Podgorica et al. 2021), often due to a lack of ethical and legal education or knowledge, or otherwise unethical attitudes or practice (Tuominen et al. 2016). Lindwall and Lohne (2021) found that nurses fulfil their ethical responsibility by seeing, listening, and being a part of the time and place experienced by the older person. This is also in line with respectful nursing care manifesting itself as "doing for" and "being with" an older individual with respect (Koskenniemi et al. 2015).

Dignity is often tied with vulnerability, especially in nursing home settings. A study by Holmberg and Godskesen (2022) showed that older residents in nursing homes typically suffer from multiple long-term health conditions and illness-related concerns, inhibiting their possibilities to live a dignified life. Older individuals' failing bodies were found to be the most significant threat to perceived dignity, as loss of abilities was constantly progressing. Such vulnerability together with a fear of becoming more and more dependent and losing independence requires sensitivity and respectful care, as well as time for interaction, not only in taking care of daily routines and responding to care needs. Holmberg and Godskesen (2022) highlighted that because older individuals cherish autonomy and self-determination while still needing much help, these circumstances place them in a very vulnerable situation. Older individuals are aware of this loss of independence, and it requires sensitive, ethically informed nursing to protect the autonomy of elderly people facing these realities and burdens of deteriorating bodies and minds. This is nursing care where respect for the person is a fundamental value for those nurses providing care (Koskenniemi et al. 2015), which maintains respectful behaviours and attitudes within nursing care of older people.

"Seeing Individuals" as an Ethical Issue

Autonomy can be promoted with individualised care practices (Moilanen et al. 2022). Person-centred, patient-centred, or individualisation of care and services is typically and frequently suggested as the best framework or gold standard for the provision of high-quality, ethically sensitive care (Suhonen et al. 2019). According to Rogers (1961), person-centred care respects personhood. Personhood is a standing, or a status, bestowed on someone in the context of a relationship. This relationship should include interpersonal communication, listening to and hearing the person's narrative, and having a dialogue with the person. When nurses focus on the older individual as a person, the older individual can share their knowledge and experiences in a safe relationship (Öhlen and Friberg 2023). Interaction with an older individual requires time and sensitivity. It also required the ability to put yourself in someone else's position. All interaction takes place in a particular situation and context. In caring for older people, devoting nurses' time in this type of interaction should be a key nursing activity. However, it should be noted that in the current work organisation, a different approach is required in home care as compared to a nursing home context. This is the case due to time constraints. These differences warrant different and multiple variations in activities from nurses. In the case study, the nurse assesses Anneli's care needs and conditions in the home context with the aim of assessing Anneli's circumstances and individual needs, and deciding whether Anneli's needs can be taken care of in the home environment.

Person- or patient-centredness is often espoused to be at the heart of the health service system and care. Individualisation of care puts that promise into action. The need for such an approach has been highlighted in providing nursing care to older people. It may be clear that with individualisation of care when treating a patient, a person, the service system must be tuned to each patient so that their care pathway, with all its events, is flexible, guided, and informed. However, based on the examples discussed above, questions can be raised as to whether care, including the nursing care of older people, fulfils these promises. For example, an ethical analysis of person-centred care by Hansson and Fröding (2020) questioned the possibilities of providing person-centred or individualised care. They framed their discussion considering healthcare in general, but some of their arguments are highly relevant when analysing the nursing care of older people.

Hansson and Fröding (2020) identified several conflicts related to the themes of patient-centred care, three examples of which will be raised next. Hansson and Fröding (2020) firstly argued that holistic, comprehensive care includes far more of the patient's needs, characteristics, perceptions, sensations, life circumstances, and health/health problem issues than can be treated, assessed, or even brought to light in a visible way. And even if it were possible to assess and bring these issues to light, how would this information be transferred between professionals, at the interface of organisations, and, on the other hand, how would the security of information and the privacy of the patient be guaranteed? These are tricky questions in the care of older individuals living at home, with care and services provided by different professionals from different parts of the care system, including nursing care.

Another example of compromised issues in providing person-centred care is the personal relationship that requires reciprocity and focusing in the moment, time, and place on the part of both the professional and the patient. This requires exchange of information, "give and take" in discovering the care required and preferred by the older person (and the care the nurse considers it necessary/desirable to give). It assumes a strong element of mutual respect and care in the relationship. If we consider, for example, the interactions between older individuals being cared for in different care settings and their care providers in the changing situations, it is unclear whether the required reciprocity is even possible. However, it is positive that in caring for older people, the care settings, and likely time periods involved, enable the building of relationships between staff and patients/residents to a degree where there can be real knowledge regarding the will and preferences of the elderly person/resident among members of staff. In this sense, focusing on developing and learning from nursing care for older people could take a very positive step forward in supporting autonomy and self-determination.

Finally, Hansson and Fröding (2020) raised shared decision-making as a key element of individualised and patient-centred care. As indicated above shared decision-making involves the participation of both the professional and the patient in the decision-making process, sharing information and achieving a common understanding of the issue, participation in making the decision itself, the expression of preferences, and the implementation of the decision. This is, of course, aimed at supporting relational autonomy and self-determination (Denier and Gastmans 2022). On the other hand, looking at the whole picture, the question immediately arises as to whether the information and preferences of the professional and the patient correspond and whether the conditions for decision-making are met. Legislation supporting self-determination and assisted decision-making has been enacted, for example, in Ireland (Assisted Decision-Making (Capacity) Act 2015 2023)[2] or is under preparation in many countries. In care settings for older people, these questions can be resolved by implementing models and procedures for advanced care planning, shared decision-making, and daily care need assessment. Advance care planning (ACP) encompasses a process by which individuals may express and record their values and preferences for care and treatment should they lose the capacity to communicate these in the future (Martin et al. 2016). Whilst ACP has been especially linked to end-of-life care (Reitjens et al. 2017), such procedure would be beneficial in wider use. Older individuals living in nursing homes and residential or long-term care settings may benefit from expressing and recording their will. Nurses can initiate similar procedures for older individuals' comprehensive needs assessment, to decrease missed care and missed opportunities. This would be especially important in the home care context, as comprehensive assessment, which is included in procedures such as ACP, may provide guidance for respectful care. Such a comprehensive approach and shared decision-making may also decrease hospitalisations (Martin et al. 2016).

---

[2] Please see Chap. 6 for further discussion of assisted decision-making legislation.

Ethical Issues in Using Technology in Caring for Older People

Technology is believed to be useful in many healthcare contexts, including in supporting older people to remain in their own homes for as long as possible.[3] Several initiatives have been taken, and much expectation has been generated in the developing technologies, especially for home care. Whilst there has been a rapid increase in the use of technology in nursing care as a response to increasing needs, the move to investigate the ethical issues involved in the use of such technology has been slower to gain traction. In terms of the provision of nursing care, technology and technological devices can be used for different purposes (e.g. Sundgren et al. 2020). First, technology can be used to assess and detect deficits in motor, cognitive, and other abilities. Second, surveillance technology can be used to monitor the performance and health status of older people living at home using wearable systems. Third, technology can be used to compensate for possible deficits, especially at home. Finally, technology has been developed for social purposes or care relations, including the use of care robots (Ide et al. 2023). However, inclusion of technology in nursing care, and the issues involved, gives rise to several ethical issues (Ibuki et al. 2023). Ethical issues in this context include issues of consent and privacy, advocacy, accountability, and caring. Ibuki et al. (2023, p. 1) stated that "among the components of advocacy, safeguarding and apprising can be more easily implemented, while elements that require emotional communication with patients, such as valuing and mediating, are difficult to implement". In the caring domain, more difficulties can be expected in care-receiving than in caregiving (Ibuki et al. 2023). This clearly points out the need for a balanced evaluation of the use of technology and the ethical issues involved, including understanding different views, involvement of all stakeholders including nurses, and older individuals and their family members.

The use of technology and care robots requires ethical awareness, for example, of the implications of use of personal information, privacy protection (Felber et al. 2023; Ide et al. 2023), and safety (Fasoli et al. 2023). From the perspective of the older individual concerns regarding the potential dehumanisation of care have been raised (Sundgren et al. 2020; Fasoli et al. 2023), reflecting fears of being left alone or without human caring contact. The quality of interaction is known to be a difficult issue, regarding the value of human versus artificial interaction—including the use of social robots (Felber et al. 2023). This gives rise to issues of moral responsibility (Fasoli et al. 2023) and trust (Felber et al. 2023). Older individuals with frailty require special consideration when incorporating technology into their care because of their vulnerability, complex health needs, and social status (Wang et al. 2023).

However, strong potential has been identified, in supporting autonomy, independence, and active ageing, using technology in the home and in other care contexts (Fasoli et al. 2023; Felber et al. 2023). Whilst many of the technological solutions developed may be beneficial for supporting older individuals to age in place and live

---
[3] For an in-depth discussion of the ethics of communication technologies in the provision of remote, home-based nursing care, please see Chap. 16.

in their own homes, we need to be cognisant of the nuance, from a nursing care perspective, that the use of such technology puts on ethical issues such as patient autonomy or self-determination, consent, privacy, dignity, and many more. The use of technology as a joint initiative from service providers and service users to replace, for example, a home visit with remote tablet communication is different from that initiated by individuals, in this case, older individuals. Older individuals may not be familiar with these technologies, and they tend to be more cautious or critical of the use of technology in nursing care. Older people are also more powerless to influence and are vulnerable to the potential to replace human care with such technology. It appears that care has a very low priority in contemporary society, and a human workforce has become expensive. If there is a cheaper way of meeting physical needs, it is likely to be unstoppable, unless we have nurses who can influence this development in constructive ways that lead to the integration of such technology as an adjunct to nursing care, rather than as a replacement of the nurse.

Holistic, individualised, or person-centred nursing care, where the presence of the other person, the professional nurse, is special, has a profound impact on patient outcomes. There has not been much discussion to date regarding how well older individuals' needs and health issues can be assessed or recognised when care is delivered using digital solutions for communication. Currently there is also not much research evidence about the ethics, rights, and responsibilities regarding health communication when using digital technologies to replace onsite examination and assessment. Other issues such as loneliness, isolation, and concerns about losing human contacts have been raised by older individuals. In home nursing care, this requires taking care that no one is left behind.

Conclusions

Nursing care is delivered in the prevailing socio-political context. The ethical issues arising in the nursing care of all individuals and especially in the care of older individuals are context-bound. This context sets the framework for the resources available and for their allocation. However, it should be noted that nursing has its own ethical foundation that needs to be cherished and brought into discussion at a deeper level. The ethical competence of nursing professionals, as well as the education of nursing students, should be based on a more comprehensive discussion about ethical issues and the necessary tools and interventions required to safeguard the patient or client role and to protect the person-centredness of nursing care for vulnerable groups.

The person-centred approach can offer fruitful circumstances for holistic nursing care. The competence and natural inclinations of professionals (in addition to access to the resources required to implement patient-centred care and relevant legislation where it exists) influence how the individuality and holistic approach mentioned above can be made visible and whether all these issues, which can only partially be brought to light, can then be dealt with in the healthcare system. In care of the older people contexts, nurses normally have enough time to get to know the individual. In care of the older people settings, interactions and relations provide room for deep communication and relationship. The question arises as to how to fully support older individuals in their variable situations in a dignified and meaningful way.

> **Key Learning Points**
> - Ethical issues in caring for older people are multidimensional and complex.
> - Fundamental values including autonomy, respect, and dignity are particularly central in the nursing care of older individuals.
> - The use of technological solutions is evolving rapidly in the care of older people, introducing ethical issues such as access to care, privacy, trust, and autonomy.
> - The ethical competence of nursing professionals is the basis for providing dignified care to older individuals in different care settings and may be deeply compromised by the cultures in which nurses work.

References

Assisted Decision-Making (Capacity) Act 2015 (2023) https://revisedacts.lawreform.ie/eli/2015/act/64/revised/en/html. Accessed 2 Oct 2023

Bartlett VL, Finder SG (2018) Lessons learned from nurses' requests for ethics consultation: why did they call and what did they value? Nurs Ethics 25:601–617

Bollig G, Gjengedal E, Rosland JH (2016) Nothing to complain about? Residents' and relatives' views on a "good life" and ethical challenges in nursing homes. Nurs Ethics 23:142–153

Denier Y, Gastmans C (2022) Relational autonomy, vulnerability and embodied dignity as normative foundations of dignified dementia care. J Med Ethics 48:968–969

European Commission (2021) Total population size, and numbers and percentages of people in vulnerable categories in EU member states in 2017. https://knowledge4policy.ec.europa.eu/health-promotion-knowledge-gateway/health-inequalities-vulnerable-2_en. Accessed 29 Sept 2023

European Network of National Human Rights Institutions (2017) We have the same sights: the human rights of older persons in long-term care in Europe. http://ennhri.org/IMG/pdf/ennhri_hr_op_web.pdf. Accessed 28 Sept 2023

Fasoli A, Beretta G, Pravettoni G et al (2023) Mapping emerging technologies in aged care: results from an in-depth online research. BMC Health Serv Res 23:528. https://doi.org/10.1186/s12913-023-09513-5

Felber NA, Tian YJA, Pageau F et al (2023) Mapping ethical issues in the use of smart home health technologies to care for older persons: a systematic review. BMC Med Ethics 24(1):24. https://doi.org/10.1186/s12910-023-00898-w

Gómez-Vírseda C, de Maeseneer Y, Gastmans C (2019) Relational autonomy: what does it mean and how is it used in end-of-life care? A systematic review of argument-based ethics literature. BMC Med Ethics 20:76. https://doi.org/10.1186/s12910-019-0417-3

Hammouri A, Taani MH, Ellis J (2022) Ageism in the nursing care of older adults: a concept analysis. Adv Nurs Sci 46:441. https://doi.org/10.1097/ANS.0000000000000472

Hansson SO, Fröding B (2020) Ethical conflicts in patient-centred care. Clin Ethics 16:55–66

Hirt J, Adlbrecht L, Heinrich S et al (2022) Staff-to-resident abuse in nursing homes: a scoping review. BMC Geriatr 22:1–14

Holmberg B, Godskesen T (2022) Dignity in bodily care at the end of life in a nursing home: an ethnographic study. BMC Geriatr 22:593. https://doi.org/10.1186/s12877-022-032

Husted GL, Scotto CJ, Wolf KM et al (2015) Bioethical decision making in nursing, 5th edn. Springer, New York

Ibuki T, Ibuki A, Nakazawa E (2023) Possibilities and ethical issues of entrusting nursing tasks to robots and artificial intelligence. Nurs Ethics. https://doi.org/10.1177/09697330221149094

Ide H, Suwa S, Akuta Y et al (2023) Developing a model to explain users' ethical perceptions regarding the use of care robots in home care: a cross-sectional study in Ireland, Finland, and Japan. Arch Gerontol Geriatr 116:105137. https://doi.org/10.1016/j.archger.2023.105137

International Council of Nurses, ICN (2021) The ICN code of ethics for nurses. https://www.icn.ch/sites/default/files/2023-06/ICN_Code-of-Ethics_EN_Web.pdf. Accessed 26 Sept 2023

Kalánková D, Stolt M, Scott PA et al (2021) Unmet care needs of older people: a scoping review. Nurs Ethics 28:149–178

Kangasniemi M, Papinaho O, Moilanen T et al (2022) Neglecting the care of older people in residential care settings: a national document analysis of complaints reported to the Finnish supervisory authority. Health Soc Care Community 30:e1313–e1324

Kelly F, Innes A (2013) Human rights, citizenship and dementia care nursing. Int J Older People Nurs 8:61–70

Koskenniemi J, Leino-Kilpi H, Suhonen R (2015) Manifestation of respect in the care of older patients in long-term care settings. Scand J Caring Sci 29:288–296

Lindwall L, Lohne V (2021) Human dignity research in clinical practice—a systematic literature review. Scand J Caring Sci 35:1038–1049

Mabel H, Myers G, Gorecki J et al (2023) The ethics resource caregiver program: equipping nurses as ethics champions. J Clin Ethics 34:27–39

Martin RS, Hayes B, Gregorevic K et al (2016) The effects of advance care planning interventions on nursing home residents: a systematic review. J Am Med Dir Assoc 17:284–293

Moilanen T, Kangasniemi M, Papinaho O et al (2021) Older people's perceived autonomy in residential care: an integrative review. Nurs Ethics 28:414–434

Moilanen T, Suhonen R, Kangasniemi M (2022) Nursing support for older people's autonomy in residential care: an integrative review. Int J Older People Nurs 17:e12428. https://doi.org/10.1111/opn.12428

National Institute on Ageing (2017) Ageing in place: growing older at home. https://www.nia.nih.gov/health/aging-place-growing-older-home. Accessed 27 Sept 2023

Nemiroff L (2022) We can do better: addressing ageism against older adults in healthcare. Healthc Manage Forum 35:118–122

OECD (2023) Health at a glance 2023: OECD indicators. OECD Publishing, Paris. https://doi.org/10.1787/7a7afb35-en

Öhlen J, Friberg F (2023) Person-centred conversations in nursing and health: a theoretical analysis based on perspectives of communication. Nurs Philos 24:e12432. https://doi.org/10.1111/nup.12432

Paananen J, Lindholm C (2023) Discussing physical restrictions in care plan meetings between family members of residents with dementia and nursing home staff. Dementia (London) 22:1530–1547

Pennestrì F, Villa G, Giannetta N et al (2023) Training ethical competence in a world growing old: a multimethod ethical round in hospital and residential care settings. J Bioeth Inq 20:279–294

Podgorica N, Flatscher-Thöni M, Deufert D et al (2021) A systematic review of ethical and legal issues in elder care. Nurs Ethics 28:895–910

Reitjens JAC, Sudore RL, Conolly M et al (2017) Definition and recommendations for advance care planning: an international consensus supported by the European Association for Palliative Care. Lancet Oncol 18:e543–e551

Rogers C (1961) On becoming a person: a therapist's view of psychotherapy. Houghton Mifflin Company

Rush KL, Hickey S, Epp S et al (2017) Nurses' attitudes towards older people care: an integrative review. J Clin Nurs 26:4105–4116

Spasova S, Baeten R, Coster S et al (2018) Challenges in long-term care in Europe. A study of national policies. European Social Policy Network (ESPN), Brussels. https://doi.org/10.2767/84573

Suhonen R, Stolt M, Launis V et al (2010) Research in ethics of nursing care for older people. A literature review. Nurs Ethics 17:337–352

Suhonen R, Stolt M, Habermann M et al (2018) RANCARE consortium COST Action—CA15208. 2018. Ethical elements in priority setting in nursing care—a scoping review. Int J Nurs Stud 17:25–42

Suhonen R, Stolt M, Papastavrou E (2019) Individualised care—theory, measurement, research and practice. Springer International Publishing AG, Cham

Sundgren S, Stolt M, Suhonen R (2020) Ethical issues related to the use of gerontechnology in the care of community-dwelling older people: a scoping review. Nurs Ethics 27:88–103

Sworn K, Booth A (2020) A systematic review of the impact of 'missed care' in primary, community and nursing home settings. J Nurs Manag 28:1805–1829

Tuominen L, Leino-Kilpi H, Suhonen R (2016) Older people's experiences of their own free will in and its actualisation, promoters and barriers in nursing homes. Nurs Ethics 23:22–35

United Nations (2020) UN decade of healthy ageing: plan of action. https://cdn.who.int/media/docs/default-source/decade-of-healthy-ageing/decade-proposal-final-apr2020-en.pdf?sfvrsn=b4b75ebc_28. Accessed 21 Sept 2023

Wang RH, Tannou T, Bier N et al (2023) Proactive and ongoing analysis and management of ethical concerns in the development, evaluation, and implementation of smart homes for older adults with frailty. JMIR Aging 6:e41322. https://doi.org/10.2196/41322

World Health Organization (2016) Framework on integrated, people-centred health services. Report by the secretariat. http://apps.who.int/gb/ebwha/pdf_files/WHA69/A69_39-en.pdf?ua=1. Accessed 23 Sept 2023

World Health Organization (2022) Abuse of older people. https://www.who.int/news-room/fact-sheets/detail/abuse-of-older-people. Accessed 21 Sept 2023

Yon Y, Mikton CR, Gassoumis ZD et al (2017) Elder abuse prevalence in community settings: a systematic review and meta-analysis. Lancet Glob Health 5:e147–e156

Yon Y, Ramiro-Gonzalez M, Mikton C et al (2019) The prevalence of elder abuse in institutional settings: a systematic review and meta-analysis. Eur J Public Health 29:58–67

Ethical Issues at the End of Life

14

Janet Holt

Abstract

This chapter explores the ethical, legal and professional issues that healthcare professionals face when caring for individuals at the end of life. Contemporary guidance will be drawn upon along with an evolving case study and legal judgments to illustrate and discuss the issues raised. Beginning with an exploration of the concept of the good death and the role of palliative care in facilitating a good death, the process of advance care planning and making advanced decisions is discussed. This is followed by a consideration of the withdrawal of treatment and draws on English and Irish cases to illustrate the legal and ethical aspects of futile treatment. The classification of artificially administered nutrition and hydration and the controversy surrounding the use of the Liverpool Care Pathway are also considered. The final sections of the chapter consider the difficult subject of assisted dying, suicide and physician-assisted suicide. The discussion is informed by cases in the English and Irish Courts and the most recent attempts to change legislation in the UK. Euthanasia, arguably the most controversial aspect of assisted dying, is examined. Insight from countries such as the Netherlands, where active voluntary euthanasia is lawful, informs the debate.

Keywords

Good death · Palliative care · Withdrawing treatment · Assisted dying · Euthanasia

J. Holt (✉)
School of Healthcare, University of Leeds, Leeds, UK
e-mail: hcsjh@leeds.ac.uk

Introduction

The care of the dying person is a fundamental and important part of nursing in critical, acute and continuing care as well as in community, hospital, and other institution settings. While death and the process of dying are of importance to everyone, healthcare professionals face particular challenges in ensuring that high-quality care is delivered in accordance with the patients' wishes and in their best interests. Some of these challenges are of a practical nature, but others pose significant ethical dilemmas and problems for practitioners striving to do the best for their patients, while being mindful of their legal and professional duties. Beginning with an examination of the concept of the good death, this chapter explores the ethical issues of withdrawing treatment, including nutrition and hydration, assisted suicide, physician-assisted suicide and euthanasia. Contemporary guidance will be drawn upon along with an evolving case study and legal judgments to illustrate and discuss the issues raised.

The Concept of a Good Death (Including Case Study)

While death may be an event, dying is a process which due to technological advances allows patients to be resuscitated, given new treatments and kept alive using artificial means. In some instances, instead of asking 'can we treat the patient?', a more appropriate question may be 'should we treat the patient?' The concept of the good death has been a matter of debate for centuries. For example, discussion of the subject can be found in ancient writings such as Plato's Dialogues from the fifth century BC. In the Phaedo, for example, Plato recounts the 'good death' of Socrates who, having been convicted of impiety and corruption of the young, chooses to die by taking hemlock rather than escape his prison cell (Plato 1969). For some the idea of a swift and relatively pain-free death, such as that resulting from a catastrophic brain injury, might be considered a good death; while for others, a more protracted process that gives time for the person to see friends and relatives say goodbye or 'put their house in order' is more preferable. The quest for a universal definition of a good death therefore may seem futile and instead should perhaps be recognised as dependent on individual preferences and culturally determined (Goldsteen et al. 2006).

Towards the end of life, many individuals receive palliative care, which is defined by the World Health Organization (2020) as 'an approach that improves the quality of life of patients (adults and children) and their families who are facing problems associated with life-threatening illness. It prevents and relieves suffering by the early identification, correct assessment and treatment of pain and other problems, whether physical, psychosocial or spiritual'. The United Kingdom (UK) is recognised as a leader in the development of palliative care as a speciality particularly through the work of Dame Cecily Saunders and the introduction of the hospice movement in 1967. Changes to the Health and Care Act in 2022 included palliative care in the section detailing the legal responsibilities of integrated care boards to commission services to meet the needs of their populations (NHS England 2022). There are also a number of policy and guidance documents specifically addressing palliative and end of life care, such as the National Institute for Health and Care Excellence (NICE) quality standard *End of Life Care for Adults* (National Institute for Health and Care Excellence 2021), comprising of quality statements to ensure that the best care can be offered to individuals through the NHS. While patients may prefer to die in their own homes or in a hospice, opportunities for exercising choice regarding the place of death are limited. In England, for example, around half of all deaths occur in hospital (Office for National Statistics 2015) where care may not always be given by palliative care specialists. It is therefore possible that some patients may not receive optimum care. A survey of over 8000 members of the public showed that respondents identified being pain-free, with loved ones, dying with dignity, having access to a trained carer and privacy as key priorities in palliative and end-of-life care (Marie Curie 2021). The importance of our understanding of the good death was brought sharply into focus during the COVID pandemic in 2020/2021, as many of the customary rituals and practices associated with death were prohibited. At the height of the pandemic, thousands of people died in circumstances far removed from what they or their family and friends might have anticipated at the end of life, as they were not allowed to hold or attend funerals, make hospital visits, or be present with someone in the final hours of their life.

While there have been clear improvements in end-of-life care, there are still inequalities in access to good-quality care and support. This is further exacerbated, in the UK for example, by the complex funding arrangements for end-of-life care, where only around 30% of funding comes from the NHS and statutory sources. The remainder is provided through voluntary sector organisations. Ensuring patients have a choice regarding their place of death, as well as access to expert care irrespective of the place of death, according to policy documents, is a key priority in the UK. However, this means that sufficient resources need to be provided to support families and healthcare professionals to put this into practice. A report from authors at the London School of Economics for Sue Ryder estimates that the number of patients in need of palliative care services is likely to rise from 47 to 66% by 2031/31 (Von Petersdorff et al. 2021). The following short case study may help us identify and work through some of the relevant issues here.

> Susan is a 58-year-old single woman with end-stage ovarian cancer. She lives on her own but has a 30-year-old son Peter who lives 200 miles away and a 35-year-old daughter Clare who lives with her family in Australia. Susan understands her diagnosis and knows that she is expected to die in a few months. She would prefer to be at home but cannot rely on her children to support her. Having been brought up in the Roman Catholic faith, Susan no longer has any religious beliefs and describes herself as agnostic. Susan values her independence and until recently has been very active in her local community. She has served as a Town Councillor and as a School Governor and volunteers in the local food bank. Through these activities Susan has enjoyed a good social life and developed a wide group of friends.
>
> Susan's situation is complicated by the fact that she lives on her own and neither of her children is in a position to help to care for her in her own home. She would therefore need support from community nursing services and possibly organisations such as Marie Curie,

which she may be fortunate enough to access. But in a publicly funded health system with competing priorities, despite the best intentions, the goal of high-quality care in a place of the patient's choice may well remain aspirational.

Advance Care Planning

Everyone receiving treatment and care from healthcare professionals is entitled to decide what should and what should not happen to them, and individuals should expect to have the decisions they make respected. The ethical justification for this is explained by the principle of autonomy. Being free to make autonomous decisions is a key principle in ethics and underpins legally valid consent. However, to exercise an autonomous decision, a person must be able to understand the choices available, be free from any controlling influences, and make the decision based on accurate information.[1] Under the terms of the Mental Capacity Act 2005 (Department of Health (DoH) 2005), capacity is assumed, and incapacity needs to be proven through the use of tests for competence (Pattinson 2020). The Mental Capacity Act came into force in England and Wales in 2007 and provides a framework for decision-making for those no longer able to do this themselves. The remit of the Act is far-reaching, but the underlying principles are particularly relevant when caring for people at the end of life. For example, a person should not be treated as lacking capacity simply because they make what is thought to be an unwise decision. People are allowed lawfully to refuse treatment or procedures, in what may seem to others to be an irrational decision. An example of this would be a Jehovah's Witness refusing a lifesaving blood transfusion. While preferring to die rather than have a relatively simple procedure may seem irrational to someone who does not share that faith, as long as the person has capacity and their decision is unquestionably autonomous, then they have both an ethical and legal right to have their decision respected.

The link between autonomy and capacity is important, as it is only by having capacity that a person can exercise an autonomous decision, which consequently places others under an obligation to respect the person's freedom of choice. At this stage in her illness, Susan has capacity, and as death is foreseen, she has the opportunity to make some plans about her preferences. For example, she could prepare an advance statement, a written statement that sets out a person's preferences, wishes, beliefs and values regarding their care. Such a statement can be written by any person at any time. And while not legally binding it is designed to ensure any preferences can be recorded, so that should capacity be lost in the future the advance statement could help others, such as Susan's family, in making decisions on her behalf. In the statement Susan could let her family know her preferences about where she would like to die, who she would like to be present, or that she definitely would or would not like to be visited by a priest.

The advance statement is different to an advance decision. An advanced decision is a means by which a person may make decisions about the treatment they would

---

[1] See Chap. 6 for a discussion of the concept and principle of autonomy.

not like to receive, should they lose capacity and be unable to communicate their wishes. Typically, this would include life-sustaining treatments such as mechanical ventilation or cardiopulmonary resuscitation (CPR). Advance decisions are sometimes know by other terms such as an advance directive, advance decision to refuse treatment, or living wills. Such advance decisions are legally binding in England and Wales under the terms of the Mental Capacity Act (MCA) 2005 (Department of Health (DoH) 2005). The MCA also makes provision for proxy decision-making through lasting powers of attorney (LPA). This means that a patient can appoint someone of their choice to make treatment decisions they consider to be in their best interests once they lose capacity (Pattinson 2020). There are a number of conditions that have to be met for an LPA to be lawful, but even if these are met, it does not mean that they are without problems in practice.

Suppose that Susan, towards the beginning of her illness, made an advance decision that she did not want to have CPR. Later on as Susan's condition starts to deteriorate, Clare her daughter returns from Australia and finds out about the advance decision. Clare is very unhappy about this and tells the health professionals caring for her mother that she wants everything possible done for her. If Susan still has capacity, she will of course be able to explain her decision to Clare herself, and it is recommended that family members or carers be involved in or at least be aware of advance decisions. But if Susan is no longer able to communicate, then it will be up to the health professionals to explain. If Susan has made a fully autonomous decision about the CPR, then there can be no ethical justification to override her wishes just to appease her daughter. This will undoubtedly result in a difficult conversation between the health professionals and Clare, but this is more an issue of effective communication skills rather than one of ethics. Hence in England and Wales, an advance decision for refusal of treatment, if valid and applicable, is considered to have the same force in law as if Susan was making the statement contemporaneously.

Withdrawing Treatment

There are situations when rather than making a decision to refuse treatment, the patient themselves insists on being treated against the advice of the health professionals. The patient may understand that there is little chance of success but decide they still want to receive treatment. For example, suppose that Susan decides that she wanted to continue with her cancer treatment against medical advice because she wants to stay alive until Clare and her family were able to travel from Australia. Even if she understands there are no guarantees that this will happen if the treatment continues, she thinks it's worth the risk. If Susan's autonomous wish is to be respected, then the treatment should continue, but this could be an ethical problem for the health professionals treating Susan, if they believe that the treatment will be of no benefit and not in Susan's best interests. If respecting the patient's autonomy is the best way in which Susan's best interests are protected, then ethically, giving the treatment is justified. But there may be other competing interests or demands such as appropriate utilisation of resources and practising according to best evidence that also need to be taken into consideration. In a publicly funded healthcare system, it is important to ensure that best use is made of the resources available and the National Institute for Health and Care Excellence (NICE) provides national guidance and advice to improve health care with resources that make best use of available evidence.

As noted above, the aim of palliative care is to achieve the best quality of life for patients and their families, through the process of diagnosis, treatment and care through the trajectory of their illness. Administering treatment that is both costly and ineffective cannot be of benefit on an individual level for a patient like Susan, nor does it demonstrate good use of resources for society as a whole. While there may be justification for the withdrawal of medical treatment towards the end of life, there is some disagreement regarding what actually constitutes medical treatment and whether the administration of nutrition and hydration falls within the scope of this definition. A legal interpretation of nutrition and hydration can be found in Airedale NHS Trust v Bland. Tony Bland was a young man severely injured in the Hillsborough football disaster in 1989. He was left in a permanent vegetative state with no hope of recovery and although breathing spontaneously and was fed through a nasogastric tube. Mr. Bland's parents and treating physician believed that the withdrawal of treatment was in his best interest and so applied to the Court for permission to withdraw all treatment, including artificially administered nutrition and hydration. Following a lengthy court case, in 1993, five Law Lords ruled that the artificial hydration and nutrition could lawfully be removed. The Law Lords did not draw a distinction between the provision of nutrition and hydration by artificial means and medical treatment and consequently held that tube feeding was part of the regime of treatment and care (Pattinson 2020).

In Ireland a similar case, Re a Ward of Court, was heard in the Supreme Court in 1995. The case concerned a woman described as being in a near persistent vegetative state for over 23 years. She had experienced three cardiac arrests while under anaesthetic for minor gynaecological surgery in 1972 and suffered brain damage from which she did not recover. Consequently the woman was unable to communicate, move or swallow and was fed initially by a nasogastric tube and later via a gastrostomy. The Ward's family asked the court to have the gastrostomy tube removed, but the hospital where she was being cared for objected to discontinuing feeding which they saw as a means of hastening death. The Ward received excellent nursing care, any infections were treated with antibiotics and the nurses described in court the special relationship that had developed between them and the Ward. However, the Supreme Court did rule in favour of discontinuing feeding considering that as the woman lacked capacity, the decision should be made on the basis of best interests. Similar to, and possibly influenced by, the Bland case, the Court considered the administration of nutrition and hydration through the gastrostomy tube to be medical treatment. As the treatment was of no net benefit to the Ward, it could be lawfully withdrawn (Dooley and McCarthy 2005).

Therefore, as seen in both of these cases, nutrition and hydration administered by artificial means are classed in law as medical treatment that can in some circumstances be withdrawn. But this classification of feeding as medical treatment is not without its critics, and for some, food and fluids constitute ordinary care that should not be withdrawn. In a study 51 individuals with experience of relatives in either a vegetative or minimally conscious state were interviewed. Kitzinger and Kitzinger (2015) found that even when the respondents thought their relatives would no longer want to be alive, they were 'horrified by the idea of causing death by starvation and dehydration' (p. 157). Some even thought that administering a lethal injection would be more humane and dignified than death by neglect.

The provision of nutrition and hydration is usually considered to be a fundamental aspect of nursing care, but while nutrition and hydration are necessary for life, the evidence that they are also a requirement for a comfortable death is less clear-cut. An important distinction needs to be drawn here between the legality of withdrawing fluids and nutrition and a requirement to do so. If discontinuing fluid and nutrition through clinically assisted means is not considered by all involved in their care, including the patient themselves, as being in the patient's best interests, then there is both a legal and ethical justification to support their removal. However, this does not mean that it has to be done. The guidance from the Royal College of Physicians and the British Medical Association (2018) specifically addresses this point, recommending that practitioners have dialogue with the patient and those important to them, consider their views and explain the benefits, risk and burdens of providing fluids and/or nutrition on an individual basis. Nevertheless, the removal of clinically assisted nutrition and hydration remain controversial and as noted by Szawarski and Kakar (2012) likely to be defined by those opposed to assisted dying as a form of killing or at least as a pragmatic but inhumane practice.

Sometimes, the appropriate course of action will be to withdraw or withhold treatment including fluids or nutrition if there appears to be of no net benefit to the patient. But it may be questioned whether it is possible to be objective about the futility of treatment. Such judgements may be value laden, with patients, relatives and health professionals not necessarily sharing a common understanding of the concept of futility. So while judgements about what is in a patient's best interests are made from the patient's perspective, judgements made with reference to futility inherently assume there is an objective standard for determining benefits and burdens. But this is not the case due to differences not only in values but also in the probabilities of clinical outcomes. As noted by Wilson and Savulescu (2011), even if a treatment is judged futile by healthcare professionals because the chances of recovery are very small, such as 0.5%, some patients would still think this was a chance worth taking if the alternative is death.

Withdrawing treatment was the focus in the debate of the controversy surrounding the Liverpool Care Pathway (LCP). Developed in the 1990s, the LCP was based on end of life care developed in hospices and intended as a mechanism to share good practice to other palliative care settings. Hence, it was considered to be the gold standard in end of life care. However, a highly charged public condemnation of the LCP began to emerge in the media, and an independent review concluded that while there were examples of good use, in a number of cases, the LCP had become a generic protocol, often used without recognition of the individualised care needs of patients—resulting in a tick box exercise (Neuberger 2013). The review found that one of the key problems with the implementation of the LCP was a failure to accurately recognise the point at which some patients approached the last few days or hours of their lives, with the implication that the care prescribed by the LCP was commenced at too early a point in the process. This led to accusations of treatment, including fluids and nutrition, being withdrawn too early, in addition to accusations of an over use of sedative medication. Subsequently, the LCP was withdrawn in the UK (although is still in use in other European countries), and the Leadership Alliance for the Care of Dying People, a coalition of 21 national organisations with an interest in end of life care, took forward the recommendations of the Neuberger review and published new guidance in *One Chance to Get it Right* (Leadership Alliance for the Care of Dying People 2014). However, the problems with the LCP occurred because of the inability of some healthcare professions to accurately assess how close to death patients were. This resulted in commencing a regime of care too soon, with insufficient provision for individualised care or room for adjustments to be made to that care. It was not a failure of the pathway itself. Further criticism of the LCP suggested that there was a lack of a gold-standard evidence base supported by randomised controlled trials. In a detailed analysis of the rise and fall of the LCP, Seymour and Clark (2022) note that the replacement guidelines from LACPD and NICE also have a *flimsy evidence base* and are *long on values and aspirations but short on a practical course of actions. They replaced one set of deficiencies with another.* Therefore, what is crucially important for the revised guidelines to be effective and not repeat the same mistakes is a commitment at the highest level to provide resources to ensure comprehensive education and training for practitioners especially for those not working in specialised palliative care facilities.

While across all four nations of the UK, there is evidence of the recognition of the importance of palliative care services in the reports and recommendations produced, there is wide variation in state-funding to palliative care services. A substantial amount of care is provided through charitable organisations. By definition this gives rise to ethical issues of disparity and inequality in care provision. Susan therefore may be fortunate enough to live in an area with sufficient funding for palliative care to allow her to die at home supported by community services. Alternatively, she may not, and the burden of care will fall upon her family. If they are unable to provide this, Susan may be faced with no alternative than to receive institutionalised care, for example, in a nursing home. Hence the ethical problem that arises is not necessarily one of recognition of individualised care in accordance with the patient's wishes. The ethical problem, despite government aspirations, may be one of implementation and appropriate resource allocation in putting recommendations into effective practice to ensure the provision of individualised care.

Assisted Dying: Suicide and Physician-Assisted Suicide

Let us develop the scenario regarding Susan and her illness a little further.

As Susan's cancer progresses, she feels pessimistic about being able to die at home and is worried about needing institutional care. She is less worried about pain or the other symptoms she is experiencing as these are largely under control. What is concerning her is the thought of losing her independence and having to be cared for by nurses for fundamental needs. Susan discusses the possibility of taking her own life with her son Peter and asks him if he would be willing to help her take some medication that will result in her death.

While choice is important, autonomy cannot be considered to be an absolute ethical principle that will take precedence in every case. A person's autonomous choice can be legitimately constrained by the rights of others, as demonstrated in the assisted dying debate. One of the key issues in discussions about assisted dying is confusion in the way that the terms are used. Assisted dying is when a terminally ill person, with capacity, obtains assistance from a third party to help them die. If the assisting person is a doctor, then this is described as physician-assisted dying. Under the terms of the Suicide Act 1961 in England and Wales, a legal right to suicide is recognised. However, assisting someone to take their life by aiding, abetting, counselling or procuring the suicide of another is an offence and therefore unlawful in the UK (Pattinson 2020). So while Susan can take her own life, her doctor cannot lawfully prescribe medication for her, nor can someone lawfully administer medication to her with the intent of aiding her suicide.

Suppose that Peter understands the choice Susan has made and recognises this as a rational, autonomous decision. This does not necessarily mean that he is obliged to respect her wishes and assist her suicide. Susan may have a well thought-out plan upon which she wants to act, but in doing so she is asking Peter to act unlawfully, and he too must make an autonomous decision. Of course he may agree to do this and accept the consequences of his actions, or he may choose not to. Whatever course of action he chooses should be made on the basis of his own autonomous decision not simply because he feels obliged to act according to his mother's wishes. So rather than being an absolute principle, respecting autonomy is described as a prima facie principle. That is one that must be fulfilled unless it conflicts with an equal or stronger claim. Even if he agrees with his mother's decision in principle, Peter might consider the need to keep within the law a stronger claim than Susan's claim to have her autonomy respected.

Physician-Assisted Suicide

There have been a number of so-called 'right to die' cases brought before the courts in the UK such as that of Tony Bland, Dianne Pretty and Tony Nicklinson. The Nicklinson case is particularly interesting in drawing out the similarities and differences in judgments made in law and ethics. Mr. Nicklinson was a 58-year-old man suffering from locked-in syndrome and paralysed from the neck down following a stroke in 2005.

In 2012, Mr. Nicklinson's case to allow doctors to end his life without fear of prosecution was rejected by the High Court. The case was not considered to be one of assisted suicide as Mr. Nicklinson would have been unable to take lethal drugs, even if they were prepared by someone else. Lord Justice Toulson stated that a decision to allow the case would have far-reaching consequences and that to carry out Mr. Nicklinson's request meant that the court would be making a major change in the law. He added that 'It is not for the court to decide whether the law about assisted dying should be changed and, if so, what safeguards should be put in place. Under our system of government these are matters for Parliament to decide' (R (Nicklinson) v Ministry of Justice 2012). Mr. Nicklinson subsequently refused food and fluids and died of pneumonia 2 weeks after the judgment. While undoubtedly a correct legal judgement, authors such as Savulescu (2014) have questioned the ethics of this course of action, suggesting that if someone in Tony Nicklinson's position has a right to refuse to eat, then he also should be able to exercise a right to die by quickly and painlessly being relieved of his suffering. Mr. Nicklinson was clearly determined to end his life irrespective of the decision in law. But the action he subsequently took in refusing nutrition and fluids does challenge the concept of a good death and illustrates the complexity of deciding if this was a good ethical judgment, even if it was a correct legal one.

The question of rights was also an issue in a recent case brought before the Supreme Court in Ireland (Marie Fleming v Ireland, Attorney General and the Director of Public Prosecutions 2013). Marie Fleming, a woman with multiple sclerosis, sought permission for her partner to assist her to die at a time of her choice without fear of prosecution. Ms. Fleming claimed that not allowing assistance with her suicide breached her constitutional rights. However, echoing the judgement in the Dianne Pretty Case in the UK, the Supreme Court did not agree and found that there was no constitutional right to die or be assisted to do so. The attitudes of health professionals to assisted dying do appear to be changing as the Royal College of Nursing. British Medical Association, Royal College of Physicians and the Royal College of Surgeons currently all hold a neutral stance on assisted dying. Although surveys have been carried out to determine members view in each of these organisations, the response rates do not always reflect the proportion of members, and it is difficult to interpret a clear mandate of professionals in either favouring or being opposed to assisted dying. Hence, a statement of neutrality is possibly the most appropriate way to represent the diversity of view of members.

In the UK, there have been attempts to bring about a change in law to allow assisted dying in different forms, all of which have to date been unsuccessful. The most recent of which was Baroness Meacher's Assisted Dying Bill which received a second reading in the House of Lords in October 2021. But despite reaching the committee stage, the Bill ran out of time and was unable to complete all the necessary stages before the end of the 2022 parliamentary session. However, the issue has not gone away, and the Westminster and Scottish Parliaments, Dail Éireann in the Republic of Ireland, Parliaments in Jersey and the Isle of Man are all at the time of writing giving further consideration to making changes to the law. In December 2022, the Health and Social Care Committee of the Westminster Parliament launched an enquiry into assisted dying. An initial report of findings from public engagement has been published (House of Commons Select Committees 2023), and the Committee is still hearing oral evidence. Once completed, this committee of

Members of Parliament (MP) will make recommendations to the Government on next steps which may include recommendations for new legislation. Changes to the law in Scotland are also being explored by the Scottish Parliament. The Assisted Dying Scotland Members Bill proposed by Liam McArthur in June 2021 has gained enough support from Members of the Scottish Parliament to allow it to be introduced and is currently being drafted. In November 2021, Jersey in the Channel Islands became the first area of the British Isles to allow assisted dying. As a British Crown Dependency, Jersey is able to legislate independently, and the States Assembly agreed to the proposal in principle, with legislation being prepared for a final vote in 2024.

Of particular interest to nurses is the approach to medical assistance in dying (MAID) in Canada which was legalised in 2016. The situation in Canada is unique as it is the first country to allow nurse practitioners to determine if a person is eligible for MAID and to administer the medication to end the person's life. Barbara Pesut and her colleagues from the University of British Columbia have interviewed over 100 nurses about their experiences of MAID, the legalisation of which has profoundly influenced Canadian nursing practice, in the form of provoking deep personal experiences in providing the perfect death and the impact of MAID on their personal and professional relationships (Pesut and Thorne 2022). The current activity in the UK and its near neighbours could result in legislation that follows the Canadian example, giving an active role to nurses in carrying out assisted dying. Any such legislation would inevitably contain a conscience clause, meaning that practitioners objecting to the procedure would not have to participate. However, Pesut and Thorne (2022) discuss the much deeper and more nuanced implications for nursing practice as a consequence of MAID. They suggest that now 'the person decides when their life as a social being has crossed from life into death and that nurses now bear much more responsibility for promoting a good death as the person remains cognitively and biologically intact until the very end'. These are important matters to consider irrespective of whether as a nurse you support or object to the legalisation of assisted dying.

Assisted Dying: Dignitas

The new attempts to bring about changes in the law across the devolved nations of the UK, Jersey, the Isle of Man and the Republic of Ireland, even if successful, will take time to go through the stages of drafting legislation and approval through the various parliaments. If and until assisted dying is deemed lawful, the other option open to people determined to end their lives is to use the services of Dignitas. This Swiss-based organisation describes itself as a not-for-profit society that advocates, educates and supports improving care and choice at the end of life. Unlike the UK, the law governing suicide is less strict in Switzerland, where only people who personally gain from assisting a suicide are liable to prosecution and doctors are allowed in some circumstances to provide assistance when patients are terminally ill. In July 2023, representatives from Dignitas gave evidence to the Health and

Social Care Committee mentioned above. Stating that they though it was time to legalise assisted dying in the UK, members of Dignitas told the committee that the organisation had assisted in the deaths of 540 people and described the current rules in the UK as 'inadequate and incoherent' (Booth 2023).

Let us develop our scenario with Susan and her progressive illness a step further.

Peter has said he won't help Susan take her own life, but she has found out about Dignitas and thinks that perhaps ending her life this way at the time of her choosing may be more preferable. But she is reluctant to travel alone and would like Peter and Clare to be with her when she dies. So she asks them both to accompany her to Zurich.

The Suicide Act 1995 prohibits aiding and abetting suicide (Pattinson 2020), but what of the legal status of relatives or friends accompanying someone to use services of Dignitas? Clarification of this point is associated with Debbie Purdy, a woman with multiple sclerosis, who in 2009 won a case in the High Court seeking assurances that her husband would not be prosecuted if he accompanied her to Switzerland. The Law Lords agreed that the law was unclear and subsequently the Director of Public Prosecutions published new guidelines in 2010 (updated in 2014) clarifying the factors that would be taken into account when making a decision about prosecution. These include consideration of the person's ability to make a clear informed decision about their suicide and the motivation of the person accompanying them (Pattinson 2020). However, it is important to note that the guidelines are neither embodied in nor change the law. If Peter and Clare decide to accompany Susan to Switzerland, they may still be questioned by the police on their return, and therefore there is still a chance that they could face prosecution. The latest figures from Crown Prosecution Service (CPS) indicate that in the 6 years leading up to March 2023, the police have referred 182 cases of assisted suicide to the CPS. Of these, the CPS did not proceed with 125 cases, 35 were withdrawn by the police and 4 are ongoing. The report states that four cases have been successfully prosecuted and a further nine cases referred on for prosecution for homicide or other serious crime, leaving three cases unaccounted for. However, there are no further details available, making it unclear what the circumstances of the assisted suicide were or if any involved using Dignitas (Director of Public Prosecutions 2023).

Assisted Dying: Euthanasia

Despite the fact that assisted suicide remains unlawful in the UK, there is still a debate about the morality of assisted dying. Proponents of euthanasia (such as members of the UK organisation Dignity in Dying) campaign for changes to be made in the law to allow not only physician-assisted suicide but for health professionals to administer medication to terminally ill patients with the explicit intention of killing them, so called active voluntary euthanasia.

Returning to Susan and her family:

Peter and Clare tell Susan they don't want to accompany her to Switzerland, and while they have sympathy with her view, they don't think they should have to take the risk of facing prosecution. Together they decide to approach Dr Ahmed, Susan's GP, to ask her if, when the time comes, she will help Susan to die and administer a dose of lethal medication if necessary.

Administering lethal medication with the intent to kill a person is, in the UK, considered to be murder, irrespective of the motive or whether it is at the person's request. Therefore, should Dr. Ahmed agree to Susan's request, she will be liable to prosecution and face a mandatory life sentence if found guilty.

Euthanasia is one of the most emotive and controversial ethical subjects facing practitioners. While the law and professional body guidance is clear, the shift in focus to assisted dying rather than voluntary active euthanasia makes it difficult to interpret data measuring the attitudes of the general public to euthanasia, complicated by the use of different terms with a variety of meanings in published reports and research in this area. Dr. Ahmed does have some options available to her, in that she may prescribe and administer medication to control Susan's pain which may have the unintentional effect of hastening her death. The argument used to justify this draws on the Doctrine of Double Effect[2] whereby a doctor may legitimately use strong analgesics or sedatives even if this might risk hastening death, provided their intention is to relieve suffering and the prescription is in keeping with that intention (General Medical Council 2022). This is not only permissible in law, but along with withholding and withdrawing treatment (defined as passive euthanasia) is considered to be good practice by experts in palliative care.

However, some ethicists, most notably James Rachels (1997), raise moral objections to permitting one practice (e.g. the prescription of strong analgesics or sedatives to relieve pain but which is also very likely to hasten death) while forbidding the other (i.e. the administration of a dose of lethal medication in order to hasten death). Discussing this in terms of active and passive euthanasia, Rachels famously asks his readers to engage in a thought experiment regarding Smith and Jones who both stand to gain if their 6-year-old cousin dies. Smith sneaks into the bathroom while his cousin is in the bath and drowns the child. Jones is going to do the same thing, but on entering the bathroom, he sees his cousin hit his head and fall face down in the water. The child drowns and Jones does not intervene.

For Rachels, the actions of Smith cannot be described as morally worse over the omissions of Jones because Smith deliberately drowned the child. Nor can Jones's failure to act be considered to be morally more preferable than the actions of Smith, because Jones did not deliberately drown the child but simply failed to rescue him when he could easily have done so. The key to this dilemma for Rachels is that the intention of both Smith and Jones was the same. Rachels extrapolates from this that to condemn active euthanasia while condoning passive euthanasia is illogical. Of course the most obvious objection to this example is that we cannot compare the

---

[2] The doctrine of double effect means that while it is always wrong intentionally to perform a bad act for the sake of the good consequences that may arise, it may be permissible to perform a good act in the knowledge that unintended bad consequences will arise.

intention of a healthcare professional intent on helping their patient to that of someone whose intention is based on monetary gain. But the point that Rachels makes focuses more on the concept of intent, rather than the specifics of the example itself. Therefore, if the intention is the same, we may question whether it makes any difference how it is achieved. Intent is crucially important for the Doctrine of Double Effect, where the intention of the health professional administering potentially life-shortening medication is to alleviate suffering. While it may be argued that this is entirely different to the scenario posed by Rachels, using the Doctrine of Double effect to justify distinctions between acts and omissions has been criticised as encouraging health professionals to engage in hypocrisy rather than being honest about their actions (Begley 1998).

Even if you are persuaded by Rachels's argument regarding acts and omissions, it does not necessarily follow that you are committed to accepting that active euthanasia is morally permissible. For others, the fear of allowing active voluntary euthanasia is the worry that we will slide down a slippery slope to permitting involuntary euthanasia. So while active voluntary euthanasia in itself may be ethically justified, the concern is that it will lead to complacency and result in euthanasia without consent where the person lacks capacity, for example, through brain injury or progressive conditions such as dementia. The existence of a slippery slope is disputed, but for some further insight, we can look to the experience of Belgium, Luxembourg, and the Netherlands where active voluntary euthanasia is permissible in law. The Netherlands has had formal legislation permitting euthanasia since 2001, but the practice was common for several years before this, if carried out according to the professional guidelines of the Royal Dutch Medical Association. Cases of euthanasia are reported to regional review committees in the Netherlands, and data is freely available. However, the data is open to interpretation with proponents of euthanasia citing the Netherlands as an example of good practice, while those who condemn the practice question the true voluntariness of the decisions. Whether this is evidence of complacency and sliding down the slippery slope is also open to debate. However, the practice does appear to be increasing as the most recent published data shows that in 2021 7666 cases were reported, which equates to 4.6% of all deaths in the Netherlands and is an increase of 10.6% (0.4% of all deaths) from the previous year (Regional Euthanasia Review Committee 2022). Considering the slippery slope argument while developing their own legislation, the Canadian judges examined data from The Netherlands but concluded that the Dutch evidence did not indicate abuse or a greater risk for vulnerable people (Downie and Schuklenk 2021).

In Susan's case it is highly unlikely, although not impossible, that Dr. Ahmed will agree to Susan's request and deliberately give her lethal medication with the express intent of ending her life. To do so would be very risky for both Dr. Ahmed's professional registration and perhaps more importantly her liberty. This is not to say of course that Dr. Ahmed necessarily disagrees with active voluntary euthanasia in principle. It simply indicates that she is not prepared to carry it out, even if it seems to be in Susan's best interests, and she is convinced that Susan has the capacity to make the decision. While the subject remains highly controversial and permissible in other European countries, in the UK the focus has shifted towards legalisation of assisted dying, and it seems unlikely that any of the UK parliaments will even debate, let alone approve, the more radical step of legalising euthanasia in the near future.

Conclusion

The ethical issues that arise when caring for patients at the end of life pose a challenge for healthcare professionals. There are numerous advisory documents produced by charitable and professional organisational on the provision and delivery of palliative care showing a clear commitment to ensure good-quality care irrespective of the place of death. Despite complex funding arrangements, the UK is considered to be a leader in the development of this speciality particularly through the hospice movement. While practitioners will undoubtedly want to deliver care commensurate with the very highest standards, for some individuals there appears to be a discrepancy between the care they would like, and perhaps feel entitled to receive, and the reality of what services can be provided. This is particularly noticeable in the assisted dying debate where the attitudes of the public seem to be at odds with health professionals. Without changes to the legal position to allow people to make lawful decisions about the place and time of their death, some will take matters into their own hands and use the services of Dignitas. But ensuring the provision of a good death will in many cases fall to health professionals across a broad spectrum of care services, not just specialists in palliative care. Therefore it is crucially important that lessons are learned from the failure of the LCP and that adequate funding for education and training is made available to make certain that the principles and guidance in *One Chance to Get it Right* are a reality and not merely aspirational.

> **Key Learning Points**
> - Ensuring patients have a choice regarding their place of death and access to expert care is essential to facilitate a good death.
> - New guidance *One Chance to Get it Right* published in 2014, focusing on individualised care and good communication in end of life care, replaced the discredited Liverpool Care Pathway.
> - Treatment that is costly and ineffective is of no benefit to a patient on an individual level, nor does it demonstrate good use of resources.
> - The withdrawal of nutrition and hydration administered by artificial means remains a controversial issue, despite being classed as medical treatment that can in some circumstances be lawfully withdrawn.
> - Attempts to bring about changes to the law to allow physician-assisted dying in the UK, the Republic of Ireland, Jersey and the Isle of Man are currently being pursued, although this is allowed in other countries including Canada and Switzerland.
> - The Suicide Act 1995 prohibits aiding and abetting suicide, but several individuals travel each year from the UK, to use the services of Dignitas, accompanied by relatives who risk prosecution.

References

Begley A (1998) Acts, omissions, intentions and motives: a philosophical examination of the moral distinction between killing and letting die. J Adv Nurs 28(4):865–873

Booth, R (2023) Dignitas has helped 540 British people die, MPs told. The Guardian. https://www.theguardian.com/society/2023/jun/27/assisted-dying-dignitas-h. Accessed 5 Dec 2023

British Medical Association (2018) Clinically assisted nutrition and hydration (CANH) and adults who lack the capacity to consent. BMA, London

Department of Health (DoH) (2005) Mental capacity act, 2005. Her Majesty's Stationary Office, London. http://www.legislation.gov.uk/ukpga/2005/9/pdfs/ukpga_20050009_en.pdf. Accessed 5 Dec 2023

Director of Public Prosecutions (2023) Latest assisted suicide figures [online]. http://www.cps.gov.uk/publications/prosecution/assisted-suicide. Accessed 23 Aug 2023

Dooley D, McCarthy J (2005) Nursing ethics Irish cases and concerns. Gill & Macmillan, Dublin

Downie J, Schuklenk U (2021) Social determinants of health and slippery slopes in assisted dying debates: lessons from Canada. J Med Ethics 47(10):662–669. https://doi.org/10.1136/medethics-2021-107493

General Medical Council (2022) Treatment and care towards the end of life. GMC, London

Goldsteen M, Houtepen R, Proot IM, Abu Saad HH, Spreeuwenberg C, Widdershins G (2006) What is a good death? Terminally ill patients dealing with normative expectations around death and dying. Patient Educ Couns 64:378–386

House of Commons Select Committee (2023) What are the key considerations in the debate around assisted dying/assisted suicide

Kitzinger C, Kitzinger J (2015) Withdrawing artificial nutrition and hydration from minimally conscious and vegetative patients: family perspectives. J Med Ethics 41:157–160

Leadership Alliance for the Care of Dying People (2014) One chance to get it right. LACDP, London

Marie Curie (2021) Public attitudes to death and dying in the UK. Marie Curie, London

Marie Fleming v Ireland, Attorney General and the Director of Public Prosecutions (2013). https://ie.vlex.com/vid/fleming-v-Ireland-and-793748649. Accessed 5 Dec 2023

National Institute for Health and Care Excellence (2021) End of life care for adults. NICE, London

Neuberger J (2013) More care less pathway: a review of the Liverpool care pathway. https://assets.publishing.service.gov.uk/media/5a75153340f0b6397f35d87c. Accessed 5 Dec 2023

NHS England (2022) Palliative and end of life care: statutory guidance for integrated care boards. NHS England, London

Office for National Statistics (2015) Mortality statistics. National Survey of bereaved people (Voices): England 2015. Accessed 23 Aug 2023

Pattinson S (2020) Medical law and ethics, 6th edn. Sweet and Maxwell, London

Pesut B, Thorne S (2022) Reflections on the relational ontology of medical assistance in dying. Nurs Philos 24:e12438. https://doi.org/10.1111/nup.12438

Plato (1969) The last days of Socrates. Penguin Books, London

R (Nicklinson) v Ministry of Justice (2012) EWHC 2381 (Admin), (2012) MHLO 77

Rachels J (1997) Can ethics provide answers? Rowan & Littlefield, London

Regional Euthanasia Review Committee (2022) Annual report 2021. RERC

Savulescu J (2014) A simple solution to the puzzles of end of life? Voluntary palliated starvation. J Med Ethics 40(2):110–113

Seymour J, Clark D (2022) The Liverpool care pathway for the dying patient: a critical analysis of its rise demise and legacy in England. Wellcome Open Res 3:15. https://doi.org/10.12688/wellcomeopenres.13940.2

Szawarski P, Kakar V (2012) Classic cases revisited: Anthony bland and withdrawal of artificial nutrition and hydration in the UK. J Intensive Care Soc 13(2):126–129

Von Petersdorff C, Patrignani P, Lanszaat W, Jones S (2021) Modelling demand and costs for palliative care services in England. Sue Ryder, London

Wilson DJC, Savulescu J (2011) Knowing when to stop: futility in the intensive care unit. Curr Opin Anaesthesiol 24(2):160–165

World Health Organization (2020) Palliative care. https://www.who.int/news-room/fact-sheets/detail/palliative-care

Pandemic Ethics and Nursing Practice: When Will We Learn?

15

Dónal P. O'Mathúna

Abstract

The COVID-19 pandemic brought many challenges for nursing practice, including many ethical challenges. These have deeply impacted nurses and continue to have deep emotional and psychological consequences. Nurses and other healthcare workers need support and resources as they continue to grapple with various consequence of dealing with the moral challenges during the pandemic. We also need to learn from these experiences and use this learning to prepare better for the next pandemic or other crisis.

Pandemic ethics for nursing practice can learn from past pandemics and the relatively new field of humanitarian ethics. Many of the same types of ethical issues are faced regularly in humanitarian and disaster settings. For example, humanitarian workers regularly deal with scarce resources and frequently work in the midst of unjust or insecure environments. Humanitarian ethics includes other principles such as solidarity and impartiality which can contribute to broader ethical deliberations about pandemics.

Humanitarian ethics points to some limitations in standard approaches to ethics education which can help improve education for the types of ethical issues faced in pandemics. This includes acknowledging that sometimes in ethics no option is completely ethically satisfactory and requires identifying the best of a number of bad options. Such situations often have emotional consequences and point to the importance of addressing emotions in ethics. Both reason and emotions should be engaged in ethical decision-making. Situations and cases which reflect the complex, emotional, relational and cultural dimensions of ethics should be used or developed for pandemic ethics education.

D. P. O'Mathúna (✉)
College of Nursing, The Ohio State University, Columbus, OH, USA
e-mail: omathuna.6@osu.edu

© The Author(s), under exclusive license to Springer Nature Switzerland AG 2024
P. A. Scott, S. M. Scott (eds.), *Key Concepts and Issues in Nursing Ethics*,
https://doi.org/10.1007/978-3-031-54108-7_15

Keywords

Pandemic · Humanitarian ethics · Emotions · Dilemma · Solidarity

Introduction

Nursing practice during a pandemic is difficult and stressful. The restraints imposed by a pandemic make it challenging for nurses to provide good care. Since nurses and nursing organisations view the provision of excellent care as central to nursing, being unable to provide good care is seen as a serious ethical problem (Oh and Gastmans 2023). Hence, moral distress, moral injury[1] and post-traumatic stress disorder (PTSD) have been reported as relatively common among nurses caring for patients during the COVID-19 pandemic (Rushton et al. 2021).

To examine the nature of these ethical issues during COVID-19, a systematic review was conducted of qualitative research studies that involved such nurses and that collected data on ethical issues those nurses encountered (Oh and Gastmans 2023). They included 26 studies and the analysis identified 2 key themes. The first was the role of nurses' moral character in their willingness to respond to and care for vulnerable human beings. This theme included a strong belief that caring for people in medical need is a core ethical responsibility of nurses. At the same time, nurses often experienced conflicting emotions about acting on this commitment, but this tension generally resulted in a renewed sense of the importance of altruism and themselves as moral agent. The review concluded that "Compassion 'won out' over anxiety, moving the nurses to concentrate on caring for their patients" (p. 13). While the ethical struggles of nurses during COVID-19 have been described, positive stories can also be found, particularly around the moral courage demonstrated by many nurses (O'Mathúna et al. 2023).

The second theme identified by Oh and Gastmans (2023) focused on the ethical issues experienced as barriers to providing excellent care. These barriers were organised around three issues. The first type of barrier related to situations where the dignity of patients or other healthcare providers was threatened, such as through lack of resources, incompetence or policies like visitation restrictions without exceptions. These situations led to nursing care which was perceived as undignified and highly problematic ethically. The second type of barrier was difficulty dealing with ethical dilemmas where nurses saw they had incompatible ethical obligations. An example here was balancing care for patients against care for self and one's family. The third type of barrier was dealing with ethical uncertainty where nurses felt completely unsure about how to address an ethical situation or even whether one existed or not. The reviewers concluded that this issue stemmed from nurses being poorly prepared to apply good ethical reasoning to practice and/or having unclear ethical guidance.

The COVID-19 pandemic generated many ethical challenges for which many people in general, and healthcare practitioners in particular, felt unprepared.

---

[1] See Chap. 4 for further discussion of the notion of moral injury and nursing practice.

"Pandemic ethics" will be used here as a summary term for the ethical issues that arise during pandemics. Some of these ethical issues are not unique to pandemics, but pandemics have a number of distinct features that raise ethical challenges that fall within "pandemic ethics". Hirose (2023) identifies five challenges, noting that his list is not exhaustive. His five are:

- A sudden rise in cases that almost always leads to acute scarcity and requires rationing.
- Extraordinary measures such as restricting basic freedoms.
- A high level of uncertainty when the disease is new.
- A balancing of short-term and long-term consequences of responses and policies.
- The global dimension, particularly as it relates to global disparities.

Pandemic ethics seeks to address these and other pertinent ethical issues, providing analysis and options to guide responses to pandemics. Pandemic ethics has been actively discussed since the 2002–2004 severe acute respiratory syndrome (SARS) outbreak, though "within a relatively small circle of public health ethicists" (Hirose 2023 p. 1). Yet pandemic ethics are not new. Martin Luther wrote in 1527 about whether it was ethical for people to flee from the Black Death rather than stay and help those afflicted by the illness (Luther 1527). In 1722, Daniel Defoe published a fictionalized account of one man's experience of the Great Plague of London in 1655 (Dafoe 1969). Many of the ethical dilemmas faced in the book by individuals, families, communities and public authorities are very familiar after experiencing the COVID-19 pandemic.

Those same ethical dilemmas and issues have exacted a large toll on nurses around the world. They have contributed to what has been called the "parallel pandemic" (Dzau et al. 2020) or the "shadow pandemic" (Iserson 2020). The SARS-CoV-2 virus directly caused one pandemic; but a second pandemic has developed related to the harmful effects of the first on clinician wellbeing, a global impact which continues. One empirical study of nurses during the pandemic did not aim to assess their wellbeing but concluded that their most significant finding was the extent of the psychological burden born by nurses during the pandemic (Dellasega and Kanaskie 2021). Foremost among the contributing factors identified in that study was the moral distress resulting from the ethical issues reported by nurses. The study authors also noted that while the American Nurses Association Code of Ethics was viewed as relevant and helpful, it did not provide guidance on how to address these lingering effects. The participants expressed a strong sense of ethical obligation and commitment to their patients, but the ethical challenges they faced continued to weigh heavily on them.

The lasting emotional and psychological effects of the ethical dilemmas and challenges faced by nurses during COVID-19 have been reported frequently. A qualitative research study conducted eight focus groups in four sites across the USA in the second half of 2020. Ethics was identified as a cross-cutting theme which was associated with the three other major themes: challenges, feelings and coping (Kelley et al. 2022). Further analysis of the ethical concerns raised by participants led to six subthemes: moral dilemma, moral uncertainty, moral distress, moral injury, moral outrage and moral courage (O'Mathúna et al. 2023). The first two subthemes relate to classes of ethical issues encountered and were also identified by Oh and Gastmans (2023) as key difficulties for ethical practice during the pandemic. We will return to these later in the chapter.

Many different terms have been used to describe and distinguish the multiple and complex ethical issues experienced by nurses during the COVID-19 pandemic, many of which led to various forms of moral suffering. These moral terms are defined in varying ways, and consensus is lacking on the boundaries between them. "Despite the overlapping definitions of the various types of moral suffering in health care, each illuminates important dimensions of the moral landscape that are essential to protecting and preserving clinicians' basic goodness, wholeness, and capacity to serve, especially in such complex, uncertain, and changing times" (Rushton et al. 2021 p. 125). This chapter does not aim to provide conceptual clarity on these terms.[2] Instead, the focus here will be on showing how these experiences can help us learn from this pandemic. Many reports show that nurses regularly felt poorly prepared to address the distressing ethical situations they encountered. We need to learn from the COVID-19 pandemic so that we can be better prepared and better able to serve those we care for during the next one.

Lack of Preparation

The need to prepare for the ethical issues that arise during pandemics had been identified long before COVID-19. The 2002–2004 SARS outbreak highlighted to the world the importance of preparing for pandemics. In particular, the need to pay closer attention to pandemic ethics was highlighted (Peter et al. 2022). Toronto was one of the cities hit hard by SARS, and a report conducted by the University of Toronto's Centre for Bioethics concluded:

> "*SARS showed there are costs of not having an agreed-upon ethical framework, including loss of trust, low morale, fear, and misinformation. SARS taught the world that if ethical frameworks had been more widely used to guide decision-making, this would have increased trust and solidarity within and between health organizations*" (University of Toronto Joint Centre for Bioethics Pandemic Influenza Working Group 2005 p. 4).

In 2005, the World Health Organization (WHO) published recommendations to assist countries in preparing their own plans for a global influenza pandemic (Thomas et al. 2007). In the USA, a federal strategy and national plan were published later that year, with calls for all state and local authorities to develop their own plans. In 2006, all federal and state plans available online were analysed for evidence of their ethical guidance. All plans recognized that pandemic responses have ethical dimensions and identified some ethical issues. However, the federal plan did not call for preparations in or training for ethical decision-making. The state plans reflected "a belief that ethics are self-evident or of little practical

---

[2] For a discussion of some of these moral concepts, see Chap. 4.

relevance" and implied that the guiding principles were "trust us and do as we say" and "just do what is needed to preserve lives" (Thomas et al. 2007 p. S29). The authors concluded that given the lack of attention to ethics in the existing plans, if a pandemic was to occur, "we risk making unjust and indefensible decisions that will affect thousands of people" (p. S31).

Following the 2009 H1N1 pandemic, the US Institute of Medicine (IOM) was asked to develop guidance that would help health officials establish and implement standards of care during disasters, including pandemics (Romney et al. 2020). The IOM identified five key elements in state plans, one of which was "strong ethical grounding". Further guidance on such plans was published in 2014 by CHEST, the US professional body for chest medicine, with ethics/culture and triage being 2 of the 11 core elements. However, a systematic review of US state plans available up until 2020 found that 19 states had no publicly available pandemic plan and only 5 states had plans that addressed all five of the IOM's key elements. Eighteen plans (covering about one third of US states) had strong ethical grounding. The authors concluded that there "may be inadequate guidance to inform providers and policy-makers about the most effective strategies for allocating scarce resources during a time of crisis" (Romney et al. 2020 p. 6), especially given the void in federal guidance. This was certainly borne out during COVID-19.

A lack of ethical preparedness for public health emergencies and disasters was also identified among nurses. Johnstone and Turale (2014) published a systematic review of studies using qualitative methods to report nurses' direct experiences of being prepared for and managing ethical issues during public health crises and disasters. All included papers (published between 1973 and 2010) identified a lack of clinical and emotional preparedness in nurses for public health emergencies and disasters. The reviewers concluded that there was "a failure to directly address the issue of ethical considerations in planning, preparedness, and response to public health emergencies and disasters by nurses" which "leaves both the nursing profession and the public vulnerable to the otherwise preventable harms of … 'unjust and regrettable decisions'" made during crises (Johnstone and Turale 2014 p. 72–73). They presciently stated that nurses who would find themselves on the frontlines of public health emergencies would have little preparation for the ethical quandaries they would face.

During the first year of the COVID-19 pandemic, questions were still being raised about the ethics education and preparation of nurses for the complex ethical challenges they were facing. Even at that point, "Relevant ethical frameworks need to be revised or developed and adopted widely in nursing practice" (Turale et al. 2020 p. 167). Previous pandemics like SARS, H1N1, Ebola virus disease and Middle East respiratory syndrome coronavirus (MERS-CoV) should have helped us learn about pandemic ethics and help us prepare for the related ethical challenges. Now the question before us is whether we will learn from the painful, tragic experiences that COVID-19 has pushed upon us.

Humanitarian Ethics for Nursing in Pandemics

In addition to learning from earlier pandemics, this chapter aims to show that key features of humanitarian ethics can assist nurses and other healthcare professionals as they prepare for and grapple with the ethical issues in pandemics. Humanitarian ethics, according to Slim (2015), holds that "every human life is good and that it is right to protect and save people's lives whenever and wherever you can" and that people should have a "profound feeling of compassion and responsibility towards others who are living and suffering in extremis" (2015 pp. 26–27). This approach has much in common with nursing and points to both the principled aspect of ethics (the good and the right) as well as the emotional aspect (the feelings) which will be developed in this chapter for pandemic ethics.

No one wants to go through another experience like COVID-19, but living and practicing through another pandemic is very likely (Hirose 2023). Preparing for pandemic ethics is important and an ethical responsibility in itself. Planning and preparing for disasters, mass casualty events and humanitarian crises is now seen as part of our public responsibility. All of these situations include difficult ethical issues and dilemmas that are similar to those faced in pandemics. Therefore, it is important that nursing ethics education, at all levels, include attention to pandemic ethics, especially how it is distinct from or involves changes from nursing ethics in more "normal" situations.

Each of the following subsections identifies areas within humanitarian ethics which can be usefully applied to some of the ethical issues that have arisen for nursing during the COVID-19 pandemic. The set of themes is not exhaustive, as each pandemic is likely to have distinct aspects and challenges. But these provide a core set of issues that can form the basis for pandemic ethics applied to nursing practice.

From Individual Ethics to Public Health Ethics

A key distinctive of practicing in a pandemic is the shift from individual ethics to public health ethics. This shift can be particularly stressful for nurses at any time, such as when healthcare policies on cost or effectiveness are oriented towards maximizing benefit for the common good.[3] This is because "nursing care is often oriented towards the individual good", and it is difficult to shift to a focus on the common good (Lützén et al. 2003). These same types of ethical decisions are faced regularly in all sorts of disasters (Iserson 2020). Among humanitarian healthcare workers, this shift to the common good was found to underlie many of their ethical struggles. Schwartz et al. hypothesized that this was ".. likely in part because Western-schooled health care professionals are enculturated in an ethical tradition that prioritizes the individual over the general. They are accustomed to promoting respect for individual autonomy enacted via informed consent, or protecting the vulnerable by attending to the patient's best interests" (2010 p. 52).

---

[3] For a discussion of maximizing benefit for the greatest number, please see Chap. 8.

Individual autonomy is an important ethical principle in healthcare. However, it can sometimes become viewed as a principle that "trumps" other principles when they conflict (Gordon et al. 2011 p. 297). In Western healthcare ethics, the four principles approach (or principlism)[4] has been widely taught in professional schools as a way to resolve ethical dilemmas. Hardin (2018) states that it is the approach to ethics most familiar to nurses. Resolution of an ethically challenging situation can be seen as a balancing of ethical principles until the most ethical solution becomes apparent. The chapter on autonomy in this volume[5] reviews philosophical and practical problems with a highly individualised approach to autonomy in healthcare ethics. It has been found to reduce the importance of relationships in ethical decision-making and also to minimise concerns about social justice (Hardin 2018). The latter is especially relevant for pandemics and will be addressed below.

Ethical issues related to decisions that favoured common good over individual good were particularly problematic for nurses during COVID-19. These included decisions over how to allocate scarce resources, such as personal protective equipment (PPE), staff or interventions typically viewed as standard of care (Oh and Gastmans 2023; Peter et al. 2022) and also decisions over public health restrictions. For example, institutional policies that restricted visitor access to patients or nursing home residents were viewed as particularly troublesome. Such decisions and policies were justified on the basis that one approach promoted an ethical value to a greater degree, or for a greater number of people, than a different approach. Nurses' commitment to the dignified care of all individual patients raised serious questions about such approaches, or left nurses feeling distressed or guilty when they implemented them. Even when such decisions can be ethically justified, more attention was needed to communicate those justifications to nurses left to implement them and to support nurses with the resulting emotional aftermath. Having pandemic ethics and relevant cases in nursing ethics education could prepare nurses better for these situations.

In their systematic review, Oh and Gastmans (2023) found that the second key barrier to nurses providing dignified care were the ethical dilemmas they faced. Nurses could see that they had incompatible ethical responsibilities which could not all be satisfied at the same time. No decision was going to satisfy all ethical principles, and nurses found themselves with little guidance on how to balance such incommensurate duties. Being left with no good resolution left nurses distressed and with feelings of uncertainty, guilt, regret and others. Part of the problem is that a principles-based approach to ethics can lead to the perception that every ethical dilemma can be "resolved or overcome" (Hardin 2018 p. 467). But by definition, ethical dilemmas are those where "no option is obviously preferable" (O'Mathúna et al. 2023 p. 5). Humanitarian ethics shows that even when people clarify the ethical principles that are in tension in a situation, the principles alone will not assist the individual to identify a satisfactory solution. All options will be problematic and

---

[4] For a discussion of principlism and nursing ethics, please see Chap. 7.
[5] Please see Chap. 6 for an in-depth discussion of patient autonomy in nursing and healthcare contexts.

thereby emotionally challenging. The pandemic has shown that such realities can suddenly become a part of everyday nursing. Therefore, more preparation is needed to develop ways of reflecting on and living with the ethical issues that do not allow options that satisfy everyone. That is a big part of the terrain pandemic ethics addresses.

Emotions and Ethics

Nurses have regularly described how the ethical issues with COVID-19 have left them with bad feelings and negative emotions. In Oh and Gastmans (2023) systematic review of nursing ethics during COVID-19, emotions were central in both of the two key themes their analysis identified in the literature. Nurses' emotional faculties allowed them to detect ethical problems and also to express emotions within ethical and caring relationships. Humanitarian ethics has identified that many decisions made in humanitarian contexts will result in negative emotions and bad feelings— even if the best possible decision has been made. When there are insufficient resources to provide everyone with everything they need, some will be "left out", and that should leave us with bad feelings. When liberties and activities carry high risks of spreading infections, public health restrictions will involve curbing commonly held freedoms. Many will struggle with those and disagree over whether they can be justified. As a result, many ethical decisions will not be ideal but will be the "lesser evil" where violating one ethical ideal is required to uphold another (Slim 2015 p. 163). Such choices inevitably leave people with a sense of moral loss or pain. Even when the decisions can be ethically justified, "they do not erase the moral residue that accompanies them" (Rushton et al. 2021 p. 124). Living with the consequences of such decisions, and seeking to make peace with them, is part of the ethical challenge of practicing in humanitarian settings—and in pandemics. This also places an ethical responsibility on organisations to help practitioners with those feelings and emotions.

However, a broader challenge exists with emotions and ethics. The role of emotions has been neglected in much of contemporary healthcare ethics. "Yet many clinical ethicists are ignorant, suspicious or critical of the role of emotions in making moral decisions and reflecting upon them. Emotions are often referred to as irrational or subjective" (Molewijk et al. 2011, p. 383). As a result, healthcare ethics "has tended to focus on rationality and rational reasoning" (ibid.) and has contributed to an emphasis on learning about ethical principles. This can lead to ethics being seen as a detached engagement with rational principles and theories and emotions as interfering with ethical deliberation. Some empirical research has demonstrated that nursing ethics education that focuses on abstract principles leads to a disconnect between theory and practice and inconsistency in ethical decision-making (O'Mathúna 2022).

Throughout the history of ethics, different philosophical schools have either emphasised or dismissed the role of emotions. Alasdair MacIntyre described ethical thinking since the Enlightenment as a "catastrophe" where ethical decision-making has been characterised in binary terms as either rule-based "calculations" or emotional "preferences" (Slim 2015 p. 126). Instead, a longer history seeks to integrate reason and emotion in ethical decision-making. Virtue ethics since Aristotle, feminist ethics, care ethics and philosophers such as Martha Nussbaum have argued for the importance of emotions in ethical decision-making (for an overview, see O'Mathúna 2022). This approach has been taken up in Slim's humanitarian ethics and other discussions of disaster ethics. Philosophical reasons support this approach, and so do the experiences reported by those working in humanitarian crises and pandemics. Humanitarian settings are filled with tragedy, and in those settings tragic choices must be made where no good decision exists. As a result, even ethical decisions can have bad outcomes, and those result in bad feelings for those who care. We should similarly not be surprised when ethical decisions made during pandemics leave us with negative emotions.

Social Justice

One of the challenges of working in humanitarian settings is the visibility of social injustices. The field hospital or aid station might be an oasis of refuge or resources but all around the poverty or destruction or violence screams. Writing about an earthquake he lived through, theologian Jon Sobrino stated: "The earthquake is not just a tragedy, it is an X-ray of the country... The tragedy is largely the work of our own hands. We shape the planet with massive, cruel, and lasting injustice... This ubiquitous inequality is evident even in normal times, and even more in an earthquake" (Sobrino 2004 p. 3–4). Pandemics and disasters may have natural origins, but the vulnerable in societies are disproportionately impacted. The pandemic showed this clearly in the morbidity and mortality caused and how "vaccine nationalism" was used to justify allocation of scare resources.

Humanitarian healthcare workers have described how working within environments where social injustice is transparent raises intense ethical challenges (Schwartz et al. 2010). Arriving in an unfamiliar setting or culture can quickly show existing social injustices, inequities or exploitative relationships. Many workers become ethically burdened by participating in such arrangements. Triage systems can be particularly difficult to implement when healthcare workers are aware of injustices that influence who reaches the facilities first. Humanitarian workers found it ethically difficult to have comfortable living arrangements with sufficient food and water, while the communities they were serving lived in poverty or insecurity. "The tension between knowing you can only do so much, perceiving much more was needed, and wanting deeply to do more, was common" (p. 51).

The COVID-19 pandemic exposed social injustice, inequity and discrimination in ways that had previously been overlooked. In the USA, the deaths of African Americans in police custody led to widespread protests that raised questions of social justice that had been ignored for years. Instances of anti-Asian racism and threats also occurred. The pandemic X-ray pointed out social injustices that impacted many clinicians as they saw evidence of these injustices in their own clinics or added to the burdens carried by clinicians from vulnerable populations. Such "recalcitrant societal ills" added to the "grief, guilt, shame, and trauma that health care clinicians carry" (Rushton et al. 2021 p. 123) as they witnessed firsthand "the disproportionate burden of sickness and death because of systemic injustice across generations" (p. 125).

Humanitarian ethics does not provide easy solutions to practicing ethically in the midst of social injustices. Clinical practice in the moment is unlikely to change widespread social practices. Yet by bringing attention to underlying social problems and injustices, efforts can be initiated to address those problems. Steps can be taken such as taking available pandemic resources to marginalized communities rather than assuming those people will find a way to the clinic. Small steps can be initiated right away, while acknowledging resource limitations. But having become aware of the ethical problems, efforts can be undertaken to address them more fully as the pandemic wanes.

Solidarity

Solidarity is an ethical commitment long promoted within humanitarian ethics. In spite of this, there has been little consensus on a precise definition (Domingo-Osle and Domingo 2022). The concept includes having an attitude of concern for others, especially those in need, and a willingness to help or promote the interests of others, even at personal cost. The COVID-19 pandemic led to much interest in solidarity within healthcare and particularly within nursing. Domingo-Osle and Domingo state that "Solidarity is at the heart of nursing practice" (p. 652). They trace the origins of the concept to Roman law where it "captures the idea of one for all and all for one" (p. 653). The idea is that certain obligations bind groups of people, even if only some are directly involved. Solidarity refers to the joint responsibility for an action shared by two or more people and applies to both good and bad actions. It presupposes interdependence among those who share responsibility. For example, environmental solidarity would refer to the responsibility of all humans to steward planet Earth on the basis that all benefit from the protection of the Earth. Solidarity can be viewed as a virtue by which people have a persevering commitment to the common good of each and every other human. A commitment to solidarity goes beyond commitments to individuals but sees the responsibility as arising from individuals as members of communities to other individuals who similarly are members of their respective communities.

Solidarity has a number of implications for nursing and nursing ethics. Nurses are not simply individuals who care for individual patients, but both are members of interconnected communities of various sizes. Solidarity affirms that nurses are members of nursing teams, healthcare systems and public health systems. These bring varying levels of responsibilities that nurses must take into account and make patients aware of. At the same time, patients should be seen as not only individuals but members of families, broader communities and society at large. This provides support for family-centred care and also raises challenges for pandemic policies that severely restrict visitation by families at healthcare facilities. In this way, the principle of solidarity adds a counter-balancing principle to that of individual autonomy and can contribute to a more relational approach to ethical decisions where public health restrictions are being considered during pandemics. Rather than simply enforcing a no-visitor policy, solidarity calls for consideration of the importance of relationships to patients' and residents' well-being and efforts to balance infection control with relational contact. Such efforts are particularly important for dying patients, where notions of dying alone were found to be particularly distressing on patients, families and nurses. Much was learned during Ebola about balancing relational and cultural values with infection control that could have helped during COVID-19.

Resistance Humanitarianism

The final topic here is another way that pandemic nursing ethics can benefit from humanitarian ethics and requires a longer introduction. An important humanitarian principle is that of neutrality. Accordingly, many humanitarian organisations "may not take sides in hostilities or engage at any time in controversies of a political, racial, religious or ideological nature" (Slim 2015 p. 66). Many international humanitarian organisations, including the International Committee of the Red Cross and United Nations agencies, insist on neutrality as a guiding principle for humanitarian action. However, abiding by neutrality can be a source of ethical dilemmas as individuals and organisations seek to provide aid in defiance of unjust ruling authorities or military powers. This leads to some humanitarian aid being provided that is not neutral, involving people taking sides against an unjust situation to help others and save lives. Such forms of aid have been called "humanitarian resistance".

Hugo Slim has argued that humanitarian resistance has frequently been practiced throughout history and that it can be justified ethically and under international humanitarian law. Slim defines humanitarian resistance as:

> "*the rescue, relief and protection of people suffering under an unjust enemy regime. It is specifically organised by individuals and groups who are politically opposed to the regime and support resistance against it because of their political commitments or personal conscience. Humanitarian resistance takes sides and is carried out without enemy consent, often covertly and at great personal risk*" (2022 p. 8).

Slim gives several examples, including many from the war in Ukraine as individuals and organisations help and rescue Ukrainians from the invading Russian forces as a way to resist Russia's actions.

Slim (2022) views humanitarian resistance as a specific instance of civil resistance, and his justification is based on how it upholds other important ethical and humanitarian principles. Within humanitarianism, what is called the "principle of humanity" is a commitment to protect the life and health of humans and to promote respect for all humans (Slim 2015). Another principle is impartiality, which is the requirement to uphold the principle of humanity fairly and without discrimination by basing one's actions on the needs of others. Important support is also provided by the way humanitarian resistance seeks to promote justice in the midst of unjust situations and by its commitment to responding to the suffering of others. In this way, humanitarian resistance goes beyond solidarity (seen as an attitudinal response to others' suffering) and leads to actions that seek to redress unjust suffering.

Humanitarian resistance can inform pandemic nursing ethics through an analogy between the humanitarian principle of neutrality and the ethical principle of autonomy. Neutrality and autonomy are important ethical principles and should be respected and promoted in many situations. But problems arise when these principles are held up as non-negotiable and used as trump cards to make decisions about complex ethical dilemmas. Ethical dilemmas involve balancing competing ethical principles and values, and in some cases any ethical principle may have to secede to other principles.

For example, as noted earlier, sometimes autonomy is seen as the deciding ethical principle (even if not necessarily an absolute principle). Nurses play an important role in advocating for their patient's wishes. This has led to situations where nurses see their role as promoting those wishes.[6] This can create challenging ethical dilemmas when those wishes are not based on the best available evidence, or violate nurses' own professional responsibilities, or simultaneously put others at risk of harm. Just as humanitarians have felt constrained to address injustices by a commitment to neutrality, nurses can feel constrained to resist a patient's wishes by their commitment to autonomy. Humanitarian ethics acknowledges that neutrality is not an essential component of humanitarian action, and there are times when helping others requires violating neutrality. Analogously, pandemic ethics can support situations where nurses resist patients' wishes that violate other ethical commitments. Examples would include speaking out against disinformation which promotes ineffective therapies or which disparages evidence-based vaccines or therapies.

In his argument for humanitarian resistance, Slim raises an important point which is also relevant for pandemic ethics. He argues that impartiality continues to require that resistance humanitarians continue to meet the needs of their enemies and their supporters. He views this as "the acid test" (2022 p. 13) that distinguishes legitimate humanitarianism from other approaches where groups do humanitarian work in collaboration with unjust regimes and also become complicit with the inhumanity of their militaries and political authorities. In an analogous way, pandemic nursing ethics would insist that nurses continue to care for their patients even if they disagree with their positions or wishes on pandemic-related beliefs and practices. Just as a nurse has moral obligations to care for a patient whose actions contributed to their health needs, even if a patient's needs can be traced to their refusal to be vaccinated or abide by evidence-based pandemic restrictions, nurses should care for those patients as they would others. Even if such patients are characterized by some as "enemies", they should not be treated as such but as fellow humans who are still in need to care.

---

[6] For further discussion of advocacy and nursing, please see Chap. 2.

Conclusion

The COVID-19 pandemic has highlighted the multiple and complex ethical challenges faced by nurses around the world. The emotional and psychological toll on healthcare workers has been documented in terms of moral distress, moral injury and other impacts. Nurses and other healthcare workers need support, assistance and resources as they grapple with the moral residues they are experiencing. Many have been shaken to the core of their nursing identity. One nurse reflected, "I feel a fracture between who I want to be and who I sense I am becoming" (Rushton et al. 2021 p. 119. These same types of experiences were reported by humanitarian healthcare workers, one of whom said, "I felt all of the sudden as if I was not a nurse anymore" (Schwartz et al. 2010 p. 51).

Part of the problem has been uncertainty over how to address the ethical issues with pandemics. Oh and Gastmans (2023) identified a third type of barrier to dignified care which was uncertainty about ethical issues. This went beyond initial doubt over how to decide about an ethical issue to the point where nurses were completely unsure how to address an ethical problem or even if it was an ethical issue. One nurse reported, "we have a basic idea of what's ethical and what's not ethical. COVID has really just blown my mind when it comes to ethics. I don't know what's ethical and what's not anymore" (O'Mathúna et al. 2023 p. 10). Another stated, "I don't know anymore and wonder where I lost my moral compass" (Rushton et al. 2021 p 119).

Nurses felt unprepared for COVID-19 and must be helped prepare for the next pandemic or other crisis. Given globalisation activities, the risk of infectious disease outbreaks becoming pandemics has increased and is expected to continue to increase (Hirose 2023). Pandemic planning includes better organisational and resource planning by healthcare systems and institutions. All healthcare professionals need ethics education that addresses pandemic ethics. Those working to develop pandemic ethics for nursing practice can learn from the field of humanitarian ethics. Humanitarian ethics addresses many of the same types of ethical issues faced in pandemics. Hirose (2023) five distinct challenges in pandemics also occur in humanitarian settings: scarce resources, restrictions on basic freedoms (from the coercive regimes regularly found in humanitarian settings), much uncertainty, balancing short-term and long-term consequences and disparities. Humanitarian ethics has already been addressing such issues and provides direction and practical guidance for education in pandemic ethics. This includes careful analysis of and reflection on the ethical issues faced in pandemics.

Humanitarian ethics also points towards general changes in teaching ethics. Healthcare ethics education must go beyond principlism and include other ethical and humanitarian principles and other theoretical approaches to ethics.[7] The way emotions are deeply involved in ethics must be discussed, including how emotional and rational aspects contribute to making ethical decisions. Inclusion of the arts and

---

[7] See as examples of other theoretical approaches Chap. 8 on utilitarian approaches, Chap. 9 on virtue ethics and Chap. 10 on care ethics and nursing practice.

humanities in ethics education is one way this can be done (O'Mathúna 2022). Situations and cases which reflect the complex, emotional, relational and cultural dimensions of ethics should be included. Cases should be used or developed that reflect the reality that sometimes good solutions cannot be found. Sometimes the best option available may be the least worst one. Realising this will not take away the bad feelings when people find themselves in those situations. But it can provide a glimmer of hope that they have done the best that was possible in terrible circumstances. And that others know how they feel because they have faced similar tragic dilemmas. That is the nature of pandemic ethics.

> **Key Learning Points**
> - The COVID-19 pandemic revealed a complex mix of ethical issues for which many nurses felt unprepared.
> - Nurses and other healthcare workers are experiencing various negative consequences from the ethical issues faced during the pandemic.
> - Pandemic ethics education should be developed for nurses, and humanitarian ethics can provide useful input into these materials.
> - Pandemic ethics education must address the tragic nature of many ethical dilemmas where no solution satisfies all ethical requirements.
> - Ethics involves a complex interplay between reason, emotions and relationships which should be reflected in ethics education.

References

Dafoe D (1969) A journal of the plague year. Oxford University Press, Oxford
Dellasega C, Kanaskie ML (2021) Nursing ethics in an era of pandemic. Appl Nurs Res 62:151508
Domingo-Osle M, Domingo R (2022) Redefining nursing solidarity. Nurs Ethics 29(3):651–659
Dzau VJ, Kirch D, Nasca T (2020) Preventing a parallel pandemic—a national strategy to protect clinicians' well-being. N Engl J Med 383(6):513–515
Gordon J-S, Rauprich O, Vollmann J (2011) Applying the four-principle approach. Bioethics 25(6):293–300
Hardin J (2018) Everyday ethical comportment: an evolutionary concept analysis. J Nurs Educ 57(8):460–468
Hirose I (2023) The ethics of pandemics: an introduction. Routledge, Abingdon
Iserson KV (2020) Healthcare ethics during a pandemic. West J Emerg Med 21(3):477–483
Johnstone M-J, Turale S (2014) Nurses' experiences of ethical preparedness for public health emergencies and healthcare disasters: a systematic review of qualitative evidence. Nurs Health Sci 16(1):67–77
Kelley MM, Zadvinskis I, Miller PS, Monturo C, Norful AA, O'Mathúna D, Roberts H, Smith J, Tucker S, Zellefrow C, Chipps E (2022) United States nurses' experiences during the COVID-19 pandemic: a grounded theory. J Clin Nurs 31(15–16):2167–2180
Luther M (1527) Whether one may flee from a deadly plague. In: Lull TF, Russel WR (eds) (2012) Martin Luther's basic theological writings, 3rd edn. Augsburg Fortress, Minneapolis, pp 475–487
Lützén K, Cronqvist A, Magnusson A, Andersson L (2003) Moral stress: synthesis of a concept. Nurs Ethics 10(3):312–322

Molewijk B, Kleinlugtenbelt D, Widdershoven G (2011) The role of emotions in moral case deliberation: theory, practice, and methodology. Bioethics 25(7):383–393

O'Mathúna DP (2022) Nursing ethics education: thinking, feeling and technology. Nurs Clin N Am 57(4):613–625

O'Mathúna D, Smith J, Zadvinskis I, Monturo C, Kelley MM, Tucker S, Miller PS, Norful AA, Zellefrow C, Chipps E (2023) Ethics and frontline nursing during COVID-19: a qualitative analysis. Nurs Ethics 30(6):803–821

Oh Y, Gastmans C (2023) Ethical issues experienced by nurses during COVID-19 pandemic: systematic review. Nurs Ethics 31(4):521–540

Peter E, Variath C, Mohammed S, Mitchell M, Killackey T, Maciver J, Chiasson C (2022) Nurses' experiences of their ethical responsibilities during coronavirus outbreaks: a scoping review. Can J Nurs Res 54(3):246–260

Romney D, Fox H, Carlson S, Bachmann D, O'Mathúna D, Kman N (2020) Allocation of scarce resources in a pandemic: a systematic review of U.S. state crisis standards of care documents. Disaster Med Public Health Prep 14(5):677–683

Rushton CH, Turner K, Brock RN, Braxton JM (2021) Invisible moral wounds of the COVID-19 pandemic: are we experiencing moral injury? AACN Adv Crit Care 32(1):119–125

Schwartz L, Sinding C, Hunt M, Elit L, Redwood-Campbell L, Adelson N, Luther L, Ranford J, DeLaat S (2010) Ethics in humanitarian aid work: learning from the narratives of humanitarian health workers. AJOB Prim Res 1:45–54

Slim H (2015) Humanitarian ethics: a guide to the morality of aid in war and disaster. Hurst and Oxford University Press, London and Oxford

Slim H (2022) Humanitarian resistance: its ethical and operational importance Humanitarian Practice Network Paper. https://odihpn.org/publication/humanitarian-resistance-its-ethical-and-operational-importance. Accessed 30 Oct 2023

Sobrino J (2004) Where is god? Earthquake, terrorism, barbarity, and hope, translated by Margaret Wilde. Orbis, Maryknoll

Thomas JC, Dasgupta N, Martinot A (2007) Ethics in a pandemic: a survey of the state pandemic influenza plans. Am J Public Health 97(S1):S26–S31

Turale S, Meechamnan C, Kunaviktikul W (2020) Challenging times: ethics, nursing and the COVID-19 pandemic. Int Nurs Rev 67(2):164–167

University of Toronto Joint Centre for Bioethics Pandemic Influenza Working Group (2005) Stand on guard for thee. Ethical considerations in preparedness planning for pandemic influenza. https://jcb.utoronto.ca/wp-content/uploads/2021/03/stand_on_guard.pdf. Accessed 30 Oct 2023

16

The Ethics of Communication Technologies in the Provision of Remote, Home-Based Nursing Care

Alan J. Kearns

Abstract

This chapter examines the utilisation of communication technologies to assist in the delivery of remote, home-based nursing care—and health care more broadly—from an ethics perspective. The chapter begins by outlining some of the terms that have come to be used to describe the application of communication technologies within the digitalisation of health care. Second, some of the common ethical concerns and ethical questions regarding the application of communication technologies are set out. Finally, it is proposed that on a macro level, an adapted Equivalence of Care (Charles and Draper, J Med Ethics 38:215–218, 2012) should be an overarching principle for supplying nursing care and that on a micro level, technomoral virtues (Vallor, Oxford University Press, New York, 2016) should be fostered in nurses providing care remotely to home-based patients, using communication technologies.

Keywords

Communication technologies · eHealth · Equivalence of care · mHealth · Technomoral virtues · Telehealth · Telemedicine · Telenursing

Introduction

As John and Mary are putting their 2-year-old daughter Claire to bed, they notice that her belly is covered in spots. They begin to panic. Without too much thinking, they rush off to the nearest emergency department (ED). After undergoing a triage assessment, they end up waiting several hours before they are seen. Claire plays

A. J. Kearns (✉)
School of Theology, Philosophy, and Music, Dublin City University, Dublin, Ireland
e-mail: alan.kearns@dcu.ie

© The Author(s), under exclusive license to Springer Nature Switzerland AG 2024
P. A. Scott, S. M. Scott (eds.), *Key Concepts and Issues in Nursing Ethics*,
https://doi.org/10.1007/978-3-031-54108-7_16

around in the waiting room having a great time. When they are eventually brought into an examination cubical, the spots are almost gone. Probably a heat rash, but all is fine with Claire as she sleeps soundly on the journey home; her parents are relieved.

Now imagine a similar hypothetical situation, but this time instead of rushing off to the ED, John and Mary can log on to a hospital's website that enables them to have a triage consultation with a nurse via a video link. Imagine the nurse could do an initial assessment and be a reassuring presence. The nurse could then instigate the next steps such as whether a video call back by a medic was appropriate or advise them to come to the hospital, for example. In such a situation, John and Mary may be saved from a wasted journey, from having to spend a long time in a waiting room as well as from adding to an already overcrowded ED. In such a situation, the use of communication technologies could save on time and resources for patients, nurses and health-care systems more generally.

Communication technologies[1] have become ubiquitous in health-care settings and continue to transform the supply and provision of nursing care. This chapter examines the utilisation of communication technologies to assist in the delivery of remote, home-based nursing care—and health care more broadly—from an ethics perspective. The chapter begins by outlining the various terms that have come to be used to describe the application of communication technologies in the domain of distant health care such as telemedicine, telehealth and telenursing. Given the impressive array of cutting-edge contemporary technological devices, wearables and online video platforms, it is not possible to examine each one individually in any meaningful depth and provide a more targeted ethical analysis. Instead, the common ethical concerns and ethical questions regarding the application of communication technologies are set out. Finally, it is proposed that, on a macro level—following in the thought of Charles and Draper (2012)—an adapted Equivalence of Care[2] should be an overarching principle for supplying nursing care, and that on a micro level, following in the thought of Vallor (2016), technomoral virtues[3] should be fostered in nurses providing care remotely to home-based patients, using communication technologies.

---

[1] Given the various terms including telemedicine, telehealth and telenursing as well as others, I use 'communication technologies' in a broadly conceived way to capture that facilitation of the remote interaction between health-care workers and patients and the transmission of health information that is made possible through technology.

[2] We will return to this principle in more detail below. Primarily, the Principle of Equivalence of Care advocates that those who are in prison should receive an equivalence of health care to those who are on the outside (Charles and Draper 2012 p. 215).

[3] Technomoral virtues is a term used by Vallor (2016), which refers to virtues that can enable us to flourish in our world that is shaped by technologies that are new and still emerging (p. 1, p. 10, p. 119). We will come back to this term towards the end of this chapter.

Communication Technologies for Remote Care

The convergence of communication technologies and nursing practice is not new. Indeed, the recognition of the importance of communication can be seen in the work of Florence Nightingale, who not only saw the value of gathering statistical data but also saw the value of the communication of that evidence for policy change, as can be seen in the development of the coxcomb chart (see Florence Nightingale Museum 2020, p. 18). Today, the advancements in digitalisation and the proliferation of new, ingenious, communication devices, online video platforms, monitoring systems and wearables can assist in the provision of care at a distance by providing remote interaction between health-care workers and patients and providing remote transfer of health information (see Nittari et al. 2020, p. 1427). The possibilities of supplying and providing care and gathering health data remotely (e.g. at home rather than in a hospital) have greatly increased which has enabled a shift from the hospital to the home, potentially freeing up beds, especially in overstretched hospitals focused on providing acute services.

In the context of nursing, the following question could be asked: Should the provision of nursing care be thought of as a primarily online activity in the first instance (see Duffy and Lee 2018)? This may seem, at first glance, an odd question for nurses to consider, given that perhaps their usual experience of providing care is that of a person-to-person encounter, within the confines of a physical building such as a clinic or a hospital. Yet, given that our lives are impacted by a variety of online activities—whether it be communicating through emails and keeping in contact through social media, or perhaps participating in online education and training, or purchasing and selling products online—it may not seem that farfetched to wonder whether nursing should also be thought about first within the context of this digitised world of providing remote care to patients primarily at home. Certainly, the dominant model of in-person, nurse-to-patient experience has evolved alongside technological innovation. The development of mass communication through radio, telegraph, telephone, television and the Internet and its close connection to the delivery of medicine and health care have had a long history (see Barbosa and Silva 2017, p. 929; Craig and Patterson 2006, pp. 6–7). Indeed, it has been pointed out that the necessity to be able to gather medical information on astronauts while they are in space—the ultimate delivery of remote health assessment—formed the springboard for future progress in the area of care at a distance (Barbosa and Silva 2017, p. 929; Nesbitt and Katz-Bell 2018). The possibility of providing health care online compels us to rethink what type of nursing care should be provided and how those services should be supplied remotely, informed by a theoretical perspective and governed by a competent and ethical practice.

Telemedicine, Telehealth and Telenursing

Terms such as telemedicine, telehealth and telenursing, for example, have been used to capture the various uses of communication technologies that provide assessment, monitoring and care remotely in cases where patients and health-care workers are physically distant to each other. Regarding the etymology of 'telemedicine' as a word, it is derived from the Greek term for distance, which is *tele*, and from the Latin for heal, which is *Mederi* (Kumar 2011, p. 1). Khandpur (2017) defines telemedicine as 'the use of electronic information and communications technologies to provide and support healthcare when distance separates the patient and the doctor' (p. 1). The remote communication between the health-care worker and the patient, together with the exchange of health information, can be either synchronous (i.e. in real time), or it can be store-and-forward (i.e. recorded in advance) (Craig and Patterson 2006, p. 5).

Telehealth has been defined as:

> "*the utilization of telecommunications technology to link two or more end-user sites by any interactive electronic means, such as telephones, computers, e-mail, fax, and interactive video transmissions, for the purpose of transfer and/or exchange of information and data in any health-related application*" (Sharpe 2001, p. 3).

Yet these terms—i.e. telemedicine and telehealth—are frequently employed in an interchangeable manner, and the literature in this area often acknowledges that (e.g. Kaplan 2022, p. 106; Sharpe 2001, p. 2). Whereas telemedicine is focused mainly on the medical needs of a patient, telecare (another term used) is focused on the broader care needs of a patient so that they can remain at home (Draper and Sorell 2013, p. 365).

Telenursing is the coming together of communication technologies and nursing practice for patient care, which enables the remote delivery of nursing care. Based on a systematic search and review of the literature, McVey (2023) defines it as 'the delivery of care at a distance, using information and communication technologies within the nursing scope of practice' (p. 276). Although telenursing has been around since the telephone (Sharpe 2001, p. 4), it is contended that 1974 marked the advent of telenursing care, as understood today, when it was given at Logan International Airport through its link to the telemedicine division of Boston Hospital (Martich 2017, p. 9).

There is an array of other terms to denote the variety of possible remote services offered by the use of communication technologies, including teleconsultation, telemonitoring, telediagnostics, teletreatment (which is medical experts—at one location—advising others, at another location, of a programme of treatment) (Khandpur 2017, pp. 3–4). Other terms include mHealth, which involves the use of mobile phones and a range of wireless devices, which can be used to assist the monitoring of an individual's health conditions at home, as well as to assist public health initiatives, whereas eHealth involves the electronic means of communicating health care and information through the Internet (Khandpur 2017, p. 6 and p. 8).

Telemedicine, telehealth and telenursing provide a means to access health care remotely, especially in contexts that otherwise would not be possible to access care (see Botrugno 2019, p. 358; Bidmead and Marshall 2020, p. 18). Although that may still remain the case, there is no doubt that the COVID-19 pandemic broadened that out as it wasn't necessarily geographical barriers that prompted the use of communication technologies but rather the pressing necessity to provide a protective barrier, as it were, between patients and other patients, between patients and health-care workers and between health-care workers and other health-care workers, in terms of being infected by, or transmitting, SARS-CoV-2 (see Campbell et al. 2021, p. 69; Bidmead and Marshall 2020, p. 18; Kaplan 2022, p. 105).

Ethical Concerns and Questions

Beyond the COVID-19 pandemic, from the perspective of health systems, communication technologies can provide solutions to supplying health care when facing issues of geographical distance, overstretched bed capacity and overcrowded EDs, to name just a few. From the perspective of the patient, communication technologies can enable them to stay at home and be provided with care, for example, in the case of a discharge after surgery/treatment or in the case of receiving palliative care. All of this can bring benefits to both the health-care system supplying a service and to the patients being provided care.

From surveying the academic literature on the ethics of telemedicine, telehealth and telenursing, it can be said that in the main, the ethical concerns tend to focus on issues pertaining to equitability of access, patient autonomy and consent, privacy and confidentiality, quality of care and the relationship between the patient and the health-care worker (e.g. see Kaplan 2022; Kumar 2011; Fleming et al. 2009, pp. 798–800). The four standard principles of bioethics, i.e. beneficence, nonmaleficence, respect for autonomy and justice (Beauchamp and Childress 2019),[4] have provided a framework to examine the ethical concerns[5] and promote ethical questions for this area.

Starting with beneficence, one concern of using communication technologies is to ensure that high-quality care is maintained and not lost or reduced. For some, certainly the doctor-patient interaction can be altered (Kaplan 2022, p. 107). A similar concern about the nurse-patient relationship is not only understandable but is of utmost importance. There are concerns regarding how new forms of communication technologies will affect the relationship of care between nurses and their patients and whether warning signs of a decline in a patient's health will be identified (Pols 2012, p. 46). It has been argued that physical presence is important to fostering a trusting relationship between the health-care worker and the patient, which can be

---

[4] For a fuller treatment of the principles, see Chap. 7 on Principles and Nursing Ethics.
[5] See Keenan et al. (2021) for their review of papers that examine telehealth with reference to these principles.

part of the healing process and that technology should assist rather than replace traditional person-to-person meetings (see Fleming et al. 2009, pp. 799).

From the perspective of beneficence, the following ethical question can be raised: Does the use of communication technologies serve the best interest of the patient in a home-based setting (see Campbell et al. 2021, p. 69)? In terms of positive beneficence, do communication technologies contribute to the welfare of the patient (see Beauchamp and Childress 2019, p. 217)? In terms of utility of beneficence, does the balance of the benefits of communication technologies outweigh any negatives (see Beauchamp and Childress 2019, p. 217)? Two clear benefits can be proposed: the possibility of patients not needing to travel to a clinic or a hospital and receiving remote care in their homes and the possibility of avoiding exposure to an infectious airborne virus such as SARS-CoV-2 (see Campbell et al. 2021, p. 70).

The challenge is to secure the benefits that come with communication technologies without putting at risk the quality and standard of care or without leading to opportunities for care to be missed. From the standpoint of the principle of nonmaleficence, it would seem that if patients can receive continuous remote monitoring at home, then the occasion for harm is reduced (see Keenan et al. 2021, p. 6). Then again, the presence of technological devices in a patient's home may generate risks of harms too, for example, if those devices are experienced as being intrusive (Keenan et al. 2021, p. 6; also see Fleming et al. 2009, p. 798). Remote monitoring could lead certain patients to become more focused on their health condition (Stowe and Harding 2010, p. 196). With communication technologies, the hospital or clinic can 'enter' the home. For some patients, this may provide a reassurance to them if they know that their health is being constantly monitored. For other patients, it may be more difficult for them to focus on other things in their lives, and therefore the lines between being at home and being at a hospital/clinic may become blurred. In many ways, the same can be said for work and life: working from home is made possible in some occupations because of communication technologies. The difference is that for some people, being able to 'leave behind' a hospital or clinic may be important to them; it may even be part of their own therapeutic journey to recovery.

From the perspective of nonmaleficence, the following ethical question can be asked: Does the use of communication technologies cause any unjustified setbacks to the patient (see Beauchamp and Childress 2019, p. 158)? One concern that could be raised is the lack of physical examination, in the traditional sense. Although some examinations can take place through videoconferencing, the traditional type of physical assessment can spot issues that may not be entirely visible through a screen (see Campbell et al. 2021, p. 71). For example, a patient may visit their doctor because of one particular ailment that is bothering them, but through a physical examination, the doctor may pick up on something else that the patient may not even be aware of. The use of video for consultations has not been deemed to be apt in all cases (Bidmead and Marshall 2020, p. 20). Whereas obligations to prevent harms arises from the principle of beneficence, obligations not to place patients at risk of harm arises from the principle of nonmaleficence (Beauchamp and Childress 2019, pp. 157–159). Nonetheless, it is also recognised that although it may not be the perfect medium for some medical issues, the use of some forms of communication technologies may be the only route for some patients to obtain medical care (Chaet et al. 2017, p. 1137), which brings us to the principle of justice.

Given the originating context of providing access to care to geographically remote regions, the question of patients having access to communication technologies that is fair and equitable is another pressing ethical concern (see Keenan et al. 2021, pp. 6–7). Patients can remain in their homes without having to attend a clinic or hospital to receive medical or nursing care (see Botrugno 2019, p. 363). From the perspective of the principle of justice, the following ethical question can be asked: Does the use of communication technologies contribute to the provision of equitable and fair access? The main driving force behind the development and implementation of telemedicine was to provide more accessibility to the supply of health-care service (Botrugno 2022, p. 107). However, whether it has been successful in attaining this for deprived regions has been questioned (see Botrugno 2022, p. 107).

The impact on the autonomy of patients is a major point of discussion in the academic literature (see Botrugno 2019, p. 363; Keenan et al. 2021, p. 5).[6] While the possibility of receiving care at home may seem to contribute to safeguarding or indeed fostering autonomy, it can also lead to less autonomy if the patient begins to feel alienated from others; there can therefore be a double-edged sword effect (see Keenan et al. 2021, p. 5). Given that one of the roles of consent is to protect autonomy (Beauchamp and Childress 2019, pp. 118–119), consent also needs to be suitable for the context of home-based care that utilises technical devices and online platforms, either as a synchronous live event or as an asynchronous means of data exchange, as it remains a 'clinical intervention' (Fleming et al. 2009, p. 799). Appropriate information about diagnosis and prognosis needs to still continue where communication technologies are used. In addition, appropriate information about the medium of videoconferencing and the use of other technologies should also be given to patients (see Chaet et al. 2017, p. 1138). The same applies to privacy and confidentiality. In fact, given the ethical concerns pertaining to cybersecurity and other potential compromises to IT systems, privacy and confidentiality take on a particular significance in the use of communication technologies to provide remote health care (see Chaet et al. 2017, p. 1138). Unsurprisingly, maintaining privacy of data is a key issue (Nittari et al. 2020, p. 1436). In addition, there may be issues of achieving privacy within the home, which may be out of the control of the health provider: a patient may not feel completely at ease to disclose something to a nurse through a video link, for example, because of other family members being present. Overall, from the perspective of respect for autonomy, the following ethical question can be asked: Does the use of communication technologies support autonomous choices and actions by the patient (see Beauchamp and Childress 2019, pp. 104–105)?

In the final part of this chapter, two proposals are advanced regarding the use of communication technologies in the context of nursing care: First, on a macro level, an adapted Equivalence of Care should be a guiding principle for supplying remote,

---

[6] For an in-depth discussion of patient autonomy in nursing and health-care contexts, please see Chap. 6

home-based nursing care and second, on a micro level, technomoral virtues should be fostered in nurses providing remote care to patients at their home.

Principle of Equivalence of Care

The Principle of Equivalence of Care is normally applied in the context of the issue of supply of health care to those who are incarcerated (Charles and Draper 2012, p. 215). The principle advocates that those who are on the inside of prison should receive an equivalence of health care as those who are on the outside, because there is no moral difference between the two groups when addressing their health needs (Charles and Draper 2012, p. 215). According to Charles and Draper (2012), the Principle of the Equivalence of Care can apply to the process (i.e. how health-care services are supplied) and to the outcome of care (i.e. the health outcomes stemming from the care that is supplied) (pp. 215–217). Yet there are issues with seeking equivalence of care in terms of process, given the context of a prison and the particular medical needs of certain prisoners (Charles and Draper 2012, p. 216): for instance, it may seem equitable to have the same waiting times for a prisoner and a non-prisoner to access a drug-related service; however, access may be more pressing in a prison context compared to a non-prison. Therefore, pursuing an equivalency in terms of process may not lead to an equivalency in terms of health outcomes for prisoners (Charles and Draper 2012, pp. 216–217). Charles and Draper (2012) therefore argue for the modification of obtaining equivalency of care through a health outcome model (pp. 217–218).

When adapted to the context of remote supply of home-based nursing care through communication technologies, the Principle of Equivalence of Care would advocate for the morally equal treatment of patients at home as those who are in-patients or out-patients. In terms of supplying nursing care at home through communication technologies, the Principle of the Equivalence of Care in terms of process would refer to how remote, home-based nursing care is supplied, whereas in terms of outcomes, it would refer to patient's health outcomes due to remote, home-based nursing care that has been facilitated by communication technologies. A similar claim can be made in the context of supplying remote, nursing care at home through communication technologies: equitability may be obtained not in terms of process only (i.e. patient X, based at home, getting the same time with nurse Y as patient Z based in a clinic) but in terms of health outcomes (i.e. patient X not having a less favourable health outcome as patient Z because they are not in a clinic). Following in the thought of Charles and Draper (2012), the Principle of Equivalence of Care understood as a process regarding the supply of nursing care, may not be suitable depending on the home-based situation and the care needs of the patient. The Equivalence of Care would need to be complemented in terms of a focus on health outcomes. Clearly, numerous variables can impact on a patient's health outcome; however, on a macro level, should it turn out to be the case that those who are in receipt of remote nursing care have less favourable health outcomes than those who are not, then this would raise policy questions as well as ethical ones. In sum, an adapted Equivalence of Care could be an overarching principle for the supply of remote, home-based nursing care using communications technologies on a macro level.

Those receiving remote, home-based forms of nursing care through communication technological means should receive a health-care service that is not of a lesser standard because the patient is not physically present in a hospital or clinic. However, this would be based on the premise that the level of care that is provided in a hospital or clinic conforms to nursing standard and ethical practice. If it does not, then there would be an argument for a supply of remote nursing care to a greater standard and ethical practice and therefore not equivalent.

Technomoral Virtues

In this book, Sellman provides an informative explanation of the theory of virtue ethics and its relevance for the practice of nursing.[7] As a follow on to that, it is pertinent to consider Vallor's (2016) seminal work on technomoral virtues. However, given the restraints of this chapter, it is not possible to provide a full synopsis and a critique of Vallor's (2016) work. What follows, therefore, is a proposed brief adaption of some of Vallor's (2016) technomoral virtues for nurses in the context of their provision of remote, home-based care through the medium of communication technologies. These virtues are described as technomoral because they need to be fostered to enable us to flourish in our world shaped by technologies that are new and still emerging (Vallor 2016, p. 1, p. 10, p. 119). Vallor's (2016, p. 120) technomoral virtues of honesty, humility, justice, care and practical wisdom will now be highlighted for nurses engaged with communication technologies to provide remote, home-based care.[8]

Technomoral Virtue of Honesty

Given the essential link between communication technologies and the exchange of information, the technomoral virtue of honesty could not be more pertinent (see Vallor 2016, pp. 120–123). The interaction and exchange of data requires a virtue of honest communication that is suitable and proficient in an ethical sense, according to Vallor (2016, p. 121). In the context of providing remote nursing care, Vallor's (2016) definition of the technomoral virtue of honesty can be slightly rearticulated as *a commendable respect for truth, which is accompanied with a practical expertise to express that respect appropriately in the context of the provision of remote*

---

[7] Please see Chap. 9 Virtue Ethics and Nursing Practice.

[8] This does not imply that other technomoral virtues listed by Vallor (2016 p. 120) are of a lesser standing or cannot be adapted for nursing in the context of remote care. However, the chosen virtues of honesty, humility, justice, care and practical wisdom seem to be particularly apt for the provision of nursing care through communication technologies.

nursing care through the medium of communication technologies (p. 122). While the sourcing, gathering, interpretation and communication of information in general have become faster and more accessible, at the same time, the reception of information has become more and more accompanied with doubt and suspicion, often resulting in a lack of trust regarding its validity. This issue is even more significant in how a patient's health data is gathered, interpreted and transferred, with the possible impact of AI on data. Patients need to be able to trust that the information given via communication technology will be accurate and free of bias. This demands not only accuracy in terms of the gathering of the data but also an honest and expert use and communication of the same.

Technomoral Virtue of Humility

Humility, as a technomoral virtue, refers to the acceptance of the extent and constraint of knowledge using technologies (Vallor 2016, pp. 125–127). At first glance, this virtue may not seem relevant in a fast-paced world. Yet, as Vallor (2016) notes, in terms of facing the '*acute technosocial opacity*', humility is a significant virtue, as the digital world is not subjected to full human control (p. 126). Humility requires finding a balance between, what Vallor (2016, p. 127) describes as, techno-optimism and techno-pessimism: techno-optimism by nurses would be taking an unquestioning acceptance that all new forms of communication technologies are good for a patient in providing remote nursing care. Whereas the opposite would be a techno-pessimism approach. A balance in between would be nurses taking a critical stance (see Vallor 2016, p. 127) that doesn't lose sight of the intricacies of some technologies and their opacity as well as their potential impact on the lives of patients.

Technomoral Virtue of Justice

The technomoral virtue of justice would entail that nurses pursue allocating the benefits and the risks of the utilisation of communication technologies for remote care in a way that is equitable (following Vallor 2016, p. 128). In addition, nurses should be mindful of the potential effect of communication technologies could have on patients in terms of their dignity and their rights as well as their fundamental freedoms (following Vallor 2016, p. 128).

Technomoral Virtue of Care

Adapting Vallor's (2016) definition of care as a technomoral virtue for nurses, it can be said that it is *a skillful, attentive, responsible and personally responsive disposition to professionally meet the health needs of the patient in the context of the provision of remote nursing care through the means of communications technologies* (p. 138). Putting this virtue into action would mean that nurses would use communication technologies that assist the provision of remote care in a way that contributes to human flourishment (following Vallor 2016, p. 140). Vallor's (2016) work would caution against deeming technologies that are still emerging as somehow against care as a virtue, but rather they need to be incorporated well into the provision of care (see p. 140).

Technomoral Virtue of Practical Wisdom

Finally, all the technomoral virtues would need to be underpinned by practical wisdom for nurses to implement the virtues through habitual actions (following Vallor 2016, p. 154). It would imply that nurses habitually put into action the technomoral virtues of honesty, humility, justice and care, for example, when using communication technologies to provide remote patient care at their home. Honest communication, for example, by nurses needs to be accompanied by an appropriate medium to ensure that it is not only understandable to the patient but is also sensitive and compassionate. The use of video, instead of an in-person face-to-face meeting, may not be appropriate for all types of communication regarding the status of a patient's health. For instance, should a patient want to ask their nurse questions about the implications of a serious cancer diagnosis that they have received, it may be more sensitive to have this kind of meeting in person. Although rules and protocols may give specific guidance on appropriate use of communication technologies, nurses may need to use their practical judgement to assess those situations that require an in-person meeting.

It seems to me that as various forms of communication technologies continue to develop and emerge, then a range of technomoral virtues will need to be promoted and fostered in nurses using communication technologies to provide remote care at a patient's home.

Case Study

Olivia is 82 years old and lives on her own. She has been quite independent, but recently she has had bad health. Her son and daughter have their own families and live quite a distance away, but they visit her as often as they can. This has not been an issue until now, especially after Olivia nearly had a bad fall a couple of weeks ago, which is why they have found the use of telenursing service reassuring. Olivia can connect with her nurse through a video link, and aspects of her health such as her blood pressure and glucose levels can be monitored at a distance.

Nurse Tiffany has quite a few patients logged on to the virtual waiting room, and she wants to ensure that she can keep on top of things. The number of patients using the service has been increasing in recent times. She is keen to see as many patients as possible and that they would have the same wait times as the in-patients would. After seeing several patients, it is Olivia's turn to be let into the virtual clinic, and conscious of time, Nurse Tiffany begins to work her way systematically through the standard list of assessment questions. Nurse Tiffany doesn't use earphones as she feels that that might highlight more the digital aspect of clinical encounter and she wants the online experience to be as close as possible to a 'normal' in-person, face-to-face encounter.

Olivia informs Nurse Tiffany that she isn't herself today and feels a bit light-headed. Nurse Tiffany checks Olivia's blood pressure measurement but that seems fine. However, Olivia insists that her own old blood pressure device says differently. Nurse Tiffany is mystified by this as there is no obvious sign of dizziness. Suddenly, Olivia begins to become increasingly emotional and complains about her children not visiting her enough. She says she doesn't know what to think with all the new hospital equipment at home. At this point, one of the IT technicians comes into Nurse Tiffany's room to check on something. Nurse Tiffany doesn't want to stop the flow of the conversation as she sees how it is important for Olivia to express how she is really feeling. However, Olivia's screen begins to freeze, and when it returns to normal, she can't see Olivia ...

Questions to Consider

1. What are the ethical concerns raised in this case study?
2. Nurse Tiffany is keen to see as many patients as possible. Reflect on this from the Principle of Equivalence of Care as a process and as an outcome. Nurse Tiffany may be right to ensure that her patients, who are receiving remote care, have the same wait times as the in-patients. However, what about seeking equivalence of health outcomes?
3. Nurse Tiffany seems to doubt the 'old' blood pressure monitor reading as well as Olivia's experience. Does Nurse Tiffany have an uncritical trust in the remote monitor?
4. How should Nurse Tiffany react to the IT personnel? How can she uphold Olivia's dignity and privacy in the clinical encounter? Although Olivia is unaware of how 'busy' the telenursing section is, patients are aware that hospitals are busy places too.
5. What are the technomoral virtues that Nurse Tiffany displayed in this encounter? Are there any technomoral virtues that could be fostered more to reshape the experience?

Conclusion

There is no doubt that as the development and use of communication technologies continue to advance, nurses will not only need to continue to navigate their way using technological means of providing remote care to their patients; they will also be confronted with the need to negotiate the ethical and existential implications of such technologies for nursing practice. Issues such as access, patient convenience and the sustainability of services can lend great support to the continuing expansion and adoption of communication technologies for the supply and provision of remote nursing care to patients at home. In this context, an adapted Equivalence of Care as a guiding principle on a macro level as well as the technomoral virtues on a micro level should be taken into account, given nursing's concern to continue to supply and provide good quality patient care that is, equitable, accessible, competent and morally sound.

> **Key Learning Points**
> - To understand some of the differences between terms such as telemedicine, telehealth and telenursing.
> - To know some of the general ethical concerns and questions related to the use of communication technologies.
> - To reflect on an adapted Principle of Equivalence of Care for the supply of remote nursing care using communication technologies, on a macro level.
> - To consider some technomoral virtues for nurses using communication technologies to provide remote care to patients at home, on a micro level.

References

Barbosa IA, Silva MJPD (2017) Nursing care by telehealth: what is the influence of distance on communication? Rev Bras Enferm 70(5):928–934. https://doi.org/10.1590/0034-7167-2016-0142

Beauchamp TL, Childress JF (2019) Principles of biomedical ethics, 8th edn. Oxford University Press, Oxford

Bidmead E, Marshall A (2020) Covid-19 and the 'new normal': are remote video consultations here to stay? Br Med Bull 135(1):16–22. https://doi.org/10.1093/bmb/ldaa025

Botrugno C (2019) Towards an ethics for telehealth. Nurs Ethics 26(2):357–367. https://doi.org/10.1177/0969733017705004

Botrugno C (2022) The spread of telemedicine in daily practice: weighing risks and benefits. In: Ienca M, Pollicino O, Liguori L, Stefanini E, Andorno R (eds) The Cambridge handbook of information technology, life sciences and human rights. Cambridge University Press, Cambridge, pp 102–112

Campbell KA, Bosco JA, Shah MR, Bosco JA (2021) The ethics of telemedicine. Bull Hosp Jt Dis (2013) 79(2):69–71

Chaet D, Clearfield R, Sabin JE, Skimming K, Council on ethical and judicial affairs American Medical Association (2017) Ethical practice in telehealth and telemedicine. J Gen Intern Med 32(10):1136–1140. https://doi.org/10.1007/s11606-017-4082-2

Charles A, Draper H (2012) 'Equivalence of care' in prison medicine: is equivalence of process the right measure of equity? J Med Ethics 38(4):215–218. https://doi.org/10.1136/medethics-2011-100083

Craig J, Patterson V (2006) Introduction to the practice of telemedicine. In: Wootton R, Craig J, Patterson V (eds) Introduction to telemedicine, 2nd edn. The Royal Society of Medicine Press, London, pp 3–14

Draper H, Sorell T (2013) Telecare, remote monitoring and care. Bioethics 27(7):365–372. https://doi.org/10.1111/j.1467-8519.2012.01961.x

Duffy S, Lee TH (2018) In-person health care as option b. N Engl J Med 378(2):104–106. https://doi.org/10.1056/NEJMp1710735

Fleming DA, Edison KE, Pak H (2009) Telehealth ethics. Telemed J E Health 15(8):797–803. https://doi.org/10.1089/tmj.2009.0035

Florence Nightingale Museum (2020) In: Nixon K, Clark C, Sayer C (eds) Florence nightingale: celebrating her life and legacy. Pitkin Publishing, London

Kaplan B (2022) Ethics, guidelines, standards, and policy: telemedicine, COVID-19, and broadening the ethical scope. Camb Q Healthc Ethics 31(1):105–118. https://doi.org/10.1017/S0963180121000852

Keenan AJ, Tsourtos G, Tieman J (2021) The value of applying ethical principles in telehealth practices: systematic review. J Med Internet Res 23(3):e25698. https://doi.org/10.2196/25698

Khandpur RS (2017) Telemedicine: technology and applications (mHealth, teleHealth and eHealth). PHI Learning, Delhi

Kumar S (2011) Introduction to telenursing. In: Kumar S, Snooks H (eds) Telenursing. Springer, London, pp 1–3

Martich D (2017) Telehealth nursing: tools and strategies for optimal patient care. Springer, New York

McVey C (2023) Telenursing: a concept analysis. Comput Inform Nurs 41(5):275–280. https://doi.org/10.1097/CIN.0000000000000973

Nesbitt T, Katz-Bell J (2018) History of telehealth. In: Rheuban K, Krupinski EA (eds) Understanding telehealth. McGraw Hill, New York, pp 3–14

Nittari G, Khuman R, Baldoni S, Pallotta G, Battineni G, Sirignano A, Amenta F, Ricci G (2020) Telemedicine practice: review of the current ethical and legal challenges. Telemed J E Health 26(12):1427–1437. https://doi.org/10.1089/tmj.2019.0158

Pols J (2012) Care at a distance: on the closeness of technology. Amsterdam University Press, Amsterdam

Sharpe CC (2001) Telenursing: nursing practice in cyberspace. Auburn House, London

Stowe S, Harding S (2010) Telecare, telehealth and telemedicine. Eur Geriatr Med 1(3):193–197. https://doi.org/10.1016/j.eurger.2010.04.002

Vallor S (2016) Technology and the virtues: a philosophical guide to a future worth wanting. Oxford University Press, New York

Ethical Issues and Principles in Nursing and Healthcare Research

17

P. Anne Scott

Abstract

Ethical issues permeate the entire research process from the identification of the research question and selection of research participants, to dissemination of findings. This chapter identifies some of the historical influences informing the development of research ethics frameworks internationally. The author then moves to highlight some of the key ethical issues that need to be considered throughout the various elements of the research process. Some of the important principles underlying research ethics frameworks are identified and interpreted within the context of the research process.

Keywords

Nursing research · Research ethics · Respect for persons · Autonomy · Beneficence · Informed consent

Introduction

Recognition of the need to regulate research on human beings can be traced back to reactions against the abuses associated with German and Japanese research during World War II. However, as the twentieth century rolled on, it was increasingly recognised that a number of abuses, in terms of research on human subjects, continued into the post-war period in both democratic and communist countries (Mason and McCall Smith 2010). Revelations during the Nuremburg Trails, for example, of the atrocities committed in the name of medical experimentation during World War II, combined with other twentieth-century medical research scandals such as the

---

P. A. Scott (✉)
University of Galway, Galway, Co Galway, Ireland
e-mail: anne.scott@universityofgalway.ie

© The Author(s), under exclusive license to Springer Nature Switzerland AG 2024
P. A. Scott, S. M. Scott (eds.), *Key Concepts and Issues in Nursing Ethics*,
https://doi.org/10.1007/978-3-031-54108-7_17

Tuskegee Syphilis Study 1932–1972 (Adams 1996), the Willowbrook hepatitis studies (Krugman 1986) and the New Zealand cervical cancer inquiry (Cartwright 1988; Paterson 2010) have helped develop widespread resolve regarding the need to protect participants in human research projects and the need to continue to monitor the conduct of such research internationally. Dougherty and Allen (2017), reporting on psychological experimentation on detainees held by the Central Intelligence Agency, suggest that these concerns are not merely of historical relevance but continue to be live issues for societies globally. The first internationally accepted set of ethical guidelines with regard to these issues was the Nuremburg Code published in 1947 (for further comment see Moreno et al. 2017). The World Medical Association (WMA) publicly endorsed the principles expressed in the Nuremburg Code by drawing up the Declaration of Helsinki in 1964 (World Medical Association 2023). This Declaration has been revised several times since its first publication, most recently in the WMA general assembly in Brazil, October 2013. At the WMA general assembly in 2022, a working group was established to consider further revisions to the Declaration (see World Medical Association 2023).

The past 45 years has seen a number of countries and organisations highlight issues surrounding the ethics of research on human subjects: for example, the Belmont Principles (The Belmont Report: Principles and Guidelines for the Protection of Human Subjects of Research 1979), and the Irish Council for Bioethics (2004). In the nursing arena, the Nursing and Midwifery Board of Ireland (NMBI 2015), the Royal College of Nurses (Royal College of Nurses 2022), the International Council of Nurses (ICN) (Holzemer and International Council of Nurses (ICN) 2003) and the Nordic Nurses Federation (Northern Nurses Federation 2003) all published new or revised guidelines for nursing research. Issues regarding the human rights of research participants have also been underlined by the Council of Europe (Council of Europe 1997), in the European Convention on Human Rights and Biomedicine (Oviedo Convention), the only international legally binding instrument to protect human participants in biomedical research.

Guided by international instruments [such as the Nuremberg Code (Moreno et al. 2017), the United Nations Declaration on Human Rights (United Nations 1948), the United Nations Convention on the Rights of the Child (United Nations 1989), the Belmont Report (1979), the Oviedo Convention (Council of Europe 1997) and the Declaration of Helsinki (World Medical Association 2023)], in addition to various ethical theories that have become influential in healthcare ethics in general, such as Kantian ethics and the principle-based framework of Beauchamp and Childress (2019),[1] a conceptualisation of appropriate ways to treat and protect human beings, both the fully functioning adult and vulnerable human beings such as children, the older person, the cognitively impaired and the terminally ill, has emerged and continues to be modified over time.

However, as we move towards the end of the second decade of the twenty-first century, there are certain ethical principles that are seen as fundamental to the framework of ethics that guide decisions regarding the morally appropriate

---

[1] See Chap. 7 for an in-depth discussion of ethical principles and nursing practice.

consideration and treatment of human beings during research activities. For example, the Irish Council of Bioethics in 2004 commented as follows:

> *Research involving human participants should be based on a fundamental moral commitment to the individuals concerned and to advancing human welfare, knowledge and understanding. A number of guiding moral principles govern the ethical review of research proposals. These principles aim to protect the well-being and rights of research participants/volunteers.* (Irish Council for Bioethics 2004, p. 6)

Some Important Considerations

Human beings are deserving of respect and protection as inalienable rights (UNDHR 1948). This is equally the case during research activities as it is in any other circumstances. Based on the work of the philosopher Immanuel Kant, such values are expressed in the principle of respect for persons, sometimes translated as respect for autonomy. Such expressions of course raise questions of the definition of person and autonomy and when and in what set of circumstances such concepts are and are not applicable.[2] However, for the purposes of this chapter, we will take it that respect is applicable to all human participants in nursing and healthcare research. The question then arises regarding what this actually means in the case of individual participants in a particular research project. At a minimum, the considerations explored below are relevant.

Respect for the Human Person

Within the context of research activity the principle of respect for persons is frequently articulated in terms of rights—both rights to autonomous participation and welfare rights (welfare rights refer to the right to have one's support and protection needs respected). Some such rights are the following:

- The right not to be injured or mistreated.
- The right to give informed, uncoerced consent to participate in the particular piece of research.
- The right to privacy, confidentiality and/or anonymity.

In terms of protecting the participant's right not to be injured or mistreated, it is normally the duty of the research team not to expose the research participant to significantly burdensome, unreasonable, known or predictable risk. On occasion, however, when significant burden or predictable material risk is unavoidable, it is the duty of the research team to provide appropriate information on the likely burden and/or risk involved, so that the participant can determine if they fully understand and accept such burden or risk. Thus, for example, in drug trials and trials

---

[2] For a discussion of the concept of autonomy in nursing and healthcare, please see Chap. 6.

involving medical devices, the trials are phased and normally commence with non-human (laboratory and animal) trials. Such measures help to provide insight into likely effects of the particular drug or device—at least on non-human subjects. Thus by the time clinical trials (trials using human participants) commence, previous phases give insight into the actions of the agent (drug or device for example). This provides a certain level of confidence that the agent will either not cause significant physical risk to the trial participants or that any such risks, which will be explained to the participant prior to participation, can and will be managed and/or mitigated by the research team. Where discomfort, burden and/or risk cannot be avoided such discomfort, burden and/or risk must be proportionate to the anticipated gain, either directly to the individual participant and/or to humanity or society. Such considerations are directly linked to the discussion of the principles of beneficence and non-maleficence below.

Informed Consent

Respect for the individual's right to make decisions about themselves and their life (respect for autonomy) requires that research participants are adequately and properly informed regarding the nature of the research project. For example, potential participants must be informed with regard to what will be required of the individual participant, including the approximate time requirement, any procedures that will be performed on him/her, any known or predictable risks or side effects, the nature of the trial (where a clinical trial is part of the research design), whether a placebo is being used, whether the trial is blinded and so forth. Such information enables the potential research participant to give *informed consent* to participate in the particular research activity or project.

There are two other crucial elements that must be in play in order to ensure that consent is not only informed but also voluntary—and thus autonomously exercised. These elements are:

- The participant must have the capacity to both understand the information being provided regarding the particular piece of research, including the implications of participation for the individual and the (cognitive) ability to exercise consent.
- The participant must be free from coercion. Thus the participant must be assured and accept, for example, that refusal to consent will not affect her/his current care and treatment if the individual is being cared for by any member of a healthcare team; either in hospital or in the community. The individual should also be free from any other form of duress related to the research in question—from the research or healthcare team or from relatives or significant others [see HSE (2023) for a detailed discussion of the principal requirements of informed consent].

In instances where the potential research participant is a patient, practitioners should be aware of the profound influence that they may have on patients to whom they suggest participating in research. For example Kass et al. (1996), in a study on participant consent to involvement in cancer clinical trials, express it thus:

> Clinicians should be mindful of the tremendous influence they have over their patients, given that the mere suggestion of enrolment in research by a patient's personal physician was interpreted by many patients to be endorsement. (Kass et al. 1996, p.25)

Some research, within the context of health and developing the appropriate evidence base for healthcare provision, will require the participation of individuals who are temporarily or permanently deemed not to have the capacity to give consent to participate in the research activity, or who have been deemed not to have the capacity to make particular decisions. Assisted decision-making legislation, for example, the Assisted Decision-Making (Capacity) Act 2015 (2015) in Ireland requires that decision-making support be made available to enable those who are cognitively compromised to engage as fully as possible in the consent process, in research relevant to their will and preferences. People who, even with assistance, will not be capable of exercising their informed consent should only be involved in research under very clearly articulated and strictly monitored conditions. If it is impossible to carry out the particular research project with competent participants (or, e.g. to wait for the unconscious person to regain consciousness, or where such action would invalidate the study), consent must be sought from the legally authorised guardian/decision supporter of the individual involved, assuming research is listed in the relevant decision agreement. As a general rule of thumb, individuals deemed not to have the capacity to give consent, or members of other vulnerable groups, should only be involved in research when it is reasonable to expect that the individual, or the group of which they are a member, will ultimately benefit from the research in question, and where the potential participant is exposed to minimal risk and burden. This is part of protecting the welfare of these individuals. However, it is also important, from an ethics point of view, that people with various disabilities, including those cognitively compromised and those living with various vulnerabilities, are involved in high-quality research that is relevant to their care and treatment—in order to develop a relevant evidence base for this care and treatment.

Should the potential participant, identified as lacking the capacity to consent, be able to give assent to participation in research, such assent should be sought—in addition to the consent of the legal guardian/authorised decision supporter described above. In such circumstances a decision to withhold assent should be acknowledged and respected; thus this individual should not be included in the research project in question.

A corollary of informed consent is that the individual should be assured that their participation, responses, tissue samples and so forth are being used for the purposes of the identified research project only. Personal information and/or donated material, such as tissue samples, will then be destroyed under properly regulated mechanisms that are fully protective of the autonomy and privacy of the participant. If this is not the case, the potential participant should be made aware, explicitly, that it is intended to use such material for another, future study or studies. This enables the potential participant to knowingly consent, or withhold consent, to any potential future study. It clearly protects against a recurrence of cases, such as those reported in the past in both Ireland and the UK (The Royal Liverpool Children's Inquiry Report 2001; Government of Ireland 2006), where human organs were retained, postmortem, for potential use in current or future research projects.

In some, perhaps many nursing research projects private and intimate information may be sought from the research participant during data collection, for example, information on previous medical history, information on personal behaviours and habits or information on the participant's children, siblings and so forth. Intimate, personally significant information may also be discovered as a result of interventions designed into the particular research initiative—i.e. genetic screening, chromosome studies, screening for risk of cancer and cardiac disease, alcohol use, sexual activity, patient satisfaction surveys and so forth. Research participants, in order to be properly protected from unwarranted risk of such personal information becoming available publicly and thus potentially being used to the detriment of the research participant, (and to enable the participant to feel safe to participate in the particular study) should be assured that such *personal information will be kept private and confidential*. Where strict confidentiality cannot be assured, appropriate mechanisms should be designed into the study to protect participants. Participants can thus be assured that their identity will not be divulged—i.e. the *data collection, handling and storage processes protect anonymity*. In this latter case, for example, participants are normally not asked to divulge their names on self-completed questionnaires—such as when completing patient satisfaction questionnaires or when a staff member completes a staff survey.

Beneficence and Non-maleficence

Two of the internationally accepted, fundamental core principles underpinning both nursing practice and research are the principle of beneficence (do good) and the mirror principle of non-maleficence (do not harm). Thus, one should do good to and should not harm one's patients, clients or research participants. Clearly some interventions (for diagnostic, therapeutic and/or research purposes) may be uncomfortable, burdensome or painful. Some may cause a degree of harm—for example, surgical intervention, dressing of wounds and burns and so forth. However, the basic stance is that the core function of the healthcare professional is to work for the benefit of the patient or client from a health perspective. Thus the practitioner or the researcher must not cause unnecessary or avoidable harm or distress to one's patients, clients or research participants. Principle 8 of the Declaration of Helsinki states: "While the primary purpose of research is to generate new knowledge, this goal can never take precedence over the rights and interests of research subjects" (World Medical Association 2023).

In order to continue to develop the evidence base for healthcare and nursing practice, relevant, well-designed research is both important and essential. Conversely, the results of poorly designed research may, at worst, seriously harm participants or, at best, waste their time, while at the same time make misleading or detrimental contributions to the evidence base. This means that significant time and effort should be invested into research training and research oversight and governance.

At the level of the individual participant the duty to do good, and prevent harm, warrants equal vigilance. In instances where the participant is likely to experience discomfort, burden and/or risk, such discomfort, burden and/or risk must be proportionate to the expected gain from the research study—either directly to the participant or to society as a whole. Within the context of clinical trials, particularly drug trials, for example, this gives rise to a number of issues. In the first instance, in order to warrant the use of a clinical trial, there must be genuine doubt with regard to the efficacy of the drug, or treatment intervention being considered. This is often referred to as a state of *equipoise*. Such conditions exist when either the evidence is not available from which to make a judgement regarding the impact of a particular intervention or in situations where that evidence that does exist is inconclusive and/or contradictory. For a useful discussion of this concept in particular, and ethical issues underlying intervention studies in general, see O'Mathúna (2012).

As indicated above when moving to set up clinical trials, the relevant groundwork must be completed and verified, prior to introducing human trials. Appropriate oversight of the trial including close monitoring of participant responses must be assured. Furthermore, when patients are participating in experimental drug trials, they must be fully aware of this, including being made aware of the very high chance of the experimental intervention not "working". From the perspective of the ethical conduct of the clinical trial, it is good ethical practice for the research team to have a protocol in place to help determine when participation in the trial should be terminated. Such a protocol is particularly pertinent in experimental trials of new anticancer agents. The lack of this type of protocol can lead to unnecessary hardship for very ill, vulnerable patients and for the staff who care for such patients.

A corollary of the principles of beneficence and non-maleficence, in terms of clinical trials, is that a study must be stopped immediately, when the risks are found to outweigh the potential benefits. A similar imperative exists when there is conclusive evidence of positive and beneficial results from one of the agents under investigation.

Justice (Including Case Study)

Within the context of research activity, the principle of justice can be conceptualised as fairness (Rawls 1985). In Rawlsian terms fairness is achieved if the principles guiding distribution of capabilities and resources, for example, are applied so as to ensure that the "least advantaged" are benefitted and not harmed or forgotten. Thus research participants should be treated fairly. For example, if participants are being put at considerable discomfort, inconvenience or risk (it is assumed that participants are fully aware of the demands being made of them), then it may be completely reasonable to compensate a participant for such inconvenience and any expenses they may incur due to their participation in the particular research project. However, compensation should not be such as to induce financially vulnerable individuals to place themselves at significant risk for financial gain.

Another issue that emerges during discussion of the principle of justice, within the context of research activity, is who should participate in research activity? Should certain groups be excluded on grounds such as vulnerability? Over the past number of years, it has been recognised that all patient/client groups, including those identified as especially vulnerable, have the right to participate in, indeed may be necessary participants in, investigations to improve healthcare and to generate a sound evidence base for such care. For example, the 13th principle of the Declaration of Helsinki (World Medical Association 2023) states the following:

> *Groups that are underrepresented in medical research should be provided appropriate access to participate in research.*

However principle 20 qualifies this in the following manner:

> *Medical research with a vulnerable group is only justified if the research is responsive to the health needs and priorities of this group and the research cannot be carried out in a non-vulnerable group. In addition, this group should stand to benefit from the knowledge, practices or interventions that result from the research.*

Groups that come to mind are children, the terminally ill and those who are physically disabled or cognitively impaired. It is a matter of justice that such individuals are enabled to participate in relevant research as fully as possible. Such participation assists in developing our understanding of the health and illness experience of certain vulnerable groups. It helps gain insight into their perceptions of, responses to, and requirements of, interventions provided by healthcare practitioners (and the health service they encounter) over the course of their lives/illness trajectory.

However, special considerations need to come into play to ensure appropriate support and protection of such individuals. In particular specific mechanisms must be put in place to ensure that the welfare rights of vulnerable groups are recognised and protected.

> *A relevant case example concerns developing research interest in the use of a micro camera (SenseCam), to record the daily life of individuals (life-logging) with early-stage dementia (Piasek 2015). Piasek's research focuses on an in-depth analysis of the experiences of three people in early-stage dementia whilst using, over a 7-week period, an automatic camera taking photographs of the person's day-to-day life. Each participant had 14 contacts with the researcher over the 7-week period. The study is unusual in terms of the depth of analysis and the opportunity it provides for the person with dementia, and in two of the cases a family caregiver, to voice their experience of taking part in a trial of a new, potentially therapeutic, intervention. The intervention is placed in the context of how a person with dementia might maintain his/her identity in a situation where cognitive impairment may make this increasingly difficult.*

This study is enabling much needed research on a potential treatment of a vulnerable group of people—those with early-stage dementia. However, in addition to key ethical issues regarding respect for persons and information giving to enable informed consent in this study, the study also generates a requirement to acknowledge that the intervention used may generate distress in either the person with early-stage dementia or the carer—thus causing potential harm. This highlights the need to identify and put in place measures to be taken should distress occur. There are also potential ethical issues related to privacy—not only those of the participant and carer but also issues of photographing unsuspecting members of the public, should the participant have the camera on and rolling, while entertaining guests in the participant's home or while out in public places.

Working It Through: Ethical Issues and the Stages of the Research Process

As indicated above, ethical issues and considerations permeate the entire research process. This begins with the research questions that are asked (and that receive research grant funding as against those questions which do not get asked and those projects which, through lack of funding, do not proceed) and continues right through to reporting of research findings and terminating the researcher/respondent contact.

Researchers need to be sensitive to the nature of particular research agendas and the motivations, personal, political, institutional and sociocultural, which drive them. For example, the current drivers of evidence-based practice in healthcare are at least tripartite—political, economic and professional. As practitioners we are becoming more convinced that our practice must be evidence-based—and there are numerous clinical studies going on attempting to develop our evidence base. However, it is interesting to note that we are a lot less clear on what we mean by evidence or what should count as evidence in healthcare practice (Scott 2006).

It seems reasonably clear that what counts as evidence for X (healthcare practice for example) largely determines the type of evidence we should be seeking and the studies that should be funded. Despite this, little work is currently being carried out, or being funded, in relation to questions regarding the nature of the evidence base appropriate for healthcare and nursing practice. This problem has philosophical, moral and professional implications. One of the most serious is the potential impact that our lack of knowledge and understanding, regarding the nature of an appropriate evidence base, will have on patient care.

However, once the researcher has decided on the appropriate research question, it is a moral and professional requirement to ensure that the selected piece of research is necessary. Thus the researcher needs to be sure that the knowledge is required and does not already exist in a sufficiently comprehensive state. This indicates the need for the researcher to be equipped to do the required literature searching and reviewing. To do otherwise is likely to lead not only to a poorly refined research question and consequent poor research design; it is also wasteful of resources and shows a lack of respect for the study respondents and those who provide support for the researcher.

Assuming that the research question is a legitimate and useful one, the researcher must draw on personal or outside expertise in designing an appropriate study that will provide a real possibility of gaining answers to the research question posed or which will provide a firm basis for further work. This is not only a methodological issue. Sound study design is required in order to ensure that the study is ethically sound. Lack of appropriate expertise in study design is again, at a minimum, wasteful of time and other resources and indicates a lack of respect for respondents and those supporting the work of the researcher. At worst such lack of expertise may be positively damaging to the research respondents. Given that nursing researchers frequently carry out research with respondents already made vulnerable through illness, as indicated in the short case example above on the potential therapeutic use of SenseCam, lack of appropriate expertise is particularly unacceptable from an ethical perspective.

Once the researcher is confident that the design of the study is appropriate and that the data collection methods/tools will obtain the data required, ethical considerations broadly focus on ensuring respect for the participants and include the following elements:

- The role of the practitioner-researcher and the implications of the researcher identifying him or herself as a nurse, doctor, physiotherapist, clinical psychologist and so forth. The implications are potentially both positive and negative. Such self-identification may make recruitment to a study much easier—both because it may provide easier access to a participant pool and/or because a health practitioner such as a nurse is automatically seen as trustworthy by a patient or member of the public. However, it may also confuse or set up false expectations in patient-participants. Conflicts of interest are likely to arise where a practitioner is using his/her own patient group in research. Such confusion of roles should normally be avoided. Where a self-identified, qualified practitioner is carrying out a piece of research (for postgraduate work for example), it should be made clear to a participant that the researcher is not responsible for the participant's care and refusal to participate in the research will not have any impact on care provision. This should also be expressed, clearly, either on the written information participants receive regarding the research study or on the consent form. In the case of vulnerable groups—such as those cited in the case example above—the fact that the researcher is not responsible for the participant's healthcare should be repeated on each visit to/contact with the participant.
- The balance of potential inconvenience or risk to participants over potential benefit to participants and/or others. For example, with the life-logging example described above, the potential to come up with what ultimately may prove a beneficial intervention for some people with dementia must be balanced against the potential to cause distress and anxiety to study participants in current, very early-stage exploratory studies.
- Appropriate and sufficient information must be given regarding the nature of the study to enable the potential participant to make an informed choice and to give or withhold informed, voluntary consent. Taking the example of the individual

with dementia, the researcher needs to think through, very carefully, what types of information should be provided to the participant (and perhaps also to the main carer and/or the decision supporter where relevant) and in what form(s) this information should be provided. People experiencing cognitive decline and memory impairment pose particular challenges to the meaning of "being informed" and "giving informed consent" [see HSE (2023) for further detailed discussion of these matters]. In the moment of engaging with the researcher, these individuals may understand clearly what the study is about and what is being asked of them as participants. They may also agree to participate very willingly in the proposed study. However, this understanding and willingness to continue to participate will need to be reconfirmed on each occasion the researcher interacts with the participant.

In instances where the participants are unable to receive the information or to make informed decisions, for whatever reason, clear transparent processes which aim to ascertain and protect participants' interests, throughout the period of their participation, must be instituted (HSE 2023). The continued right of competent participants to withdraw from the study, without any negative consequences to the participant, must be made clear at the commencement of the study and thereafter, as the study unfolds, as required:

- Issues of anonymity and confidentiality must be given careful consideration and detailed information on these notions given to participants. As de Raeve (1996) points out, this may be particularly pertinent for health practitioner/researchers who may, for example, be used to the rather broader notion of confidentiality which is used within the healthcare team.

In empirical studies, data collection is a crucial area for research ethics. Ethical issues can be identified in the following areas:

- Obtaining permission for data collection from the organisation in question.
- Obtaining permission for data collection from the participants (patients, professionals).
- Consideration of who else may need to be approached in terms of permission—in the case example above, visitors, friends or even members of the public exposed to the SenseCam camera should be informed of the study and be given the option not to be recorded when in the vicinity of the study participant.
- Guaranteeing appropriate ethical behaviour from researchers during the data collection period.

As discussed above, in obtaining permission from individual participants, the issue of informed consent is central. It should be noted that normally practitioners directly involved in care giving do not obtain participants' consent to participate in research, as clear conflict of interest issues may arise. However, clinical nurses, in particular, may have a significant role in supporting patient-participants in making informed decisions regarding participation in a particular piece of research (NMBI 2015).

In line with the principle of respect for persons, participants' anonymity, confidentiality and willingness to participate must be ensured. Risks/benefits/burdens to respondents must be explored. The risk or burden to the participant must be weighed against the potential benefits of the research findings to the general population or specific patient populations. In the case example above, this translates into the need to balance any potential for distress to be caused to the study participants and/or their carers' with the potential to identify a useful new therapy for certain individuals with dementia. Participants in clinical trials must be as fully informed as possible regarding the nature and objectives of the trial. It should be made clear to the participants the nature of any specific risks or benefits that may accrue to trial participants. As highlighted above, particularly but not only in relation to individuals with some element of cognitive impairment, it is important to bear in mind that informed consent is an ongoing process. Research participants may have questions that arise during the data collection process, in particular, that should be addressed. Participants must also be informed and assured that they may withdraw their consent and cease participation at any point during the research process, without this negatively impacting on them or their care.

Ethics and Data Analysis

Analysis of data is an interesting issue from an ethical perspective. At a minimum the researcher and/or his or her research advisors need to have a good grasp of both the strengths and limitations of the method of analysis or any analytical tools used. This is important from an ethical perspective in order to ensure that no inappropriate claims are made, based on the analysis. The relevance of this point in terms of clinical practice and patient care is clear. A significant reason for carrying out empirical research, within healthcare, is to improve patient care and develop sound policy and practices. Inappropriate analysis is likely to lead to inaccurate results and thus potentially to poor policy and practice.

Ethics and the Relationship with Research Participants

de Raeve (1996) highlights the lack of attention to ethical issues surrounding "leaving the field" or termination of the relationship between researcher and participant. This is likely to be a particularly complex issue for researchers involved in some forms of qualitative research and in some psycho/socially focused intervention trials. It was an issue in the SenseCam intervention study (Piasek 2015) described above. Study participants and the two carers involved had come to rely on the researcher for social interaction, the hope of effective treatment and, for one of the carers, the ability to get some time to themselves while the researcher was with the participant. A researcher needs to be aware of the potential problems in this type of researcher-participant relationship. Steps should be taken to ensure that the participant does not confuse the research relationship with a therapeutic, counselling-type relationship or a friendship. Insight and personal integrity is actively required from the researcher throughout the data collection period to guard against misuse or abuse of the researcher-participant relationship (O'Mathúna 2012).

Ethics and Dissemination of Research

From an ethics perspective, if the researcher is to value and respect the contributions made by participants, funding bodies and others supportive of the research effort, it is incumbent on the researcher to report and disseminate the findings of the particular study—positive and negative—in the most effective ways available to the researcher.

In reporting the study results, the ethical issues include continued protection of the rights of, and honouring promises made to, participants (e.g. confidentiality, protection of privacy, anonymity), reporting findings truthfully, accurately and completely, citing appropriately the work of others and ensuring the authorship credits and acknowledgements are stated accurately. To do otherwise once again indicates lack of respect for the various actors in the research process. It is also wasteful of valuable resources, including those of future researchers who might have gained from the sign-posting of "blind alleys" and from insights into the findings, strengths and weaknesses of the unreported study.

Conclusion

A number of the key ethical issues and principles relevant to research with human participants are explored in this chapter. The ethical understanding thus gained is then applied to the component elements of the research process. High-quality, ethically sound research is important in developing the evidence base for healthcare practice and in the provision of effective, humane patient care. Understanding the principles guiding ethically sound research activity is thus a key component in the education and practice of healthcare professionals.

Key Learning Points
- The need to ensure a strong ethical framework to scrutinise and regulate research in healthcare has been informed, in particular, by the abuses of World War II and a number of notorious research scandals uncovered in the twentieth century.
- Within the context of research the principle of respect for persons refers to ensuring, for example, that participants are adequately informed about the research project. Such information should enable participants to give informed consent to participate in the piece of research in question. Respect for persons also requires that participants are supported in their decision-making, where this is necessary to maximise their decision-making capacity, assured of confidentiality or anonymity and that their privacy is protected.
- Two other important ethical principles underlying ethical research practices are the principles of beneficence and non-maleficence: literally this means, respectively, do good and do no harm. Within the research context, participants should be adequately protected, and researchers should avoid exposing participants to unnecessary and undue discomfort, burden or risk.
- The principle of justice demands that research participants should also be treated fairly. All sectors of the population including, where relevant, vulnerable groups and individuals should be enabled to participate in research initiatives. Such participation requires additional protections to be in place.
- Ethical issues permeate the entire research process from question identification and selection to dissemination of findings.

References

Adams M (1996) Final report on the Tuskegee syphilis study 1932–1972. http://www.hsl.virginia.edu/historical/medical_history/bad_blood/report.cfm. Accessed 23 Aug 2023

Assisted Decision-Making (Capacity) Act 2015 (2015). https://www.irishstatutebook.ie/eli/2015/act/64/enacted/en/html. Accessed 6 Dec 2023

Beauchamp TL, Childress JF (2019) Principles of biomedical ethics, 8th edn. Oxford University Press, New York

Cartwright S (1988) The Report of the Committee of Inquiry into allegations concerning the treatment of Cervical Cancer at National Women's Hospital and into other related matters. https://www.nsu.govt.nz/health-professionals/national-cervical-screening-programme/legislation/cervical-screening-inquiry-0. Accessed 23 Aug 2023

Council of Europe (1997) Convention for protection of human rights and dignity of the human being with regard to the application of biology and medicine: convention on human rights and biomedicine (Oviedo convention). European Treaty Series European Commission. https://rm.coe.int/en/web/conventions/full-list?module=treaty-detail&treatynum=164. Accessed 16 Aug 2023

De Raeve L (ed) (1996) Nursing research: an ethical and legal appraisal. Bailliere-Tindall, London

Dougherty S, Allen SA (2017) Nuremberg betrayed: human experimentation and the CIA torture programme. http://physiciansforhumanrights.org/assets/multimedia/phr_humanexperimentationreport.pdf. Accessed 23 Aug 2023

Government of Ireland (2006) Report on post mortem practice and procedures. Stationary Office, Dublin

Holzemer WL, International Council of Nurses (ICN) (2003) Ethical guidelines for nursing research. ICN, Geneva

HSE (2023) National policy for consent in health and social care research (V1.1.2). Health Service Executive, Dublin. E-version of this policy. https://hseresearch.ie/publications/. Accessed 16 Aug 2023

Irish Council for Bioethics (2004) Operational procedures for research ethics committees: guidance. Irish Council for Bioethics, Dublin. http://www.drugsandalcohol.ie/5889/1/Bioethics_Ethical_guidelines_for_research.pdf

Kass NE, Sugarman J, Faden R, Schoch-Spana M (1996) Trust: the fragile foundations of contemporary biomedical research. Hastings Cent Rep 26(5):25–29

Krugman S (1986) The Willowbrook hepatitis studies revisited: ethical aspects. Rev Infect Dis 8(1):157–162

Mason JK, McCall Smith RA (2010) Law and medical ethics, 8th edn. Butterworth, London

Moreno JD, Schmidt U, Joffe S (2017) The Nuremberg Code 70 years later. JAMA 318(9):795–796. https://doi.org/10.1001/jama.2017.10265

NMBI (2015) Ethical conduct in research: professional guidance. Nursing and Midwifery Board of Ireland, Dublin. http://www.nmbi.ie/nmbi/media/NMBI/Publications/ethical-conduct-in-research-professional-guidance.pdf?ext=.pdf

Northern Nurses Federation (2003) Ethical guidelines for nursing research in the Nordic countries. Sykepleiernes Sanarbeid i Norden, Oslo. https://ssn-norden.dk/wp-content/uploads/2020/05/ssns_etiske_retningslinjer_0-003.pdf. Accessed 8 Aug 2023

O'Mathúna DP (2012) Ethical considerations in designing intervention studies. In: Mazurek Melnyk B, Morrison-Beedy D (eds) Intervention research. Designing, conducting, analyzing, and funding: a practical guide for success. Springer Publishing, New York, pp 75–89

Paterson R (2010) The Cartwright legacy: shifting the focus of attention from the doctor to the patient. N Z Med J 123(1319):6–10

Piasek P (2015) Case studies in therapeutic SenseCam use aimed at identity maintenance in early stage dementia (Unpublished PhD thesis). Dublin City University, Dublin

Rawls J (1985) Justice as fairness: political not metaphysical. Philos Public Aff 14(3):223–251

Royal College of Nurses (2022.) Using and doing research: a novice's guide: https://www.rcn.org.uk/library/Subject-Guides/using-and-doing-research. Accessed 16 Aug 2023

Scott PA (2006) Philosophy, nursing and the nature of evidence. In: Atkinson J, Crow M (eds) Interdisciplinary research: diverse approaches in science, technology and society. Wiley, Chichester

The Belmont Report: Principles and Guidelines for the Protection of Human Subjects of Research (1979) The National Commission for the protection of human subjects of biomedical and behavioral research. US Government Printing Office, Washington, DC. http://www.hhs.gov/ohrp/regulations-and-policy/belmont-report/

The Royal Liverpool Children's Inquiry Report (2001) Report on the removal, retention and disposal of human organs and tissues at Alder hey children's hospital. HMSO, London

United Nations (1948) The universal declaration of human rights. http://www.un.org/en/documents/udhr/index.shtml. Accessed 23 Aug 2023

United Nations (1989) Convention on the rights of the child. http://www.unicef.org.uk/Documents/Publication-pdfs/UNCRC_PRESS200910web.pdf. Accessed 23 Aug 2023

World Medical Association (2023) Declaration of Helsinki: recommendations guiding physicians in biomedical research involving subjects (1964, 1975, 1983, 1989, 1996, 2000, 2002, 2004, 2008, 2013). http://www.wma.net/what-we-do/medical-ethics/declaration-of-helsinki/. Accessed 23 Aug 2023

GPSR Compliance

The European Union's (EU) General Product Safety Regulation (GPSR) is a set of rules that requires consumer products to be safe and our obligations to ensure this.

If you have any concerns about our products, you can contact us on ProductSafety@springernature.com

In case Publisher is established outside the EU, the EU authorized representative is:

Springer Nature Customer Service Center GmbH
Europaplatz 3
69115 Heidelberg, Germany

Batch number: 09458182

Printed by Printforce, the Netherlands